Hematopoietic Stem Cell: Latest Findings

Hematopoietic Stem Cell: Latest Findings

Edited by **Rex Turner**

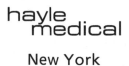

New York

Published by Hayle Medical,
30 West, 37th Street, Suite 612,
New York, NY 10018, USA
www.haylemedical.com

Hematopoietic Stem Cell: Latest Findings
Edited by Rex Turner

International Standard Book Number: 978-1-63241-250-8 (Hardback)

Contents

Preface

Hematopoietic stem cells have emerged as an area of advanced study. This book provides a complete analysis of the biology and healing possibilities of hematopoietic stem cells, and is meant for those involved in stem cell study. Beginning from primary principles in hematopoiesis, this book assembles a wealth of information related to central devices that may control separation and growth of hematopoietic stem cells in usual conditions and throughout disease. This book elucidates the functions of hematopoietic stem cells in aging and various other diseases. It also discusses diverse topics related to hematopoietic stem cell therapy. It compiles researches from renowned experts involved in this field.

The information shared in this book is based on empirical researches made by veterans in this field of study. The elaborative information provided in this book will help the readers further their scope of knowledge leading to advancements in this field.

Finally, I would like to thank my fellow researchers who gave constructive feedback and my family members who supported me at every step of my research.

Editor

Part 1

Hematopoietic Stem Cells in Aging and Disease

Insights Into Stem Cell Aging

A. Herrera-Merchan, I. Hidalgo, L. Arranz and S. Gonzalez
Stem Cell Aging Group, Foundation Spanish National Cardiovascular Research Centre
Carlos III. (CNIC), Madrid,
Spain

1. Introduction

The increase in average life expectancy in many developed countries is generating an aging society and an associated increase in age-related health problems. Mammalian aging occurs in part because of a decline in the restorative capacity of tissue stem cells. The use of stem cells in regenerative medicine promises to revolutionize the treatment of acute and chronic degenerative conditions, and stem cell research holds the key to the development of such therapies. The hallmark of adult stem cells is their ability to both self-renew and differentiate into multiple lineages. This demands a complex and still poorly understood network of molecular interactions between diverse cell-intrinsic regulators of self-renewal, such as certain Polycomb proteins and the tumor suppressor $p16^{INK4a}$, both of which are absolutely required for the maintenance of certain stem cell population. Recent studies have begun to elucidate the molecular mechanisms underlying how stem cells decide between life and death, and highlight the importance of balance in their aging pathways.

2. Aging and stem cells

Recent advances in medicine research programs, and a better health care planning, have great influences in people living in many Western countries, increasing both quality of life and average lifespan. With the extension of lifetime, there is increasing interest in slowing or reversing the negative effects of aging. The fascinating discovery of tissue-resident adult stem and progenitor cells in recent years has led to an explosion of interest in the development of novel stem cell-based therapies to improve endogenous regenerative capacity or to repair damaged and diseased tissues.

A major function of stem cells and their differentiation hierarchies may be to preserve the DNA integrity of the whole organism. When mutations occur despite certain error-prevention capacities, potent tumor-suppressor mechanisms such as senescence and apoptosis eliminate the damaged stem cell, limiting its replicative expansion. However, when unrepaired genetic lesions in stem cells are passed on to their differentiated daughters, and accumulate with aging, it is required replacement of dead and non-functional cells with newly differentiated cells derived from stem- and progenitor-cells. To date, the best-studied adult tissue stem cell type is the hematopoietic stem cell (HSC), which gives rise to all of the mature blood cells, throughout the life of the organism. Hematopoiesis in mammals occurs in distinct temporal waves shifting from the extraembryonic yolk sac and fetal liver in embryos to bone marrow in adults. Primitive HSCs are the "true" stem cells, also termed the long-term repopulating HSCs (LT-HSCs), because they replenish the pool of blood cells by both maintaining the stem cells and allowing daughter cells to differentiate into the lymphoid, myeloid, and erythroid lineages. The daily replenishment of blood cells is achieved in large part by divisions and subsequent stepwise differentiation of cells descendants of LT-HSC pool, namely short term repopulating HSC (ST-HSC), and slightly more committed hematopoietic progenitor cells (MPP-HSC). The relative quiescence of LT-HSCs pool protects their genomic integrity by reducing the rounds of DNA replication and thus the probability of acquiring DNA damage that might compromise multilineage differentiation potential and/or render them malignant over time, though they appear to age with the host (Orkin and Zon, 2008). The rapid turnover of the hematopoietic system and the availability of advanced methods to study HSCs by different markers have led to this system being widely used as a model of the effects of aging on stem cell functionality (Figure 1). It is worthy to mention that although some aspects of aging may be shared by all somatic stem cell fractions, the mechanisms of aging are likely to differ between stem cell populations located in specific tissues (for example, intestine, muscle and bone marrow).

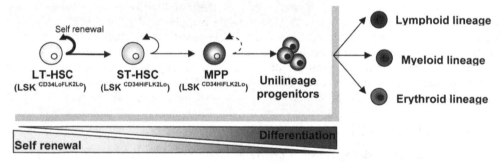

Fig. 1. The hierarchically primitive cells of the hematopoietic system. Long-Term hematopoietic stem cells (LT-HSC) maintain hematopoiesis by coordinating self-renewal, and production of short-term HSC (ST-HSC), and subsequently, the multipotent progenitors (MPP), which have an incredible capacity to divide and make other types of cells as they mature, although a limited ability to self-renew. Ultimately, this generates an array of mature blood cells with different functions: lymphoid blood cells (the B-cells; T-cells; natural killer or NK cells; plasma cells; dendritic cells and others), and erythroid and myeloid blood cells (the erythrocytes or red blood cells; megakaryocytes or platelet producing cells; granulocytes such as neutrophils, eosinophils, and basophils; and monocytes which make macrophages). The stem and progenitor cells can be purified to near-homogeneity by surface markers. For example, LT-HSCs express low levels of lineage markers, high levels of Sca1 and CD117/c-KIT receptor, and low levels of CD34 (LSK CD34 lo). With limited renewal potential, the ST-HSC pool has a similar surface immunophenotype to LT-HSC except that it has higher levels of CD34 (LSK CD34 hi). As ST-HSC in turn proliferates to form more differentiated MPP, they increase expression of another surface marker, FLK2 (LSK CD34 hi Flk2 hi).

3. The evidence for stem cell aging

A growing body of evidence shows that the capacity of stem cells to maintain tissue homeostasis declines with age, and suggests that this decline may account for many age-related phenotypes and diseases (Kirkwood and Austad, 2000). Significantly, engraftment of HSCs are capable of serial passages through a succession of mouse recipients, outliving the donor mouse (Ross et al., 1982; Siminovitch et al., 1964), though it is not possible to exceed up to five successful passages, and the recipients do not restore the hematopoietic system to the normal state (Gordon and Blackett, 1998). On the other hand, telomere length in blood cells of the transplanted recipient are 1-2 kb shorter than those in the donor, when evaluated several years following transplantation (Allsopp et al., 2003), which indicates that the level of telomerase is insufficient to prevent progressive telomere shortening in HSC. On the other hand, immunophenotypic characterization of hematopoietic stem- and progenitor-cell subsets diverges from function in old animals. The engraftment efficiency of immunophenotypically selected long-term HSCs from old mice approximately is threefold lower than that of the equivalent population from young mice (Morrison et al., 1997; Yilmaz et al., 2006). Also, age-related changes in stem-cell function include myeloid-biased differentiation and decreased homing ability (Liang et al., 2005). In conclusion, it has been extensively proved that the properties of HSCs change in several ways as they age, but still is poorly known which are the changes in the intrinsic and extrinsic factors involved that regulate the self-renewal and multilineage differentiation capacities of these regenerative cells (Huang et al., 2007).

Although the stem- and progenitor-cell proliferation guarantees tissue repair, and thereby regeneration, it can also develop hyperproliferative diseases, like cancer, risk that is moderated by tumor-suppressors mechanisms. For example, while the increased expression of tumor suppressors with age (p53, p16^{INK4a}) inhibits the development of cancer (inducing apoptosis or/and senescence) (Krishnamurthy et al., 2004; Ressler et al., 2006), over time it may have a negative effect on stem cell functionality, reducing capacity for self-renewal or differentiation, and ultimately leading to aging phenotypes (Beausejour and Campisi, 2006; Rodier et al., 2007). Thus, it is thought that many of the same mechanisms that contribute to cellular aging also act as suppressors of neoplastic growth (Campisi, 2005) (Figure 2). We will therefore need a better understanding of age-related changes in stem cell function by altering genetically the expression of tumor suppressors, which may improve effective longevity-promoting therapies.

4. Self-renewal regulators in adult HSCs

Stem cells are crucial for the homeostatic maintenance of mature, functional cells in many tissues throughout the lifetime of the animal, and this pool of stem cells must itself be maintained (Muller-Sieburg and Sieburg, 2008). This is achieved by self-renewal, a specialized cell division in which one or both daughter cells remain undifferentiated and retain essentially the same replication potential of the parent. The self-renewal program must involve the activity of dedicated regulatory genes (Gazit et al., 2008); but although the phenotypic and functional properties of HSCs have been characterized extensively, we have only just begun to understand how self-renewal is regulated.

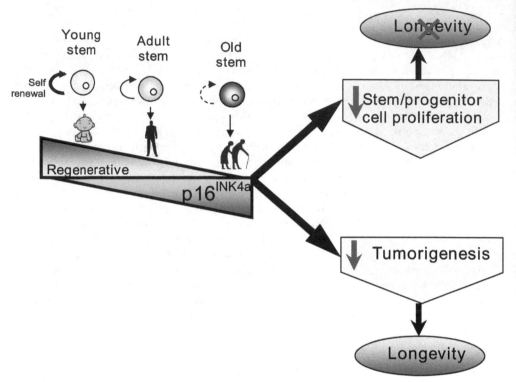

Fig. 2. Potential stem cell stage: interplay between aging and cancer. During normal aging, stem cells accumulate DNA damage as the consequence of endogenous (telomere dysfunction, oxidative stress) or exogenous (oxidative stress, g-irradiation, UV light, and others) attacks. This provokes subsequent stress-dependent changes (for example, accumulation of the products from the *INK4a/ARF* locus or telomere shortening), which activates checkpoint responses that result in apoptosis or cellular senescence. If these events occur in stem/progenitor cells, there is a decrease in the overall number and/or functionality of both stem and progenitor cells, leading an alteration of tissue homeostasis and regenerative capacity–a phenomenon that might contribute to aging and aged-related pathologies. If, instead, DNA mutations that inactivate these checkpoint pathways accumulate (for instance, loss of p16INK4a or reactivation of telomerase), then cancer can arise.

Polycomb complex in the maintenance of stemness. PcG proteins regulate self-renewal and lineage restriction in stem cells by inducing reversible chromatin modifications. PcG proteins have attracted increasing attention in stem cell and cancer stem cell research, given that it is now widely recognized that dynamic reprogramming of cells, for instance during differentiation, requires alterations to the epigenetic status of genes (Valk-Lingbeek et al., 2004). These features makes them interesting subjects for stem cell research, since it is conceivable that dynamic reprogramming of cells, for instance during differentiation, requires alterations in the epigenetic state of gene expression programs. The two major multiprotein PcG complexes identified to date, PRC1 and PRC2, function in a cooperative manner to maintain gene silencing (Pietersen et al., 2008) (Table 1). PRC2 initiates silencing, whereas PRC1 maintains and stabilizes gene repression. PRC2 contains histone methyltransferases (HMTs) that methylate lysines 9 and 27 on histone H3 and lysine 26 on histone H1. Deletion of PRC2 genes in mice results in early embryonic death, underscoring their importance in development. PRC1 recognizes the H3 lysine 27 methyl group added by PRC2 (Valk-Lingbeek et al., 2004), and subsequently the monoubiquityl-ligase activity of the PRC1 proteins Bmi1 or Ring1A/B toward histone H2A generates uH2AK119, which prevents access of the transcription machinery and facilitates chromatin compaction (Wang et al., 2004). Mouse mutants of most PRC1 members, in spite of displaying homeotic transformations, survive until birth as a result of partial functional redundancy provided by homologues, an exception being Ring1B-deficient mice (Voncken et al., 2003).

PRC2 is recruited to target genes by the cofactor jARID2 (jumonji/ARID domain-containing 2). Paradoxically, jARID2 also seems to inhibit PRC2 methyltransferase activity and may therefore regulate both the targeting and fine-tuning of PRC2 activity in stem cells and during differentiation (Panning, 2010). Once PRC1 recognizes and binds the H3K27me3 mark added by PRC2, it recruits additional proteins to establish the repressed chromatin configuration (Jones and Baylin, 2007). Gene promoters marked with H3K27me3 in ESCs are significantly more likely than other promoters to become methylated in cancer (Schlesinger et al., 2007). Moreover, the PcG targets in normal prostate cells are the same as those that become methylated in prostate cancer (Gal-Yam et al., 2008). Thus, altered chromatin structure does not always result in changes in gene expression associated with disease. Rather, disease results from the replacement of PcG repressive histone marks with methylation directly on DNA, which locks the chromatin in an inactive state, a process called epigenetic switching (Gal-Yam et al., 2008). Although the mechanism underlying predisposition of PcG targets to DNA methylation is not fully understood, the PRC1 component Cbx7 (chromobox homologue 7) was recently shown to interact directly with DNA (cytosine-5)-methyltransferase (DNMT)1 and DNMT3B at PcG target genes, establishing a link between histone and DNA methylation (Mohammad et al., 2009).

Among PcG proteins, the PRC1 component Bmi1 is a fundamental self-renewal regulator, being required for self-renewal of all postnatal stem cell populations studied to date (Molofsky et al., 2003; Park et al., 2003; van der Lugt et al., 1994). Bmi1 was originally described as a proto-oncogene that induces B and T cell leukemias (van Lohuizen et al., 1991), and is overexpressed in several human cancers, including mantle cell lymphoma, colorectal carcinoma, liver carcinomas, non-small-cell lung cancer, and cerebral tumors such as medulloblastomas (Martin-Perez et al., 2010). This evidence has strongly influenced cancer research, supporting the above-mentioned theory that cancer is essentially a stem cell disorder (Reya et al., 2001). The self-renewal function of Bmi1 in adult stem cells relies largely on the silencing of one of its targets, the locus encoding the p16INK4a and ARF tumor suppressors (Molofsky et al., 2006). Deletion of p16INK4a and/or ARF partially rescues the self-renewal defects observed in various stem cell populations from Bmi1-null mice. Nevertheless, as described by the authors, this rescue is incomplete and thus other major Bmi1 regulated genes must exist. Candidates for additional Bmi1 targets in the context of self renewal are the Hox (homeobox) genes. A subset of Hox genes has been implicated in mammalian brain development, and several of them are highly expressed in neurospheres formed in vitro from cultured neural stem cells of the subventricular zone of

PcG	Mouse	Human	Function	Hematopoietic defect
PRC1				
	Cbx2/M33 Cbx4/Mpc2 Cbx8/Pc3	CBX2/HPC1 CBX4/HPC2 CBX8/HPC3	Binds trimethylated H3K27	Hypoplasia of spleen and thymus, maturation arrest in T cell development
	Bmi1	BMI1	Co-factor of E3 ubiquitin ligase (RING1A/B) and compacts polynucleosome	Postnatal pancytopenia Impaired HSC self-renewal, hypoplasia of spleen and thymus. Maturation arrest in T and B cell development
	Ring1/Ring1a Rnf2/Ring1b	RING1/RING1A RNF2/RING1B	E3 ubiquitin ligase for H2AK119	Decreased bone marrow cells and increased myeloid progenitors
PRC2				
	Eed	EED	Stimulates histone methyltransferase activity of Ezh1/2	Myelo- and lymphoproliferative disease
	Suz12	SUZ12	Stimulates histone methyltransferase activity of Ezh1/2	Enhanced HSC activity
	Ezh1/Enx2 Ezh2/Enx1	EZH1 EZH2	Catalytic subunit of H3K27 histone methyltransferase	Maturation arrest of T cells at the early CD4, CD8 double negative stage in thymus and of B cells with impaired rearrangement of the IgH gene $Ezh2^{-/-}$ Lethal in HSC

Adapted from Takaaki Konuma et al. Develop. Growth Differ. (2010) 52, 505–516

Table 1. Principcal components of the Polycomb Group Complexes and their hematopoietic defects in mutant mice.

Bmi-null mice (Molofsky et al., 2006). More recently, Bmi1 and Ring1A were shown to play essential roles in H2A ubiquitylation and Hox gene silencing. Knockout of Bmi1 results in significant loss of H2A ubiquitylation and an upregulation of HoxC13 expression, whereas Ezh2-mediated H3-K27 methylation is not affected (Cao et al., 2005). Similar findings have been described for the HoxC5 gene. However, considering that PcG proteins modify the chromatin of large sets of genes (Kirmizis et al., 2004), a great number of additional targets are likely to exist. For instance, both PRC2 and Bmi1 have recently been shown to play roles in the repression of E-cadherin expression (Yang et al., 2010). Interestingly, PcG genes have been shown to have a tumor suppressive function. In *Drosophila*, PcG proteins repress JAK/STAT and Notch signaling activity, whose activation drives disc cell overproliferation (Classen et al., 2009). Specifically, the *Drosophila* complex Psc (posterior sex combs), which includes Bmi1, and Suz12 (suppressor of zeste 12) play a tumor suppressive role mediated by Wnt repression in follicle stem cells(Li et al., 2010). In mammals, Eed (embryonic ectoderm development protein) displays tumor suppressive activity in the mouse hematopoietic system (Richie et al., 2002). Thus, PcG genes have been suggested to behave either as proto-oncogenes or as tumor suppressors depending on the tissue, cell context, developmental stage and gene dosage.

Bmi1 is regulated by Sonic Hedgehog, providing a direct connection between PcG and a major stem cell-specific pathway (Leung et al., 2004). Furthermore, activation of either Hedgehog or Notch signaling has been shown to increase Bmi1 expression, whereas siRNA knockdown of Bmi1 abrogates the effects of Hedgehog or Notch signaling on sphere formation, a functional readout of stemness. Thus the effects of Hedgehog and Notch signaling on stem cell self-renewal appear to be largely dependent on Bmi1. A complex regulation of Bmi1 is suggested by the fact that distinct Bmi1 regulators have been found in different types of cancer, for example Twist1 in head and neck squamous cell carcinoma and the Zeb1 (zinc finger E-box binding homeobox 1) – miR-200 pathway in pancreatic cancers (Wellner et al., 2009). Furthermore, a single PcG function can be regulated by multiple factors, for example Snail1 regulates E-cadherin silencing by PRC2, whereas the action of PRC1 on this target is regulated by Twist1 (Yang et al., 2010).

In summary, PcG proteins, in particular Bmi1, are essential for self-renewal and proliferative potential, which are crucial for the maintenance of stemness, acting as a critical failsafe mechanism against loss of stem cells in response to senescence signals. In turn, Bmi1 must be finely-regulated to prevent uncontrolled replicative expansion and tumor induction. Despite the importance of PcG proteins, we are only beginning to unravel how these master regulators are themselves regulated to achieve an appropriate balance between ensuring stem cell longevity and preventing tumorigenesis.

The tumor suppressors p16^{INK4a} and ARF. Cell-cycle regulators such as the *INK4/ARF* locus appear to play an important role in the reaction of adult stem cells to stress and aging. The *INK4/ARF* locus plays a central role in tumor suppression, reflected in its inactivation in almost 50% of human cancers (Sharpless, 2005). Indeed, this locus is regarded as one of the most important anti-oncogenic defenses of the mammalian genome, comparable in importance only to p53. The remarkable feature of the *INK4/ARF* locus is that it encodes three tumor suppressors in a genomic segment of about 50 kb: *p16^{INK4a}*, its related family member *p15^{INK4b}*, and *ARF* (called *p19^{ARF}* in mice and *p14^{ARF}* in humans). The actions of p16^{INK4a}, p15^{INK4b} and ARF are well understood. Both p16^{INK4a} and p15^{INK4b} inhibit the kinase activity of CDK4/6-cycD complexes, thus contributing to the maintenance of the active, growth-suppressive form of the retinoblastoma (Rb) family of proteins. ARF contributes to the stability of p53 by inhibiting the p53-degrading activity of MDM2. Through the activation of Rb and p53, the *INK4/ARF* locus is able to induce cell senescence and cell death (Gil and Peters, 2006; Lowe and Sherr, 2003). These tumor suppressors have taken on additional importance given recent evidence that at least one product of the locus, p16[INK4a], also contributes to the decline in the replication potential of self-renewing cells during the aging of stem cells. The expression of p16[INK4a] is relatively low in the HSCs of young mice, but is upregulated with age or in response to cellular stresses (Janzen et al., 2006). Although the number of immunophenotypic HSCs increases with age in wild-type animals, HSC functionality is impaired. In particular, the HSC compartment of old animals is more rapidly exhausted by serial transplantation than that of young animals. In contrast, aging has the opposite effect on p16[INK4a]-/- HSCs, with p16[INK4a]-/- HSCs from old animals substantially outperforming young p16[INK4a]-/- HSCs in serial transplantation assays (Janzen et al., 2006). In fact, old p16[INK4a]-/- HSCs perform as well as young wild-type HSCs in this assay. Thus p16[INK4a] compromises HSC functionality in older mice. Similar results were obtained in studies of p16[INK4a]-/- neuronal stem cells and pancreatic islets (Krishnamurthy et al., 2006; Molofsky et al., 2006), revealing a general role for p16[INK4a] in the regulation of stem cell and progenitor cell aging. Therefore, on one face of this coin, p16[INK4a] acts as a potent tumor suppressor that promotes longevity by suppressing the development of cancer, while on the flipside, the increase of p16[INK4a] levels with age impairs the proliferation of stem or progenitor cells, ultimately reducing longevity. Thus, p16[INK4a] seems to balance an equilibrium reducing cancer incidence, but also contributing to aging by decreasing stem cell self-renewal and proliferation. These observations suggest the provocative but as yet unproven notion that mammalian aging results in part from the beneficial effects of tumor suppressor proteins (Figure 2).

The transcription factor p53. Besides p16[INK4a] tumor suppressor, p53 is also a tumor suppressor that influences stem cell self-renewal, tissue regenerative capacity, age-related disease, and cancer, which activity is lost in nearly half of all human cancers(Toledo and Wahl, 2006). The p53 protein is normally inactive, due in part to its rapid degradation by the specific ubiquitin ligase Mdm2. A multitude of stresses converge on p53 through complex, and partially understood, signaling pathways that stabilize and modify p53. The analysis of the effect of p53 in aging has revealed a dual role that seems to depend on the intensity of p53 activity. Overexpression of short isoforms of p53 in mice have greater protection against tumor development than wild-type mice, while at the same time they show signs of premature aging (Maier et al., 2004; Tyner et al., 2002). However, mouse models of increased wild-type p53 activity do not present premature aging. In particular, bacterial artificial chromosome transgenic mice that bear a third copy of the p53 locus show a decreased cancer incidence but normal longevity and normal onset of aging phenotypes (Garcia-Cao et al., 2002; Matheu et al., 2007; Matheu et al., 2004). An additional mouse model, the super-INK4a/ARF mice, with an extra copy of the entire *INK4a/ARF* locus (being ARF an activator of p53), show a significantly reduced incidence of cancer, although the mice aged normally (Matheu et al., 2004). To investigate whether the concomitant expression of both tumor suppressors had a synergistic effect, mice that bear a third copy of the p53 locus and a third copy of the *INK4/ARF* locus show increased longevity and delayed aging in a manner that cannot be explained by their reduced incidence of cancer (Matheu et al., 2007). Therefore, and though the effects of p53 and *INK4/ARF* locus expression in aging are context and dosage dependent, these results suggest that under physiological aging (labeled by moderate increase of still regulated p53 activity), the damaged cells are eliminated by either triggering their self-destruction (by apoptosis) or by pulling them out of the proliferative pool (by inducing senescence). In contrast, by massive DNA damage, the presence of uncontrolled activity of p53 results in excessive elimination of cells by p53 that exhausts the capacity of tissue regeneration leading to premature aging.

The *INK4/ARF* locus and age-associated phenotypes. p16[INK4a] and ARF may also be broadly important to diseases of aging beyond their function in stem cells. Specifically, three research consortia that undertook genome-wide association studies across large, carefully annotated patient samples have reported an association between single nucleotide polymorphisms (SNPs) near to *INK4a/ARF* locus and frailty (Melzer et al., 2007), atherosclerotic heart disease (ASHD)(Helgadottir et al., 2007) (McPherson et al., 2007), and type-2 diabetes (Saxena et al., 2007; Zeggini et al., 2008) in large human cohorts. However, few of the associated SNPs near the locus, and associated with these phenotypes, are not in linkage disequilibrium with each other, which suggests that more than one polymorphism near the locus influences these aging phenotypes. Therefore, although these studies do not pinpoint specific polymorphisms that affect the risks of age-related diseases, there are only four genes in the vicinity of the mapped polymorphisms: p16[INK4a], ARF, p15[INK4b], and ANRIL (a noncoding RNA). More relative data suggest specific links: p16[INK4a] expression increases with age in pancreatic β cells, and p16[INK4a] deficiency increases β-cell regenerative capacity(Krishnamurthy et al., 2006), providing a mechanism by which polymorphisms that affect p16[INK4a] expression or activity might affect risk for type-2 diabetes. It remains unclear whether these polymorphisms influence the risk of frailty and heart disease through their effects on tissue regenerative capacity or by mechanisms that are completely independent of stem/progenitor cells. Nevertheless, in light of the murine genetic studies that link *INK4a/ARF* locus and stem cell function, proteins encoded by the locus are the strongest candidates to mediate the effects of these polymorphisms on the incidence of these common diseases that are associated with aging.

5. Conclusions

The regenerative capacity of many stem cells declines functionally with age and, this decline triggers in part many age-related symptoms, and the development of certain diseases. Recent evidences have demonstrated that certain tumor suppressors, like *p16[INK4a]*, also suppresses the proliferation of stem or progenitor cells in the bone marrow, pancreas and brain. Thus, p16[INK4a] seems to balance equilibrium reducing cancer incidence, which promotes longevity, but also decreasing stem cell self-renewal and proliferation, compromising tissue regeneration and repair, which are likely to reduce longevity. These observations allow us to suggest the provocative but unproved hypothesis that mammalian aging results in part from the beneficial efforts of tumor suppressor proteins to interdict cancer. In this stage, characterization of how stem cells age, such as **the characterization of reliable biomarkers,** deregulated signaling pathways, loss of self-renewal or acquisition of defects in differentiation of stem cells, will contribute to understand the age-associated pathophysiological decline. Likewise, it is also essential to figure out the cellular and molecular components of stem cell niches, how the niche changes during aging, and whether senescent stem or support cells alter the niche. In summary, the rescue, treatment, or replacement of aged and dysfunctional adult stem and progenitor cells may provide novel avenues to treat diverse devastating premature aging and age-related disorders including hematopoietic and immune disorders, heart failure and cardiovascular diseases, neurodegenerative, muscular and gastrointestinal diseases, atherosclerosis and aggressive and lethal cancers.

6. Acknowledgement

This work was supported by the Human Frontiers Science Program Organization, the Spanish Ministries of Science and Innovation (SAF2010-15386) and Health (FIS PI06/0627). We thank Simon Bartlett for editing assistance. The CNIC is supported by the Ministry of Science and Innovation and the Pro-CNIC Foundation.

7. Abbreviatons

PcG, Polycomb Group, PRC1, Polycomb repressive complex 1, PRC2, polycomb repressive complex 2.

8. References

Allsopp, R.C., Morin, G.B., DePinho, R., Harley, C.B., and Weissman, I.L. (2003). Telomerase is required to slow telomere shortening and extend replicative lifespan of HSCs during serial transplantation. Blood 102, 517-520.

Beausejour, C.M., and Campisi, J. (2006). Ageing: balancing regeneration and cancer. Nature 443, 404-405.

Campisi, J. (2005). Senescent cells, tumor suppression, and organismal aging: good citizens, bad neighbors. Cell 120, 513-522.

Cao, R., Tsukada, Y., and Zhang, Y. (2005). Role of Bmi-1 and Ring1A in H2A ubiquitylation and Hox gene silencing. Mol Cell 20, 845-854.

Classen, A.K., Bunker, B.D., Harvey, K.F., Vaccari, T., and Bilder, D. (2009). A tumor suppressor activity of Drosophila Polycomb genes mediated by JAK-STAT signaling. Nat Genet 41, 1150-1155.

Gal-Yam, E.N., Egger, G., Iniguez, L., Holster, H., Einarsson, S., Zhang, X., Lin, J.C., Liang, G., Jones, P.A., and Tanay, A. (2008). Frequent switching of Polycomb repressive marks and DNA hypermethylation in the PC3 prostate cancer cell line. Proc Natl Acad Sci U S A 105, 12979-12984.

Garcia-Cao, I., Garcia-Cao, M., Martin-Caballero, J., Criado, L.M., Klatt, P., Flores, J.M., Weill, J.C., Blasco, M.A., and Serrano, M. (2002). "Super p53" mice exhibit enhanced DNA damage response, are tumor resistant and age normally. Embo J 21, 6225-6235.

Gazit, R., Weissman, I.L., and Rossi, D.J. (2008). Hematopoietic stem cells and the aging hematopoietic system. Semin Hematol 45, 218-224.

Gil, J., and Peters, G. (2006). Regulation of the INK4b-ARF-INK4a tumour suppressor locus: all for one or one for all. Nat Rev Mol Cell Biol 7, 667-677.

Gordon, M.Y., and Blackett, N.M. (1998). Reconstruction of the hematopoietic system after stem cell transplantation. Cell Transplant 7, 339-344.

Helgadottir, A., Thorleifsson, G., Manolescu, A., Gretarsdottir, S., Blondal, T., Jonasdottir, A., Sigurdsson, A., Baker, A., Palsson, A., Masson, G., et al. (2007). A common variant on chromosome 9p21 affects the risk of myocardial infarction. Science 316, 1491-1493.

Huang, X., Cho, S., and Spangrude, G.J. (2007). Hematopoietic stem cells: generation and self-renewal. Cell Death Differ 14, 1851-1859.

Janzen, V., Forkert, R., Fleming, H.E., Saito, Y., Waring, M.T., Dombkowski, D.M., Cheng, T., DePinho, R.A., Sharpless, N.E., and Scadden, D.T. (2006). Stem-cell ageing modified by the cyclin-dependent kinase inhibitor p16INK4a. Nature 443, 421-426.

Jones, P.A., and Baylin, S.B. (2007). The epigenomics of cancer. Cell 128, 683-692.

Kirkwood, T.B., and Austad, S.N. (2000). Why do we age? Nature 408, 233-238.

Kirmizis, A., Bartley, S.M., Kuzmichev, A., Margueron, R., Reinberg, D., Green, R., and Farnham, P.J. (2004). Silencing of human polycomb target genes is associated with methylation of histone H3 Lys 27. Genes Dev 18, 1592-1605.

Krishnamurthy, J., Ramsey, M.R., Ligon, K.L., Torrice, C., Koh, A., Bonner-Weir, S., and Sharpless, N.E. (2006). p16INK4a induces an age-dependent decline in islet regenerative potential. Nature 443, 453-457.

Krishnamurthy, J., Torrice, C., Ramsey, M.R., Kovalev, G.I., Al-Regaiey, K., Su, L., and Sharpless, N.E. (2004). Ink4a/Arf expression is a biomarker of aging. J Clin Invest 114, 1299-1307.

Leung, C., Lingbeek, M., Shakhova, O., Liu, J., Tanger, E., Saremaslani, P., Van Lohuizen, M., and Marino, S. (2004). Bmi1 is essential for cerebellar development and is overexpressed in human medulloblastomas. Nature 428, 337-341.

Li, X., Han, Y., and Xi, R. (2010). Polycomb group genes Psc and Su(z)2 restrict follicle stem cell self-renewal and extrusion by controlling canonical and noncanonical Wnt signaling. Genes Dev 24, 933-946.

Liang, Y., Van Zant, G., and Szilvassy, S.J. (2005). Effects of aging on the homing and engraftment of murine hematopoietic stem and progenitor cells. Blood 106, 1479-1487.

Lowe, S.W., and Sherr, C.J. (2003). Tumor suppression by Ink4a-Arf: progress and puzzles. Curr Opin Genet Dev 13, 77-83.

Maier, B., Gluba, W., Bernier, B., Turner, T., Mohammad, K., Guise, T., Sutherland, A., Thorner, M., and Scrable, H. (2004). Modulation of mammalian life span by the short isoform of p53. Genes Dev 18, 306-319.

Martin-Perez, D., Piris, M.A., and Sanchez-Beato, M. (2010). Polycomb proteins in hematologic malignancies. Blood 116, 5465-5475.

Matheu, A., Maraver, A., Klatt, P., Flores, I., Garcia-Cao, I., Borras, C., Flores, J.M., Viña, J., Blasco, M.A., and Serrano, M. (2007). Delayed aging through damage protection by the Arf/p53 pathway. Nature in press.

Matheu, A., Pantoja, C., Efeyan, A., Criado, L.M., Martin-Caballero, J., Flores, J.M., Klatt, P., and Serrano, M. (2004). Increased gene dosage of Ink4a/Arf results in cancer resistance and normal aging. Genes Dev 18, 2736-2746.

McPherson, R., Pertsemlidis, A., Kavaslar, N., Stewart, A., Roberts, R., Cox, D.R., Hinds, D.A., Pennacchio, L.A., Tybjaerg-Hansen, A., Folsom, A.R., *et al.* (2007). A common allele on chromosome 9 associated with coronary heart disease. Science *316*, 1488-1491.

Melzer, D., Frayling, T.M., Murray, A., Hurst, A.J., Harries, L.W., Song, H., Khaw, K., Luben, R., Surtees, P.G., Bandinelli, S.S., *et al.* (2007). A common variant of the p16(INK4a) genetic region is associated with physical function in older people. Mech Ageing Dev *128*, 370-377.

Mohammad, H.P., Cai, Y., McGarvey, K.M., Easwaran, H., Van Neste, L., Ohm, J.E., O'Hagan, H.M., and Baylin, S.B. (2009). Polycomb CBX7 promotes initiation of heritable repression of genes frequently silenced with cancer-specific DNA hypermethylation. Cancer Res *69*, 6322-6330.

Molofsky, A.V., Pardal, R., Iwashita, T., Park, I.K., Clarke, M.F., and Morrison, S.J. (2003). Bmi-1 dependence distinguishes neural stem cell self-renewal from progenitor proliferation. Nature *425*, 962-967.

Molofsky, A.V., Slutsky, S.G., Joseph, N.M., He, S., Pardal, R., Krishnamurthy, J., Sharpless, N.E., and Morrison, S.J. (2006). Increasing p16INK4a expression decreases forebrain progenitors and neurogenesis during ageing. Nature *443*, 448-452.

Morrison, S.J., Wright, D.E., Cheshier, S.H., and Weissman, I.L. (1997). Hematopoietic stem cells: challenges to expectations. Curr Opin Immunol *9*, 216-221.

Muller-Sieburg, C., and Sieburg, H.B. (2008). Stem cell aging: survival of the laziest? Cell Cycle *7*, 3798-3804.

Orkin, S.H., and Zon, L.I. (2008). Hematopoiesis: an evolving paradigm for stem cell biology. Cell *132*, 631-644.

Panning, B. (2010). Fine-tuning silencing. Cell Stem Cell *6*, 3-4.

Park, I.K., Qian, D., Kiel, M., Becker, M.W., Pihalja, M., Weissman, I.L., Morrison, S.J., and Clarke, M.F. (2003). Bmi-1 is required for maintenance of adult self-renewing haematopoietic stem cells. Nature *423*, 302-305.

Pietersen, A.M., Evers, B., Prasad, A.A., Tanger, E., Cornelissen-Steijger, P., Jonkers, J., and van Lohuizen, M. (2008). Bmi1 regulates stem cells and proliferation and differentiation of committed cells in mammary epithelium. Curr Biol *18*, 1094-1099.

Ressler, S., Bartkova, J., Niederegger, H., Bartek, J., Scharffetter-Kochanek, K., Jansen-Durr, P., and Wlaschek, M. (2006). p16INK4A is a robust in vivo biomarker of cellular aging in human skin. Aging Cell *5*, 379-389.

Reya, T., Morrison, S.J., Clarke, M.F., and Weissman, I.L. (2001). Stem cells, cancer, and cancer stem cells. Nature *414*, 105-111.

Richie, E.R., Schumacher, A., Angel, J.M., Holloway, M., Rinchik, E.M., and Magnuson, T. (2002). The Polycomb-group gene eed regulates thymocyte differentiation and suppresses the development of carcinogen-induced T-cell lymphomas. Oncogene *21*, 299-306.

Rodier, F., Campisi, J., and Bhaumik, D. (2007). Two faces of p53: aging and tumor suppression. Nucleic Acids Res *35*, 7475-7484.

Ross, E.A., Anderson, N., and Micklem, H.S. (1982). Serial depletion and regeneration of the murine hematopoietic system. Implications for hematopoietic organization and the study of cellular aging. J Exp Med *155*, 432-444.

Saxena, V., Ondr, J.K., Magnusen, A.F., Munn, D.H., and Katz, J.D. (2007). The countervailing actions of myeloid and plasmacytoid dendritic cells control autoimmune diabetes in the nonobese diabetic mouse. J Immunol *179*, 5041-5053.

Schlesinger, Y., Straussman, R., Keshet, I., Farkash, S., Hecht, M., Zimmerman, J., Eden, E., Yakhini, Z., Ben-Shushan, E., Reubinoff, B.E., *et al.* (2007). Polycomb-mediated methylation on Lys27 of histone H3 pre-marks genes for de novo methylation in cancer. Nat Genet *39*, 232-236.

Sharpless, N.E. (2005). INK4a/ARF: a multifunctional tumor suppressor locus. Mutat Res *576*, 22-38.

Siminovitch, L., Till, J.E., and McCulloch, E.A. (1964). Decline in Colony-Forming Ability of Marrow Cells Subjected to Serial Transplantation into Irradiated Mice. J Cell Physiol *64*, 23-31.

Toledo, F., and Wahl, G.M. (2006). Regulating the p53 pathway: in vitro hypotheses, in vivo veritas. Nat Rev Cancer *6*, 909-923.

Tyner, S.D., Venkatachalam, S., Choi, J., Jones, S., Ghebranious, N., Igelmann, H., Lu, X., Soron, G., Cooper, B., Brayton, C., *et al.* (2002). p53 mutant mice that display early ageing-associated phenotypes. Nature *415*, 45-53.

Valk-Lingbeek, M.E., Bruggeman, S.W., and van Lohuizen, M. (2004). Stem cells and cancer; the polycomb connection. Cell *118*, 409-418.

van der Lugt, N.M., Domen, J., Linders, K., van Roon, M., Robanus-Maandag, E., te Riele, H., van der Valk, M., Deschamps, J., Sofroniew, M., van Lohuizen, M., *et al.* (1994). Posterior transformation, neurological abnormalities, and severe hematopoietic defects in mice with a targeted deletion of the bmi-1 proto-oncogene. Genes Dev *8*, 757-769.

van Lohuizen, M., Verbeek, S., Scheijen, B., Wientjens, E., van der Gulden, H., and Berns, A. (1991). Identification of cooperating oncogenes in E mu-myc transgenic mice by provirus tagging. Cell *65*, 737-752.

Voncken, J.W., Roelen, B.A., Roefs, M., de Vries, S., Verhoeven, E., Marino, S., Deschamps, J., and van Lohuizen, M. (2003). Rnf2 (Ring1b) deficiency causes gastrulation arrest and cell cycle inhibition. Proc Natl Acad Sci U S A *100*, 2468-2473.

Wang, L., Brown, J.L., Cao, R., Zhang, Y., Kassis, J.A., and Jones, R.S. (2004). Hierarchical recruitment of polycomb group silencing complexes. Mol Cell *14*, 637-646.

Wellner, U., Schubert, J., Burk, U.C., Schmalhofer, O., Zhu, F., Sonntag, A., Waldvogel, B., Vannier, C., Darling, D., zur Hausen, A., *et al.* (2009). The EMT-activator ZEB1 promotes tumorigenicity by repressing stemness-inhibiting microRNAs. Nat Cell Biol *11*, 1487-1495.

Yang, M.H., Hsu, D.S., Wang, H.W., Wang, H.J., Lan, H.Y., Yang, W.H., Huang, C.H., Kao, S.Y., Tzeng, C.H., Tai, S.K., *et al.* (2010). Bmi1 is essential in Twist1-induced epithelial-mesenchymal transition. Nat Cell Biol *12*, 982-992.

Yilmaz, O.H., Kiel, M.J., and Morrison, S.J. (2006). SLAM family markers are conserved among hematopoietic stem cells from old and reconstituted mice and markedly increase their purity. Blood *107*, 924-930.

Zeggini, E., Scott, L.J., Saxena, R., Voight, B.F., Marchini, J.L., Hu, T., de Bakker, P.I., Abecasis, G.R., Almgren, P., Andersen, G., *et al.* (2008). Meta-analysis of genome-wide association data and large-scale replication identifies additional susceptibility loci for type 2 diabetes. Nat Genet *40*, 638-645.

From HSC to B-Lymphoid Cells in Normal and Malignant Hematopoiesis

Rosana Pelayo[1], Elisa Dorantes-Acosta[1,2],
Eduardo Vadillo[1] and Ezequiel Fuentes-Pananá[3]
*[1]Oncology Research Unit, Oncology Hospital, Mexican Institute for
Social Security, Mexico City*
[2]Leukemia Clinic, Mexican Children's Hospital 'Federico Gómez', Mexico City
*[3]Research Unit on Parasitic and Infectious Diseases, Pediatric Hospital,
Mexican Institute for Social Security, Mexico City*
Mexico

1. Introduction

Development of B-lymphoid cells is a highly ordered multi-step process that, in adult mammals, starts in bone marrow in a pool of self-renewing multipotential hematopoietic stem cells, which gradually commit to the lymphoid lineage and advance through high regulated differentiation pathways until formation of mature functional cells. Over the last few years, exceptional advances have been recorded in identifying primitive progenitors that lay the foundations of the lymphoid program while losing myeloid potential, along with patterns of transcriptional activity controlling lineage fate decisions and environmental cues that influence the differentiation pathway during normal hematopoiesis. Multicolor flow cytometry, controlled cell cultures, genetic marking systems, microarray technologies and xenotransplantation approaches are being extensively used to address fundamental questions on this regard. Of special interest is the stem cell research with relevance to hierarchy and early events in malignant lymphopoiesis, and to new insights into perspectives that may allow progress in means to protect and sustain the immune system during chemotherapy, inflammation, infection, and following hematopoietic transplantation. In this book chapter, we focus on the hierarchical structure of the early lymphoid system, the current knowledge about intrinsic and microenvironmental factors regulating the differentiation of lymphoid progenitors, and the emerging research to understand malignant lymphoid development.

2. The early steps in the lymphoid development

Mature blood cells are constantly replaced from a unique cell population of hematopoietic stem cells (HSC) residing in specialized niches within the bone marrow (BM), where the hematopoietic system is organized as a hierarchy of cell types that gradually lose multiple alternate potentials while commit to lineage fates and gain specialized functions (Baba et al., 2004; Seita & Weissman, 2010). HSC possess two major characteristics: they are capable of maintaining their constant number by self-renewal and they are in charge of producing all mature blood cells through differentiation processes (Figure 1). Furthermore, HSC are mitotically inactive (quiescent) and divide very slow and intermittently under normal conditions, but are capable of proliferation and differentiation during recovery from chemotherapy or stress circumstances (Takizawa et al, 2011; Mayani, 2010; Passegue et al., 2005; Pelayo et al., 2006b). Movement into and out of a resting state might be crucial for ensuring that the correct number of new hematopoietic cells is produced.

The lymphoid pathway proceeds through critical stages of differentiation of HSC to multipotential early progenitors (MPP), which upon progressive loss of self-renewal capacity, give rise to oligopotent progenitors. Downstream, the production of lineage-committed precursors is crucial for cell maturation. Current knowledge about development of the lymphoid system is based, in great part, on the work done in animal models, demonstrating that lymphoid specification begins in the fraction of lymphoid-primed multipotent progenitors (LMPP). A series of studies using the transgenic RAG-GFP mouse (Igarashi et al., 2002) permitted us to determine that RAG+ early lymphoid progenitors (ELP) are capable of differentiating into T, B, NK and conventional dendritic cells (cDC) (Pelayo et al., 2005a; Pelayo et al., 2006a; Welner et al., 2008a). Studies using defined co-cultures and short-term reconstitution assays have shown that ELP are also good producers of plasmacytoid dendritic cells (pDC) and of interferon-producing killer dendritic cells (IKDC), both being key components of the innate immune response to infections (Pelayo et al., 2005b; Welner et al., 2007). At the same time, ELP give rise to committed oligopotent common lymphoid progenitors (CLP), which are responsible for B- and NK- precursor cells production. CLP and lineage precursors have substantially lost the possibility of differentiating into the rest of the lineages.

Due to ethical reasons and technical limitations, human hematopoietic stem cell research has been slower than it has been in mouse models. In humans, the early hematopoietic progenitors are confined in bone marrow to a cellular compartment that expresses CD34 (Blom & Spits, 2006). The fraction of multipotent stem cells is characterized by the phenotype Lin-CD34+CD38-/loCD10-CD45RA-, whereas that of probably the earliest lymphoid progenitors is Lin-CD34+CD38-/loCD45RA+CD10+ and has been recently designated as multi-lymphoid progenitor (MLP) (Doulatov et al., 2010). According to Doulatov's studies, MLP may be directly derived from HSC. However, a precise precursor-product relationship needs to be determined (Figure 1). A description that fully matches the definition of mouse ELP is still missing, but cells with Lin-CD34+CD38+CD45RA+CD7+CD10+ phenotype seem to represent good candidates (Blom & Spits, 2006; and our unpublished observations). Lin-CD34+CD38+CD45RA+CD10+ B/NK cells, which differentiate principally into B & NK cells, are considered the counterparts of CLP in mice (Figures 1 & 2) (Doulatov et al., 2010). Of special importance is the fact that increasing levels of CD10 correspond to B-lineage specification (Ichii et al., 2010). Downstream, the differentiation of fully committed precursors gives rise to B cells that eventually are exported to peripheral lymphoid tissues (see B cell development sections below).

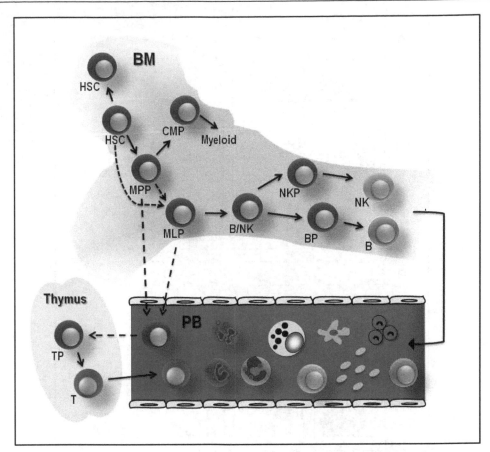

Fig. 1. Early lymphoid development in humans. Within bone marrow (BM), self-renewing hematopoietic stem cells (HSC) give rise to multipotent progenitors (MPP), which have the ability to differentiate into common myeloid progenitors (CMP) and into multi-lymphoid progenitors (MLP). MLP might alternately derive from HSC. NK and B-lymphoid cells are produced from B/NK-derived lineage committed precursors. Mature hematopoietic cells are exported to peripheral blood (PB). Early progenitor cells may colonize the thymus via circulation, and initiate the T-lymphoid development pathway. NKP, natural killer cell precursor; BP, B cell precursor; TP, T cell precursor.

The rigorous purification of human HSC and progenitor cell populations based on their surface phenotype has promoted the study of their biology in adult bone marrow, cord blood and G-CSF-mobilized peripheral blood (Figure 2). Importantly, some of their properties, including cell frequencies, developmental capacities, cell cycle status, transcription factors networks and growth factors production, show substantial differences between newborns and adults (Mayani, 2010). According to literature, we have found that most hematopoietic progenitors are more abundant in cord blood than in the adult tissues bone marrow and mobilized peripheral blood (Mayani, 2010). The implications of these discrepancies during haematological neoplastic diseases are not as yet clear.

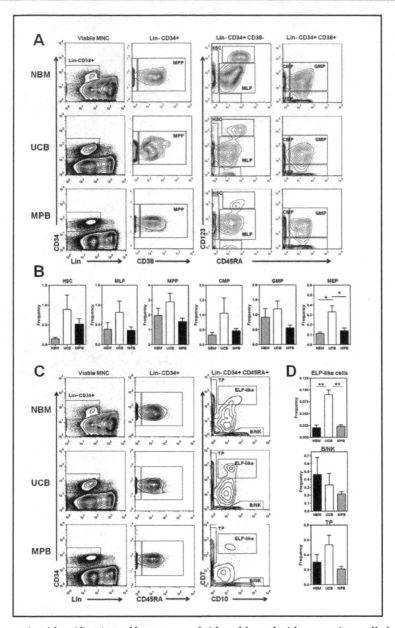

Fig. 2. Prospective identification of human myeloid and lymphoid progenitor cells by flow cytometry. HSC and early progenitor cells reside in the Lin⁻ CD34⁺ fraction of adult normal bone marrow (NBM), as well as in umbilical cord blood (UCB) and mobilized peripheral blood (MPB). Based on the surface expression of CD38, CD123 and CD45RA, multilymphoid progenitor cells (MLP) and most of the myeloid progenitors can be recognized (A). Further fractionation of Lin⁻CD34⁺CD45RA⁺ cells into CD7 & CD10-expressing cells allows the

identification of T-cell progenitors (TP), B/NK progenitors and ELP-like cells (C). Cell frequencies for each population from the different sources are shown (B and D panels). CMP, common myeloid progenitor; GMP, granulocyte & monocyte progenitor; MEP, megakaryocyte & erythrocyte progenitor. The identity and functions of Lin-CD34+CD38-CD45RA+CD123hi cells still need more investigation.

During biological contingencies -chemotherapy, infections and transplantation procedures-, the replenishment of the innate immune system from hematopoietic stem/progenitor cells appears to be critical. Interestingly, these seminal cells can proliferate in response to stress conditions and systemic infection by using mechanisms that apparently involve interferons and tumor necrosis factors, among others (Baldridge et al., 2011). Moreover, they are capable of self/non-self discrimination through Toll-like receptors (TLR), which recognize microbial components. Mouse stem cells and early B-cell progenitors express and use TLR, a mechanism that facilitates their differentiation to the innate immune system (Nagai et al, 2006; Welner et al., 2008b; Welner et al., 2009). Recent work suggests that, as in mice, human primitive cells, including MLP, also express functional TLR (Kim et al., 2005; Sioud & Fløisand, 2007; De Luca et al, 2009; Doulatov et al, 2010). In shape with those findings, we have found that BM lymphoid progenitor-enriched fractions display TLR9 (Figure 3) and their differentiation potentials bias toward NK and DC production upon TLR9 ligation (RP & EV, unpublished observations). Thus, plasticity in primitive cells is vulnerable to extrinsic agents that can modify early cell fate decisions during infections or stress, suggesting that the stages of lineage restrictions are less abrupt than previously assumed (Welner et al., 2008a).

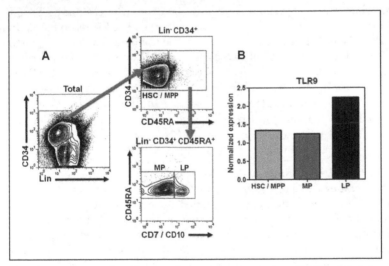

Fig. 3. Lymphoid progenitors from human bone marrow express TLR9. Adult bone marrow is fractionated according to cell surface expression of lineage markers, CD34, CD45RA and CD7/CD10 (A). Lin-CD34+CD45RA- HSC/MPP, Lin-CD34+CD45RA+CD7/CD10- myeloid progenitors (MP) and Lin-CD34+CD45RA+CD7/CD10+ lymphoid progenitors (LP) were tested for their intracellular expression of TLR9 by flow cytometry using a specific anti-TLR9 antibody (B).

3. The B cell antigen receptor (BCR) and bone marrow B cell development

The main function of mature immunocompetent B cells is to make antibodies upon recognition of particular new or recurrent antigens by the B cell receptor (BCR). The BCR is a membrane-bound complex of proteins, consisting of a heterodimer of identical pairs of immunoglobulin (Ig) heavy and light chains, which are responsible for the clonal diversity of the B cell repertoire and the antigen identification, but are unable to generate signals and trigger biological responses after antigen binding. This function is mediated by the disulfide-coupled heterodimer of Igα (CD79a) and Igβ (CD79b), which is non-covalently associated with the Ig antigen recognition unit (Figure 4A). Igα/Igβ signaling is dependent on distinct tyrosine-based activation motifs localized in the cytoplasmic tails of these proteins. It is the sequential expression and assembly of the BCR components that defines each developmental stage of the B cell pathway, and, therefore, each stage is characterized by a particular form of BCR, reflecting the progression of receptor assembly (Fuentes-Pananá et al., 2004a).

To achieve BCR clonal diversity, the Ig heavy and light chain genes are composed of constant and variable regions. The variable region is formed by a series of segments V (variable), D (diversity) and J (joining) (Figure 4B), which are brought together by a highly ordered process of VDJ recombination accomplished by the products of the recombinase-associated genes 1 and 2 (RAG1 and RAG2) occurring first in the heavy and then in the light chain loci (Thomas et al., 2009). ProB and PreB stages are characterized by rearrangements of the Ig heavy and light chains, respectively (Figure 5) (Fuentes-Pananá et al., 2004b), and further divided according to the status of the recombination. In mice, ProB-A is the sub-stage during which the heavy chain is in germ line state, whereas during ProB-B the heavy chain D and J fragments are recombined, and in ProB-C, V-DJ is recombined. In large PreB cells, the preBCR is already expressed in surface and the light chain V and J fragments are in germ line state, while in small PreB cells light chain V-J is recombined (Hardy et al., 1991). These stages are better known in humans as Early ProB or Pre-proB (A), ProB (B), PreB I (C), large and small PreB II (Figure 5). In the ProB stage Igα and Igβ are expressed at cell surface in association with chaperon proteins such as calnexin (the proBCR). As soon as the heavy chain is successfully recombined, it is assembled with Igα and Igβ and the surrogate light chains λ5 and VpreB to form the preBCR. Surface expression of this receptor marks the transition to the preB stage (Figure 5) (Fuentes-Pananá et al., 2004a; 2004b).

In addition to their VDJ recombination status and pattern of surface marker expression, ProB and PreB stages can be recognized by their proliferative state (Hardy et al., 1991). RAG-1 and RAG-2 enzymes are tightly regulated during the cell cycle, being highly active in G_0 and degraded before the cell enters S phase (Li et al., 1996). By assuring that proliferation and recombination are mutually exclusive mechanisms, the developing B cell guarantees that no events of non-homologous recombination will occur during DNA replication, thus avoiding an increase in the mutation rate.

3.1 Self-recognition and peripheral B cell development

Once the mature BCR is present in the surface of immature B cells, it is finally able to interact with conventional polymorphic ligands, and selection at this stage is designed to test the receptor-ligand interaction. Intimate contact between the immature B cell and the stromal cells of the bone marrow allows those receptors capable of recognizing self-antigens to be identified and eliminated through a variety of mechanisms collectively termed "tolerance". Non-self-reactive B cells exit to the periphery and reach the spleen where they are again tested for reactivity against self-antigens before they transition to the mature stage (Figure 5) (von Boehmer & Melchers, 2010). Three main mechanisms of B-cell tolerance are known: receptor editing, deletion of auto-reactive clones (negative selection) and anergy. Only those B cells that carry receptors without self-specificity are allowed to exit the bone marrow and become mature B cells in peripheral lymphoid organs.

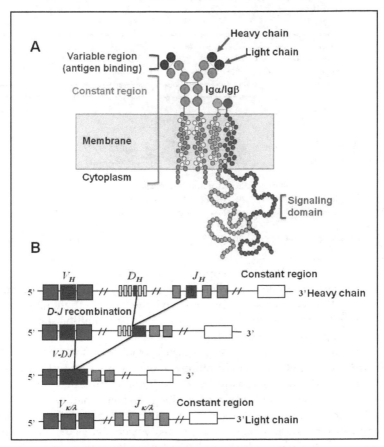

Fig. 4. The B cell antigen receptor (BCR). A) Heavy and light chains are comprised of variable regions where VDJ recombination occurs (shown in dark blue) and constant regions (green). The signaling domains are present in the cytoplasmic leaflet of Igα and Igβ. B) Variable regions are formed by a number of segments termed V (variable), D (diversity) and J (joining) within the heavy chain, and by segments V and J within the light chain, which are brought together by a VDJ recombination process. Randomly, D and J segments recombine at first, followed by V segments joining the DJ fragment (shown in dark blue squares is an example of segment choice). This mechanism is responsible for the extensive repertoire of BCR specificities.

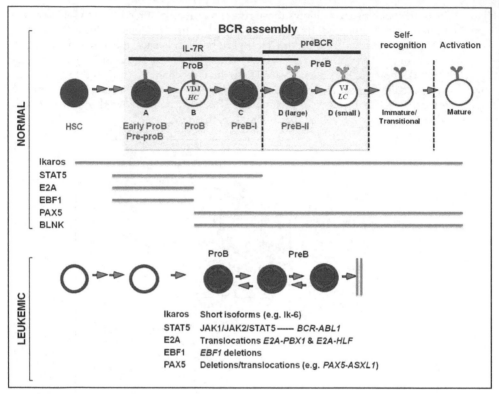

Fig. 5. Normal and leukemic B cell development. B cell stages can be divided according to the main processes guiding development: receptor assembly, self-recognition and activation (top panel). Receptor assembly occurs in bone marrow (light blue box) by VDJ recombination in the Pro-B and Pre-B stages, whereas self-recognition starts in bone marrow and ends in periphery, and activation takes place at peripheral level. Nomenclature for each sub-stage in mice is shown in black letters while the most common nomenclature for their counterparts in humans is shown in red letters. The dashed lines separating all stages indicate checkpoints at which signaling from the preBCR and BCR is required for positive selection and progression along the B-cell maturation pathway. The proBCR, preBCR, and mature receptor are also illustrated in their respective stages. Replication and recombination processes are mutually exclusive as denoted by the circular arrows and VDJ signs inside the cell. The replication stages are also frequently compromised in pediatric B cell acute leukemia. Black lines under IL-7R and preBCR indicate the stages where these receptors are most required. The differential thickness in the IL-7R line shows the sub-stages where a higher (nanograms) or lower (picograms) concentration of the IL-7 is required. Homeostatic and leukemic expression of transcription factors along the B cell pathway are shown in the middle and bottom panels. Blue bars mark normal gene expression, and the most common modified forms of the transcription factors associated with B cell acute lymphoblastic leukemia are revealed. HSC, hematopoietic stem cell.

On the basis of their cell-surface phenotype, peripheral immature B cells are further divided into transitional 1 (T1, AA4+IgMhighCD23-) and transitional 2 (T2, AA4+IgMhighCD23+). T1 cells inhabit the spleen's red pulp and give rise to T2 cells (Allman et al., 2001). There is an additional population designated T3, but it is controversial whether this is a population in line in the progression to the mature stage or whether it represents a population of anergic cells (Merrell et al., 2006).

3.2 Innate and adaptive mature B cell populations

Following antigen binding, mature B cells activate pathways that lead to proliferation and further differentiation into antibody-producing B cells (plasma cells) or memory B cells. In the spleen, mature B cells are sub-divided into follicular (FO, AA4.1-CD21intCD23high) and marginal zone (MZ, AA4.1-CD21highCD23-) B cells according to both their location and their cell-surface phenotype. A distinct subset of mature B cells is preferentially present in the peritoneal cavity; these are known as B1 cells [B220+CD11b+CD5+ (B1a) or CD5- (B1b)]. Among them, FO B cells are responsible for adaptive antibody responses, whereas MZ and B1 mature populations respond rapidly to antigenic stimulus but do not go through germinal-center reactions and thus their response can be independent of T cell help (Martin et al., 2001). Therefore, MZ and B1 B cells are thought to be part of an innate–like response. The origin of both of these populations is not well understood. While MZ B cells share part of FO pathway, the fetal liver was thought to originate a large fraction of the adult B1 B cells (Tung et al., 2006). Recently, a novel developmental model suggests that some B1 cell progenitors can be produced in bone marrow (Esplin et al., 2009).

3.3 Regulation of B lineage commitment: The critical role of preBCR tonic signaling, IL-7R and transcription factors in context

Limitation of lineage choice during development is regulated by a combination of signaling pathways and transcription factors (TF). In mice, the main receptor controlling the ProB stage is the IL-7R, which is composed of a α chain (IL-7Rα) and the common cytokine receptor γ chain (γc). Deletion of IL-7Rα or γc leads to developmental arrest at the early ProB stage (von Freeden-Jeffrey et al., 1995; Cao et al., 1995).

IL-7 activates the major signaling pathway JAK–STAT, with STAT5 being the essential mediator of IL-7 signals in early B cell development (Yao et al., 2006).

By the other hand, an important characteristic of the developmental process that distinguishes B and T lymphocytes from other cell lineages is the continuous selection of these lymphoid cells for their ability to express a competent, non-self receptor. B cells that fail to express a receptor are eliminated. Thus, BCR and BCR-like receptors must generate active permissive signals that allow differentiation through the different developmental stages. Because the preBCR lacks of the light chain and therefore of the capacity to bind polymorphic ligands, it has been proposed that this receptor is able to signal constitutively and independently on ligand, an activity also known as tonic signaling. Although there is little understanding of how tonic signals are generated, the view is supported by receptor-less B cells able to differentiate into mature B cells by expression of a chimeric construct of Igα and Igβ positioned in the cell surface membrane (Bannish et al., 2001).

Once the preBCR is expressed at the end of the proB stage, it can take over many of the functions performed by the IL-7 receptor signaling. Both receptors act individually and together to allow B cell development (Figure 5). Like IL-7R, the preBCR promotes mechanisms of positive selection, survival and proliferation (Ramadani et al., 2010; Yasuda et al., 2008). The CCND3 gene, which encodes for cyclin D3, is essential for PreB cell expansion and integrates IL-7R and preBCR signals (Cooper et al., 2006).

Downstream the IL-7 and preBCR receptors, a handful of transcription factors (TF) are critical for commitment to the B cell lineage and early development; these include E2A/TCF3 (immunoglobulin enhancer binding factors E12/E47/transcription factor 3), EBF1 (Early B cell Factor 1) and PAX5 (Paired box 5) (Figure 5). Loss of E2A and EBF1 blocks entry into the B cell lineage, while loss of PAX5 redirects B cells into other lineages (Nutt et al., 1999; O'Riordan & Grosschedl, 1999). Acting together with E2A, EBF1 and STAT5, one of the main molecular functions of PAX5 is to allow VDJ recombination (Hsu et al., 2004). Also, E2A, PAX5, IKZF1 and RUNX1, among other TF, are responsible for RAG expression (Kuo & Schlissel, 2009). Moreover, IL-7R signaling fulfills an essential role in early B cell development, with STAT5 participating in the activation of the B cell regulatory genes E2A, EBF1 and PAX5. E2A encodes two TF via alternative splicing, E12 and E47. In mice lacking the E2A gene, the B cell lineage is lost, there is no heavy chain recombination, and the expression of the B cell-restricted genes EBF1, PAX5, CD79A/B and VPREB1 (CD179A) is also affected.

Enforced expression of EBF1 and PAX5 is sufficient to overcome the developmental block in mice deficient in E2A, IL-7 or IL-7Rα, further illustrating the transcriptional hierarchy of the B cell-specific program triggered by IL-7 receptor signaling (Nutt & Kee, 2007). EBF1 acting together with PAX5 drives the expression of many genes critical for early B cell development and B cell function, including FOXO1, MYCN, LEF1, BLNK, CD79A (MB-1), RAG2, CD19 and CR2 (CD21) (Nutt & Kee, 2007; Smith & Sigvardsson, 2004).

Although PAX5 is a positive regulator of B-cell specific genes, also functions as a repressor of non B-lineage genes such as M-CSFR, NOTCH1 and FLT3 (Cobaleda et al., 2007) so B cell development is unidirectional and mostly irreversible in homeostatic conditions.

Also important for lymphoid development are members of the Ikaros family of TFs, mainly IKZF1 (which encodes Ikaros) and IKZF3 (which encodes Aiolos). Ikaros activates B cell genes and represses genes that are unrelated to the B lineage. Expression of IKZF1 and IKZF3 is regulated by alternative splicing, which produces long isoforms (Ik-1, Ik-2, Ik-3, Aio-1, Aio-3, Aio-4 and Aio-6) that efficiently bind to DNA, and short isoforms (Ik-4, Ik-5/7, Ik-6, Ik8, Aio-2, Aio-5) that are unable to bind DNA with high affinity and do not activate transcription (Liippo et al., 2001). Ikaros is activated in early stages of lymphopoiesis and is required for both early and late events in lymphocyte differentiation. Aiolos is not required during the early specification of the B and T lineages but is essential during further B cell maturation. They also act in concert to promote preB cell cycle exit and transition to small PreB stage (Ma et al., 2010).

3.4 Human B cell development

Selection processes operating on developing B cells are similar in all mammals. Thus, early B cell development in humans is also mainly guided by VDJ recombination and by the proliferative expansion of clones that have successfully completed the rearrangement of their receptors, whereas late development is led by mechanisms of tolerance to self-antigens. All these processes in humans are less well understood than are their counterparts in mice. Importantly, human B cells can still be generated in severe combined immunodeficiency (SCID) patients with mutations in the IL-7R gene, suggesting that IL-7 signaling is not essential for human B cell development (Puel et al., 1998) although a recent study has demonstrated that in vitro human B cell production is dependent on IL-7 (Parrish et al., 2009). The fine regulatory mechanism separating proliferation and differentiation might explain why the proliferating ProB and PreB sub-stages are the ones generally found to be compromised in human pediatric B-cell acute lymphoblastic leukemia (B-cell ALL) and why this disease is characterized by leukemic blast cells that are often unable to progress through the differentiation pathway. This tendency to be arrested in proliferative states might result in an increased rate of mutations, leading to formation of neoplastic cells. Supporting the later, mice expressing B cell mutants in the adaptor protein BLNK are arrested in the large PreB stage and often develop B cell malignancies (Flemming et al., 2003). Proliferative stages occur in the early ProB, PreB-I and large PreB-II fractions (Figure 5).

4. Acute lymphoblastic leukemia

Acute lymphoblastic leukemia (ALL) is a disorder characterized by the monoclonal and/or oligoclonal proliferation of hematopoietic precursor cells of the lymphoid series within the bone marrow. At present, ALL is the most frequent malignancy in children worldwide and a serious problem of public health, constituting 25% of all childhood cancers and 75%-85% of the cases of childhood leukemias (Perez-Saldivar et al., 2011). Near to 80% of ALL cases have precursor B-cell immunophenotype, while approximately 15% show T-cell immunophenotype. Even when a relatively high efficiency of therapeutic agents has been demonstrated (Pieters & Carroll, 2010), there has been a slight but gradual increase in the incidence of ALL in the past 25 years, and appears to be highest in Hispanic population, which also show superior rates of high risk patients (Fajardo-Gutiérrez et al., 2007; Abdullaev et al., 2000; Perez-Saldivar et al., 2011; Mejía-Aranguré et al., 2011). Factors such as drug resistance, minimal residual disease, cell lineage switch, and the rise of mixed lineages often put the success of treatment at risk and change the prognosis of the illness. The molecular mechanism involved in these phenomena and the identities of the target hematopoietic populations have not been completely defined, due in part, to the fact that neither the precise origin of the disease, nor the susceptibility of primitive leukemic cells to extrinsic factors, is known.

4.1 The origin of ALL

Over the last two decades, cancer stem cells (CSC) have been defined as cells within a tumor that possess the capacity to self-renew and to cause heterogeneous lineages of cancer cells that comprise the tumor (Clarke et al., 2006). According to MF Greaves, who proposed the original hypothesis for leukemogenesis, multiple consecutive carcinogenic hits in hematopoietic cells may drive the malignant transformation (Greaves, 1993; Greaves & Wiernels, 2003), where the second oncogenic event on pre-leukemic clones could be indirectly promoted by delayed infections (Greaves, 2006; Mejía-Aranguré et al., 2011). Our general current view suggests the occurring of oncogenic lesions in early development or in a primitive cell that result in the abnormal differentiation of leukemic stem cells. Among the various factors that hit the HSC fraction, anomalous microenvironmental cues may contribute to trigger and support the leukemic behaviour of precursor cells (Figure 6).

Although CSC in myeloid leukemias have been strictly depicted as the responsible cells for tumour maintenance, which clearly keep the biological hierarchy within the hematopoietic structure (Dick, 2008), identification of a rare primitive and malignant cell with intrinsic stem cell properties and the ability to recapitulate the acute lymphoblastic leukemia has been more complicated (Bomken et al.,2010), particularly due to the genetic diversity of the disease and the lack of appropriate *in vitro* and *in vivo* models.

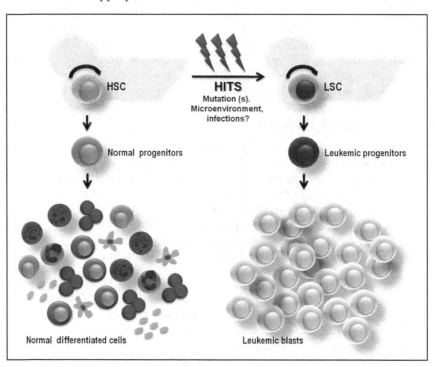

Fig. 6. Leukemic stem cell model. Normal hematopoietic stem cells (HSC) give rise to progenitors and mature blood cells within a hierarchical structure in the bone marrow. As a result of multiple and consecutive oncogenic hits on HSC including genetic and microenvironmental alterations, a malignant counterpart (the leukemic stem cell, LSC) emerge, which maintains some degree of developmental potential, generating the leukemic progenitor and blast cells.

Cell culture systems revealing alterations in early hematopoiesis, the existence of leukemic clones with unrelated DJ rearrangements and cytogenetic abnormalities on cells lacking lineage markers, have strongly suggested the participation of primitive cells in ALL. Moreover, data showing cells with immature phenotypes capable of engrafting and reconstituting leukemia in immunodeficient mice, lead to believe that, as in AML & CML, the hierarchy structure of the hematopoietic system is kept in ALL, and infant B cell-leukemia initiating cells have undifferentiated characteristics (Espinoza-Hernandez et al., 2001; Cobaleda et al., 2000; Cox et al., 2004; Cox et al., 2009). To characterize ALL progenitor cells, Blair and colleagues have purified by flow cytometry a number of cell fractions based on the expression of CD34 and the B-lymphoid marker CD19. Regardless the risk stratum of the patient, CD34+CD19- cells, but not committed B precursors, were able to reconstitute the disease in NOD/SCID models (Cox et al., 2004). Moreover, CD133+CD38-CD19- primitive cells residing in ALL BM are suggested to be the leukemia-initiating cells and responsible of drug-resistant residual disease (Cox et al., 2009). However, recent studies have remarkably shown that precursor blasts can also reestablish leukemic phenotypes *in vivo*, conferring them stem cell properties (Heidenreich & Vormoor, 2009; Bomken et al., 2010). Using novel intrafemoral xenotransplantation strategies, Vormoor's Lab has found that all differentiation stages of B precursor cells within CD34+CD19+ and CD34-CD19+ fractions are able to successfully engraft and recapitulate the original patient's disease in long-term systems, suggesting that committed cells in ALL do not lose the self-renewal stem cell property while they mature (le Viseur et al., 2008) (Figure 5), though their multi-lineage potential is uncertain.

These discordant results unveil that key questions regarding leukemic stem cells and the earliest steps of the lymphoid program in ALL still to be solved. Recently, the combination of clonal studies and alterations on genetic copies along with xenotransplant models, showed unsuspected genetic diversity, supporting multiclonal evolution of leukemogenesis rather than lineal succession (Dick, 2008). Thus, a less rigid structure of CSC models should further take account of functional plasticity and clonal evolution to understand CSC biology and to develop novel, stem/progenitor cell-directed therapies (Bomken et al., 2010).

4.2 Genes, cytogenetic alterations and transcription factors in B-cell leukemogenesis

The leukemogenic program is characterized by arrest of differentiation pathways, increased cell proliferation, enhanced self-renewal, decreased apoptosis rates and telomere maintenance. It is thought that together these alterations result in production of highly proliferative clones of immature leukemic blast cells with intrinsic survival advantage and limitless replicative potential (Warner et al., 2004).

Gain or loss of function of transcription factors such as E2A, EBF1, PAX5 and Ikaros affect homeostatic B cell lymphopoiesis in murine models, and are often associated with malignant transformation in humans, supporting conserved roles for these TFs and their activating signaling pathways (Figure 5) (Pérez-Vera et al., 2011).

A high frequency of ALL patients has genetic lesions -mostly chromosomal translocations-associated with leukemic cells. E2A is often translocated with several partners, including PBX1 [t(1;19)(q23;p13)] and HLF [t(17;19)(q22;p13)], which are detected in 5-6% and 1% of ALL children, respectively. E2A-PBX1 is a potent transcriptional activator of the WNT16 oncogene (McWhirter et al., 1999), while E2A-HLF functions as a survival factor of early B cells by activating expression of the anti-apoptotic genes SNAI2 (SLUG) and LMO2. Accordingly, gene silencing of LMO2 in an E2A-HLFpos cell line induced apoptotic cell death (Hirose et al., 2010). RUNX1 is also a frequent target for chromosomal rearrangements and mutations in ALL. 25% of children and 2% of adults of ALL patients carry the ETV6/RUNX1 fusion as a result of the translocation t(12;21)(p12;q21), which may play a role regulating the B lineage-specific transcriptional program at an early stage (Durst & Hiebert, 2004). SNP array analysis of ETV6-RUNX1 samples has recently identified multiple additional genetic alterations, but the role of these lesions in leukemogenesis remains undetermined (van der Weyden et al., 2011).

Genome-wide analysis has recorded abnormalities in PAX5 and EBF1 in up to 32% of children and 30% of adults with B ALL, and in 35% of relapsed cases (Mullighan et al., 2007). Currently, five PAX5 fusions have been identified with the gene partners LOC392027 (7p12.1), SLCO1B3 (12p12), ASXL1 (20q11.1), KIF3B (20q11.21) and C20orf112 (20q11.1), with the resulting chimeric proteins expressing lower levels of PAX5 and its target genes (An et al., 2008). EBF1 alterations are common in patients with poor outcomes and are particularly frequent (25%) in relapsed children (Harvey et al., 2010).

The MLL (mixed lineage leukemia) gene is often rearranged in leukemias with myeloid and lymphoid phenotype, probably indicating a very early multipotent progenitor origin. More than 50 fusions involving MLL have been documented. Among them, the MLL-AF4 [t(4;11)(q21;q23)] translocation is present in 80% of infant, 2% of children, and 5-10% of adult ALL (McCarthy, 2010).

The BCR-ABL1 translocation [t(9;22)(q34;q11), also known as Philadelphia chromosome] is found in 5% of pediatric and 25% of adult B cell ALL. An important consequence for this translocation is the over-expression of STAT5. STAT5 inactivation results in cell cycle arrest and apoptosis of BCR-ABL^{pos} malignant B cells and BCR-ABL1^{pos} STAT5 knockout mice do not develop leukemia (Malin et al., 2010). Interestingly, genome-wide analysis of B cell ALL has identified mutations in the STAT5 upstream regulators JAK1 and JAK2 in up to 10% of patients, and patients BCR-ABL^{pos} or with JAK1&2 mutations have a similar gene expression profile and prognosis (Malin et al., 2010). JAK2 mutations lead over-expression of CRLF2 (also known as thymic stromal lymphopoietin receptor) which forms a heterodimeric complex with the IL-7R (Harvey et al., 2010). In a subset of cases, CRLF2 promotes constitutive dimerization and cytokine-independent proliferation. Finally, high expression levels of the short Ikaros isoforms, particularly the dominant negative Ik-6, are also associated with high risk leukemia (Sun et al., 1999). Most of the BCR-ABL^{pos} B ALL patients have deletions in IKZF1 and increased levels of the short isoforms; however, Ik-6 has also been found to be elevated in BCR-ABL^{neg} patients (Mullighan et al., 2008). It has been proposed that the high level of Ikaros short isoform expression is due to genetic lesions. Supporting this idea, IKZF1 somatic deletions have been found in a number of recurrences and are strongly associated with minimal residual disease (Mullighan et al., 2009). A summary of homeostatic and leukemic expression of transcription factors along the B cell pathway is shown in Figure 5.

Despite these important advances in the definition of genetic abnormalities that are prevalent in ALL, the disease is heterogeneous at the molecular level, and possibly it is the result of combination of genetic and epigenetic alterations. Furthermore, high frequencies of ALL cases seem not to be associated to intrinsic genetic abnormalities, opening the possibility of microenvironmental cues leading to disease.

4.3 Leukemic microenvironmental cues?

The complexity of leukemogenesis increases when we consider the indubitable influence of the bone marrow microenvironment in the hematopoietic development, which is a network of cells (mesenchymal cells, osteoblasts, fibroblasts, adipocytes, endothelial cells, etc) and their products (extracellular matrix molecules, cytokines and chemokines) that support hematopoiesis. Under physiological conditions, the appropriate production of mature blood cells throughout life is sustained by special niches that provide stem and progenitor cells with regulatory signals essential for their maintenance, proliferation and differentiation (Nagasawa et al., 2011). Among secreted factors, CXCL12, FLT3-L, interleukin 7 and stem cell factor are critical for commitment to the lymphoid program and normal B cell development is supported by two stage specific cellular niches within central bone marrow: a CXCL12/SDF1 expressing niche, and a IL-7 expressing niche. B cell precursors are thought to move from one to another as differentiation progresses (Tokoyoda et al., 2004; Nagasawa, 2006). The role of the bone marrow microenvironment in carcinogenesis has been conceived through three possible mechanisms: competition of tumor cells for normal HSC niches, which may allow their maintenance and survival; manipulation of the environment to promote tumor progression and disruption of hematopoietic-niche communication that drives oncogenesis (Raaijmakers, 2011). Although these potential mechanisms are tempting, their contribution to ALL remains formally unexplored. It has been proposed by Sipkins and colleagues that the leukemic cells derived-tumor microenvironment impairs the behavior of normal hematopoietic cells (Colmone et al., 2008). Furthermore, a number of alterations have been recorded in the marrow microenvironment of ALL, including chromosomal aberrations in mesenchymal stem cells, anomalous expression of adhesion molecules, abnormal levels of CXCR4 and growth factors, as well as prevalence of pro-inflammatory cytokines (Menendez et al., 2009; Geijtenbeek et al., 1999; Juarez et al., 2009; and our unpublished results). Whether an abnormal microenvironment anticipates the leukemic stage or is a consequent fact, is still an open issue.

5. Conclusion

Much has been learned about identity, function and intercommunication of seminal cells within the hematopoietic system from animal models. However, our understanding of the hierarchy and regulation of human stem/progenitor cells is still incomplete and the hematopoietic charts have been in constant re-construction over the last few years. Furthermore, while it has long been recognized that intrinsic abnormalities in primitive hematopoietic cells may cause hematological disorders, it has also become clear that changes in both cell composition and function of the bone marrow microenvironment might govern stem cell activity and lead to disease. Future progress in these areas will be decisive to suggest novel classification, prognosis and treatment venues.

6. Acknowledgment

R.P. is recipient of funding from the National Council of Science and Technology, CONACYT (grant CB-2010-CO1-152695) and from the Mexican Institute for Social Security, IMSS (grant FIS/IMSS/852). EDA and EV are scholarship holders from CONACYT.

7. References

Abdullaev, F., Rivera-Luna, R., Roitenburd-Belacortu, V., & Espinosa-Aguirre, J. (2000). Pattern of childhood cancer mortality in Mexico. *Arch Med Res.* Vol. 31, No.5, (September-October 2000), pp. (526-31), ISSN 0188-4409

Allman, D., Lindsay, R. C., DeMuth, W., Rudd, K., Shinton, S. A., & Hardy R. R. (2001). Resolution of three nonproliferative immature splenic B cell subsets reveals multiple selection points during peripheral B cell maturation. *Journal of immunology*, Vol.167, No.12, (December 2001), pp. (6834-6840), ISSN 0022-1767

An, Q., Wright S. L., Konn Z. J., Matheson E., Minto L., Moorman A. V., Parker H., Griffiths M., Ross F. M., Davies T., Hall A. G., Harrison C. J., Irving J. A., & Stretfford J. C. (2008). Variable breakpoints target PAX5 in patients with dicentric chromosomes: a model for the basis of unbalanced translocations in cancer. *Proceedings of the National Academy of Science USA*, Vol. 105, No. 44, (October 2008), pp. (17050-17054), ISSN 0027-8424

Baba, Y. Pelayo, R.,& Kincade, PW. (2004). Relationships between hematopoietic stem cells and lymphocyte progenitors. *TRENDS in Immunology*, Vol.25, No.12, (December 2004), pp. 645-649, ISSN 1471-4906

Baldridge, MT., King, KY.,& Goodell, MA. (2011). Inflammatory signals regulate hematopoietic stem cells. *Trends in Immunology*, Vol.32, No.2, (February 2011), pp.57-65, ISSN 1471-4906

Bannish, G., Fuentes-Pananá, E. M., Cambier, J. C., Pear, W. S., & Monroe, J. G. (2001). Ligand-independent signaling functions for the B lymphocyte antigen receptor and their role in positive selection during B lymphopoiesis. *Journal of Experimental Medicine*, Vol.194, No.11 (December 2001), pp. (1583-1596), ISSN: 0022-100

Blom, B. & Spits, H. (2006). Development of human lymphoid cells. *Annual Reviews of Immunology*. Vol. 24, pp. (287-320), ISSN 0732-0582

Bomken, S., Fiser, K., Heidenreich, O., & Vormoor, J.,(2010). Understanding the cancer stem cell. *Br J Cancer*. Vol. 103 No.4, (August 2010), pp (439-45), ISSN 1532-1827

Cao X., Shores E. W., Hu-Li J., Anver M. R., Kelsall B. L, Russell S. M., Drago J., Noguchi M., Grinberg A., & Bloom E. T. (1995). Defective lymphoid development in mice lacking expression of the common cytokine receptor □ chain. *Immunity*, Vol. 2, No. 3, (March 1995), pp. (223-238), ISSN 1074-7613

Clarke, M., Dick, J, Dirks, P., Eaves, C., Jamieson, C., Jones, D., Visvader, J., Weissman, I., & Wahl, M., (2006) Cancer stem cells perspectives on current status and future directions: AACR Workshop on cancer stem cells. *Cancer Res*. Vol.66, No.19, (October 2006) pp (9339-44), ISSN 1538-7445

Cobaleda, C., Gutiérrez-Cianca, N., Pérez-Losada, J., Flores, T., García-Sanz, R., González, M., & Sánchez-García, I. (2000) A primitive hematopoietic cell is the target for the leukemic transformation in human philadelphia-positive acute lymphoblastic leukemia. *Blood* Vol.95, No.3, (February 2000) pp. (1007-1013), ISSN 0006-4971

Cobaleda, C., Schebesta, A., Delogu, A., & Busslinger M. (2007). Pax5: the guardian of B cell identity and function. *Nature Immunology*, Vol. 8, No. 4, (April 2007), pp. (463-470), ISSN 1529-2908

Colmone, A., Amorim, M., Pontier, A., , Wang, S., Jablonski, E., & Sipkins, D., (2008) Leukemic cells create bone marrow niches that disrupt the behavior of normal hematopoietic progenitor cells. *Science*. Vol.322, No.5909, (December 2008), pp. (1861-5), ISSN 1095-9203

Cooper A. B., Sawai C. M., Sicinska E., Powers S. E., Sicinski P., Clark M. R., & Aifantis I. (2006). A unique function for cyclin D3 in early B cell development. *Nature Immunology*, Vol. 7, No. 5, (May 2006), pp. (489-497), ISSN 1529-2908

Cox, CV., Diamanti, P., Evely, RS., Kearns, PR., & Blair A. (2009) Expression of CD133 on leukemia-initiating cells in childhood ALL. *Blood* Vol.113, No.14, (April 2009), pp. (3287-3295), ISSN 1528-0020

Cox, CV., Evely, R., Oakhill, A., Pamphilon, D., Goulden, N.,& Blair, A., (2004) Characterization of acute lymphoblastic leukemia progenitor cells. *Blood.* Vol.104, No.9, (November 2004), pp. (2919-25), ISSN 0006-4971

De Luca, K. Frances-Duvert, V. Asensio, M. Ihsani, R., Debien, E., Taillardet, M., Verhoeyen, E., Bella, C., Lantheaume, S., Genestier, L., & Defrance, T. (2009). The TLR1/2 agonist PAM(3)CSK(4) instructs commitment of human hematopoietic stem cells to a myeloid cell fate. *Leukemia.* Vol. 23, No. 11, pp. 2063-74, ISSN 0887-6924

Dick, J., (2008) Stem cell concepts renew cancer research. *Blood.* Vol.112, No.13, (December 2008), pp. (4793-807), ISSN 1528-0020

Doulatov, S., Notta, F., Eppert, K., Nguyen, LT., Ohashi, PS., & Dick, JE. (2010). Revised map of the human progenitor hierarchy shows the origin of macrophages and dendritic cells in early lymphoid development. *Nat Immunol*, Vol.11, No.7, (July 2010), pp.585-593, ISSN 1529-2908

Durst, KL., & Hiebert, SW. (2004). Role of RUNX family members in transcriptional repression and gene silencing. *Oncogene*, Vol.23, No.24, (May 2004), pp. (4220-4224), ISSN 0950-9232

Espinoza-Hernández, L., Cruz-Rico, J., Benítez-Aranda, H., Martínez-Jaramillo, G., Rodríguez-Zepeda, MC., Vélez-Ruelas, MA., Mayani, H. (2001) In vitro characterization of the hematopoietic system in pediatric patients with acute lymphoblastic leukemia. *Leukemia Research* Vol.25, No.4, (April 2001) pp (295-303), ISSN 0145-2126

Esplin B.L., Welner R.S., Zhang Q., Borghesi L.A., & Kincade P.W. (2009). A differentiation pathway for B1 cells in adult bone marrow. *Proceedings of the National Academy of Science USA*, Vol. 106, No.14, (April 2009), pp. (5773-5778), ISSN 0027-8424

Fajardo-Gutiérrez, A., Juárez-Ocaña, S., González-Miranda, G., Palma-Padilla, V., Carreón-Cruz, R., Ortega-Alvárez, M., & Mejía-Arangure, J., (2007) Incidence of cancer in children residing in ten jurisdictions of the Mexican Republic: importance of the Cancer registry (a population-based study). *BMC Cancer.* Vol.7, No.68, (April 2007), pp (68-82), ISSN 1471-2407

Flemming A., Brummer T., Reth M., & Jumaa H. (2003). The adaptor protein SLP-65 acts as a tumor suppressor that limits pre-B cell expansion. *Nature Immunology*, Vol. 4, No. 1, (November 2003), pp. (38-43), ISSN 1529-2908

Fuentes-Pananá, E. M. Bannish, G., & Monroe, J. G. (2004a). Basal B-cell receptor signaling in B lymphocytes: mechanisms of regulation and role in positive selection, differentiation, and peripheral survival. *Immunological Reviews*, Vol.197, No.1, (January 2004), pp. (26-40), ISSN 0105-2896

Fuentes-Pananá E. M., Bannish G., Monroe J. G. (2004b). Basal Iga/Igb signals trigger the coordinated initiation of preBCR-dependent processes. *Journal of Immunology*, Vol.173, No.2, (July 2004), pp. 1000-1011, ISSN 0022-1767

Geijtenbeek, TB., van Kooyk, Y., van Vliet, SJ., Renes, MH., Raymakers, RA., & Figdor, CG. (1999) High frequency of adhesion defects in B-lineage acute lymphoblastic leukemia. *Blood.* Vol.94. No.15, (July 1999) pp. (754-64), ISSN 0006-4971

Greaves, M., (1993) Stem cell origins of leukaemia and curability. *Br J Cancer.* Vol.67, No.3, (March 1993), pp. (413-23), ISSN 0007-0920

Greaves, M.(2006) Infection, immune responses and the aetiology of childhood leukaemia. *Nat Rev Cancer*. Vol.6, No.3, (March 2006), pp. (193-203), ISSN 1474-175X

Greaves, MF., & Wiemels, J.(2003) Origins of chromosome translocations in childhood leukaemia. *Nat Rev Cancer*. Vol.3, No.9, (September 2003) pp. (639-49), ISSN 1474-175X

Hardy, R. R., Carmack, C. E., Shinton, S. A., Kemp, J. D.,& Hayakawa, K. (1991). Resolution and characterization of pro-B and pre-pro-B cell stages in normal mouse bone marrow. *Journal of Experimental Medicine*, Vol.173, No.5, (May 1991), pp. (1213-1225), ISSN: 1932-6203

Harvey, RC., Mullighan, CG., Wang, X., Dobbin, KK., Davidson, GS., Bedrick, EJ., Chen, I M., Atlas, SR., Kang, H., Ar, K., Wharton, W., Murphy, M., Devidas, M., Carroll, AJ., Borowitz, MJ., Bowman, WP., Downing, JR., Relling, M., Yang, J., Bhojwani, D., Carroll, WL., Camitta, B., Reaman, GH., Smith, M., Hunger, SP., & Willman, CL. (2010). Identification of novel cluster groups in pediatric high-risk B-precursor acute lymphoblastic leukemia with gene expression profiling: correlation with genome-wide DNA copy number alterations, clinical characteristics, and outcome. *Blood*, Vol. 116, No. 23, (December 2010), pp. (4874-4884), ISSN 0006-4971

Heidenreich, O., & Vormoor, J., (2009) Malignant stem cells in childhood ALL: the debate continues! *Blood*. Vol.113, No.18, (April 2009), pp. (4476-7), ISSN 1528-0020

Hirose, K., Inukai T., Kikuchi, J., Furukawa, Y., Ikawa, T., Kawamoto, H., Oram, SH., Göttgens, B., Kiyokawa, N., Miyagawa, Y., Okita, H., Akahane, K., Zhang, X., Kuroda, I., Honna, H., Kagami, K., Goi, K., Kurosawa, H., Look, AT., Matsui, H., Inaba, T., & Sugita, K. (2010). Aberrant induction of LMO2 by the E2A-HLF chimeric transcription factor and its implication in leukemogenesis of B-precursor ALL with t(17;19). *Blood*, Vol.116, No.6, (August 2010), pp. (962-970), ISSN 0006-4971

Hsu L. Y., Liang H. E., Johnson K., Kang C., & Schlissel M. S. (2004). Pax5 activates immunoglobulin heavy chain V to DJ rearrangement in transgenic thymocytes. *Journal of Experimental Medicine*, Vol. 199, No. 6, (March 2004), pp. (825-830), ISSN 0022-1007

Ichii, M., Oritani, K., Yokota, T., Zhang, Q., Garrett, KP., Kanakura, Y., & Kincade, PW. (2010) The density of CD10 corresponds to commitment and progression in the human B lymphoid lineage *PloS One*. Vol.5 No9. (September 2010) pp e12954, ISSN 1932-6203

Igarashi, H., Gregory, S.C., Yokota, T., Sakaguchi, N., & Kincade, P.W. (2002). Transcription from the RAG1 locus marks the earliest lymphocyte progenitors in bone marrow. *Immunity*, Vol. 17, No. 2, pp. (117-130), ISSN 1074-7613

Juarez, JG., Thien, M., De la Pena, A., Baraz, R, Bradstock, KF., & Bendall, LJ. (2009) CXCR4 mediates the homing of B cell progenitor acute lymphoblastic leukaemia cells to the bone marrow via activation of p38MAPK. *Br J Haematol*. Vol.145, No.4, (May 2009) pp. (491-9), ISSN 1365-2141

Kim, JM., Kim, NI., Oh, YK., Kim, YJ., Youn, J., & Ahn, MJ. (2005). CpG oligodeoxynucleotides induce IL-8 expression in CD34+ cells via mitogen-activated protein kinase-dependent and NF-kB-independent pathways. *International Immunol*, Vol.17, pp.1525-1531, ISSN 0953-8178

Kuo T. C., & Schlissel M. S. (2009). Mechanisms controlling expression of the RAG locus during lymphocyte development. *Current Opinion in Immunology*, Vol. 21, No. 2, (April 2009), pp. (173–178), ISSN 0952-7915

le Viseur, C., Hotfilder, M., Bomken, S., Wilson, K., Röttgers, S., Schrauder, A., Rosemann, A., Irving, J., Stam, R., Shultz, L., Harbott, J., Jürgens, H., Schrappe, M., Pieters, R., & Vormoor, J., (2008) In childhood acute lymphoblastic leukemia, blasts at different stages of immunophenotypic maturation have stem cell properties. *Cancer* Martin F., Oliver A. M., Kearney J. F. (2001). Marginal Zone and B1 B Cells Unite in the Early Response against T-Independent Blood-Borne Particulate Antigens. *Immunity*, Vol.14, No.5, (May 2001), pp. (617–629), ISSN 1074-7613

Li, Z., Dordai D. I., Lee, J., & Desiderio, S. (1996). A conserved degradation signal regulates RAG-2 accumulation during cell division and links V(D)J recombination to the cell cycle. *Immunity*, Vol.5, No.6, (December 1996), pp. (575-589), ISSN 1074-7613

Liippo J., Nera K. P., Veistinen E., Ländesmäki A., Postila V., Kimby E., Riikonen P., Hammarström L., Pelkonen J., & Lassila O. (2001). Both normal and leukemic B lymphocytes express multiple isoforms of the human aiolos gene. *European Journal of Immunology*, Vol. 31, No. 12, (December 2001), pp. (3469-3474), ISSN 0014-2980

Ma S., Pathak S., Mandal M., Trinh L., Clark M. R., & Lu R. (2010). Ikaros and Aiolos inhibit pre-B-cell proliferation by directly suppressing c-Myc expression. *Molecular and Cellular Biology*, Vol. 30, No. 17, (September 2010), pp. (4149-4158), ISSN 0270-7306

Malin, S., McManus, S., & Busslinger, M. (2010). STAT5 in B cell development and leukemia. *Current Opinion in Immunology*, Vol.22, No.2, (April 2010), pp. (168-176), ISSN 0952-7915

Martin F., Oliver A. M., Kearney J. F. (2001). Marginal Zone and B1 B Cells Unite in the Early Response against T-Independent Blood-Borne Particulate Antigens. *Immunity*, Vol. 14, No. 5, (May 2001), pp. (617–629), ISSN 1074-7613

Mayani, H. (2010). Biological differences between neonatal and adult human hematopoietic stem/progenitor cells. *Stem Cells and Dev*, Vol.19, No.3, pp.285-298, ISSN 1547-3287

McCarthy, N. (2010). Leukaemia: MLL makes friends and influences. *Nature Reviews in Cancer*, Vol. 10, No. 8, (August 2010), pp. (529), ISNN 1474-175X

McWhirter J. R., Neuteboom S. T., Wancewicz E. V., Monia B. P., Downing J. R., & Murre C. (1999). Oncogenic homeodomain transcription factor E2A-Pbx1 activates a novel WNT gene in pre-B acute lymphoblastoid leukemia. *Proceedings of the National Academy of Science USA*, Vol.96, No.20, (September 1999), pp. (11464-11469), ISSN 0027-8424

Mejia-Arangure, JM.; (2011). *Childhood Acute Leukemias in Hispanic Population: Differences by Age Peak and Immunophenotype*, InTech, ISBN México City, México. In Press

Menendez, P., Catalina, P., Rodríguez, R., Melen, GJ., Bueno, C., Arriero, M., García-Sánchez, F., Lassaletta, A., García-Sanz, R., & García-Castro, J. (2009) Bone marrow mesenchymal stem cells from infants with MLL-AF4+ acute leukemia harbor and express the MLL-AF4 fusion gene. *J Exp Med*. Vol.206, No.13, (December 2009) pp 3131-41. ISSN 1540-9538

Merrell, K. T., Benschop, R. J., Gauld, S. B., Aviszus, K., Decote-Ricardo, D., Wysocki, L. J. & Cambier, J.C. (2006). Identification of Anergic B Cells within a Wild-Type Repertoire. *Immunity*, Vol.25, No.6 (December 2006), pp (953–962), ISSN 1074-7613

Mullighan, C G., Goorha, S., Radtke, I., Miller, CB., Coustan-Smith, E., Dalton, JD., Girtman, K., Mathew, S., Ma, J., Pound, SB., Su, X., Pui, CH., Relling, MV., Evans, WE., Shurtleff, SA., & Downing, JR. (2007). Genome-wide analysis of genetic alterations in acute lymphoblastic leukemia. *Nature,* Vol. 446, No. 7137, (April 2007), pp. (758-764), ISSN 0028-0836

Mullighan, CG., Miller, CB., Radtke, I., Phillips, LA., Dalton, J., Ma, J., White, D., Hughes, TP., Le Beau, MM., Pui, CH., Relling, MV., Shurtleff, SA., & Downing, JR. (2008). BCR-ABL1 lymphoblastic leukaemia is characterized by the deletion of ikaros. *Nature,* Vol. 453, No. 7191, (May 2008), pp. (110-114), ISSN 0028-0836

Mullighan, CG., Su, X., Zhang, J., Radtke, I., Phillips, LA., Miller, CB., Ma, J., Liu, W., Cheng, C., Schulman, BA., Harvey, RC., Chen, IM., Clifford, RJ., Carroll, WL., Reaman, G., Bowman, WP., Devidas, M., Gerhard, DS., Yang, W., Relling, MV., Shurtleff, SA., Campana, D., Borowitz, MJ., Pui, CH., Smith, M., Hunger, SP., Willman, CL., & Downing JR; Children's Oncology Group. (2009). Deletion of IKZF1 and prognosis in acute lymphoblastic leukemia. *New England Journal of Medicine,* Vol. 360, No.5, (January 2009), pp. (470-480), ISSN 0028-4793

Nagai, Y. Garrett, K. Ohta, S. Bahrun, U., Kouro, T., Akira, S., Takatsu, K., & Kincade, PW.. (2006). Toll-like receptors on hematopoietic progenitor cells stimulate innate immune system replenishment. *Immunity.* Vol. 24, No. 6, pp. 801-12, ISSN 1074-7613

Nagasawa ,T. (2006) Microenvironmental niches in the bone marrow required for B-celldevelopment. *Nat Rev Immunol.* Vol.6, No.2, (February 2006) pp. (107-16), ISSN 1474-1733

Nagasawa, T., Omatsu, Y., & Sugiyama, T. (2011) Control of hematopoietic stem cells by the bone marrow stromal niche: the role of reticular cells. *Trends Immunol.* Vol.32, No.7, (July 2011), pp. (315-20), ISSN 1471-4981

Nutt S. L., Heavey B., Rolink A. G., & Busslinger M. (1999). Commitment to the B-lymphoid lineage depends on the transcription factor Pax5. *Nature,* Vol. 401, No. 6753, (October 1999), pp. (556-562), ISSN 0028-0836

Nutt S. L., & Kee B. L. 2007. The transcriptional regulation of B cell lineage commitment. *Immunity,* Vol. 26, No. 6, (June 2007), pp. (715-725), ISSN 1074-7613

O'Riordan M., & Grosschedl R. (1999). Coordinate regulation of B cell differentiation by the transcription factors EBF and E2A. *Immunity,* Vol. 11, No. 1, (July 1999), pp. (21-31), ISSN 1074-7613

Parrish Y. K., Baez I., Milford T. A., Benitez A., Galloway N., Rogerio J. W., Sahakian E., Kagoda M., Huang G., Hao Q. L., Sevilla Y., Barsky L. W., Zielinska E., Price M. A., Wall N. R., Dovat S., & Payne K. J. (2009). IL-7 dependence in human B lymphopoiesis increases during progression of ontogeny from cord blood to bone marrow. *Journal of Immunology,* Vol. 182, No. 7, (April 2009), pp. (4255-4266), ISSN 0022-1767

Passegué, E., Wagers, AJ., Giuriato, S., Anderson, WC.,& Weissman IL (2005). Global analysis of proliferation and cell cycle gene expression in the regulation of hematopoietic stem and progenitor cell fates. *J Exp Med* Vol. 202 No. 11 (December 2005) pp (1599-1611), ISSN 0022-1007

Pelayo, R., Hirose, J., Huang, J., Garrett, KP., Delogu, A., Busslinger, M., & Kincade PW. (2005b). Derivation of 2 categories of plasmacytoid dendritic cells in murine bone marrow. *Blood,* Vol.105, No.11, (Jun 2005), pp. 4407-4415, ISSN 0006-4971

Pelayo, R., Miyazaki, K., Huang, J., Garrett, KP., Osmond, DG., & Kincade. PW.. (2006b). Cell cycle quiescence of early lymphoid progenitors in adult bone marrow. *Stem Cells,* Vol.24, No.12, (December 2006), pp.2703-2713, ISSN 1549-4918

Pelayo, R., Welner, RS., Nagai, Y., & Kincade PW. (2006a). Life before the pre-B cell receptor checkpoint: specification and commitment of primitive lymphoid progenitors in adult bone marrow. *Semin Immunol*, Vol.18, No.1, pp. 2-11, ISSN 1044-5323

Pelayo, R., Welner, R., Perry, SS., Huang, J., Baba, Y., Yokota, T,, & Kincade, PW.. (2005a). Lymphoid progenitors and primary routes to becoming cells of the immune system. *Curr Opin Immunol*, Vol.17, No.2, pp. 100-107, ISSN 0952-7915

Perez-Saldivar, M., Fajardo-Gutierrez, A., Bernaldez-Rios, R., Martinez-Avalos, A., Medina-Sanson, A., Espinosa-Hernandez, L., Flores-Chapa, J., Amador-Sanchez, R., Penaloza-Gonzalez, J., Alvarez-Rodriguez,F., Bolea-Murga, V., Flores-Lujano, J., Rodriguez-Zepeda, M., Rivera-Luna, R., Dorantes-Acosta, E., Jimenez-Hernandez, E., Alvarado-Ibarra, M., Velazquez-Avina, M., Torres-Nava, J., Duarte-Rodriguez, D., Paredes-Aguilera, R., Del Campo-Martinez, M., Cardenas-Cardos, R., Alamilla-Galicia, P., Bekker-Mendez, V., Ortega-Alvarez, M., & Mejia-Arangure, J. (2011) Childhood acute leukemias are frequent in Mexico City: descriptive epidemiology. *BMC Cancer*. Vol.11, No.1 (August 2011) In Press, ISSN 1471-2407

Pérez-Vera P., Reyes-León A., & Fuentes-Pananá E. M. (2011). Signaling proteins and trasncription factors in normal and malignant early B cell development. *Bone Marrow Research*, Vol. 2011, (no date), Article ID 502751, ISSN 2090-2999

Pieters, R., & Carroll, W. (2010) Biology and treatment of acute lymphoblastic leukemia. *Hematol Oncol Clin North Am.* Vol.14, No.1, (February 2010), pp. (1-18), ISSN 1558-1977

Puel A, Ziegler S. F., Buckley R. H., Leonard W. J. (1998). Defective IL7R, expression in T–B+NK+ severe combined immunodeficiency. *Nature Genetics*, Vol. 20, No. 4, (December 1998), pp. (394-397), ISSN 1061-4036

Raaijmakers, MH. (2011) Niche contributions to oncogenesis: emerging concepts and implications for the hematopoietic system. *Haematologica*. Vol.96, No.7, (July 2011) pp. (1041-8), ISSN 1592-8721

Ramadani F., Bolland D. J., Garcon F., Emery J. L., Vanhaesebroeck B., Corcoran A. E., & Okkenhaug K. (2010). The PI3K isoforms p110 alpha and p110 delta are essential for pre-B cell receptor signaling and B cell development. *Science Signaling*, Vol. 10, No. 134, (August 2010), pp. (ra60), ISSN 1945-0877

Seita,J. & Weissman, IL. (2010). Hematopoietic stem cell: self-renewal versus differentiation. *WIREs Systems Biology and Medicine*, Vol.2, (November/December 2010), pp. 640-653, ISSN 1939-005X

Sioud, M. & Fløisand, Y. (2007). TLR agonists induce the differentiation of human bone marrow CD34+ progenitors into CD11c+ CD80/86+ DC capable of inducing a Th1-type response. *European Journal of Immunology*. Vol. 30, No. 10, pp. 2834-46, ISSN 0014-2980

Smith E., & Sigvardsson M. J. (2004). The roles of transcription factors in B lymphocyte commitment, development, and transformation. *Journal of Leukocyte Biology*, Vol. 75, No. 6, pp. (973-981), ISSN 0741-5400

Sun, L., Heerema, N., Crotty, L., Wu, X., Navara, C., Vassilev, A., Sensel, M., Reaman, GH., & Uckun, FM. (1999). Expression of dominant-negative and mutant isoforms of the antileukemic transcription factor ikaros in infant acute lymphoblastic leukemia. *Proceedings of the National Academy of Science USA*, Vol.96, No.2, (January 1999), pp. (680-685), ISSN 0027-8424

Takizawa, H. Regoes, R. Boddupalli, C. Bonhoeffer, S.,& Manz, MG.. (2011). Dynamic variation in cycling of hematopoietic stem cells in steady state and inflammation. *Journal of Experimental Medicine*. Vol. 208, No. 2, pp. 273-84, ISSN 0022-1007

Thomas, L. R., Cobb, R. M., & Oltz, E. M. (2009). Dynamic regulation of antigen receptor gene assembly. *Advances in Experimental Medicine and Biology*. Vol.650, pp. (103-115), ISSN 0065-2598

Tokoyoda, K., Egawa, T., Sugiyama, T., Choi, BI., & Nagasawa, T. (2004) Cellular niches controlling B lymphocyte behavior within bone marrow during development. *Immunity*. Vol.20, No.6, (June 2004), pp. (707-18), ISSN 1074-7613

Tung J. W., Mrazek M. D., Yang Y., Herzenberg L. A., & Herzenberg L. A. (2006). Phenotypically distinct B cell development pathways map to the three B cell lineages in the mouse. *Proceedings of the National Academy of Science USA*, Vol. 103, No. 16, (April 2006), pp. (6293–6298), ISSN 0027-8424

van der Weyden, L., Giotopoulos, G., Rust, A., Matheson, L., van Delft, F., Kong, J., Corcoran, A., Greaves, M., Mullighan, C., Huntly, B., & Adams, D. (2011) Modeling the evolution of ETV6-RUNX1-induced B-cell precursor acute lymphoblastic leukemia in mice. *Blood*. Vol.118, No.4, (May 2011), pp. (1041-51), ISSN 1528-0020

von Boehmer, H., & Melcher, F. (2010). Checkpoints in lymphocyte development and autoimmune disease. *Nature Immunology*, Vol.11, No.1, (January 2010), pp. (14-20), ISSN: 1529-2908

von Freeden-Jeffrey U., Vieira P., Lucian L. A., McNeil T., Burdach S. E., & Murray R. (1995). Lymphopenia in interleukin (IL)-7 gene-deleted mice identifies IL-7 as a non-redundant cytokine. *Journal of Experimental Medicine*, Vol. 181, No. 4, (April 1995), pp. (1519-1526), ISSN 0022-100

Warner, J., Wang, J., Hope, K., Jin, L., & Dick, J.(2004) Concepts of human leukemic development. *Oncogene*. Vol.23, No.43, (September 2004) pp. (7164-77), ISSN 0950-9232

Welner, RS., Pelayo, R., Garrett, KP., Chen, X., Perry, SS., Sun, XH., Kee, BL., & Kincade PW. (2007). Interferon-producing dendritic cells (IKDC) arise via a unique differentiation pathway from primitive c-kit[hi]CD62L[+] lymphoid progenitors. *Blood*, Vol.109, No. 11, (Jun 2007), pp. 4825-4831, ISSN 0006-4971

Welner, RS., Pelayo, R., & Kincade, PW. (2008a). Evolving views on the genealogy of B cells. *Nat Rev Immunol*, Vol.8, No.2, (February 2008), pp. 95-106, ISSN 1474-1733

Welner, R.S., Pelayo,R., Nagai,Y., Garrett,K.P., Whest,T.R., Carr,D.J., Borghesi,L.A., Farrar,M.A., & Kincade, P.W. (2008b). Lymphoid precursors are directed to produce dendritic cells as a result of TLR9 ligation during Herpes infection. *Blood*, Vol.112, No.9, (November 2008), pp.3753-3761, ISSN 0006-4971

Welner, RS., Esplin, BL., Garrett, KP., Pelayo, R., Luche, H., Fehling, HJ., & Kincade PW.(2009) Asynchronous RAG-1 expression during B lymphopoiesis. *J Immunol*.

Yao Z., Cui Y., Watford W. T., Bream J. H., Yamaoka K., Hissong B. D., Li D., Durum S. K., Jiang Q., Bhandoola A., Hennighausen L., & O'Shea J. J. (2006). Stat5a/b are essential for normal lymphoid development and differentiation. *Proceedings of the National Academy of Science USA*, Vol. 103, No. 4, (January 2006), pp. (1000-1005), ISSN 0022-1767

Yasuda, T., Sanjo, H., Pagès, G., Kawano, Y., Karasuyama, H., Pouysségur, J., Ogata M., & Kurosaki T. (2008). Erk kinases link pre-B cell receptor signaling to transcriptional events required for early B cell expansion. *Immunity*, Vol.28, No.4, (April 2008), pp. (499-508), ISSN 1074-7613

3

Hematopoietic Stem Cell in Acute Myeloid Leukemia Development

Sérgio Paulo Bydlowski and Felipe de Lara Janz
University of Sao Paulo School of Medicine
Laboratory of Genetics and Molecular Hematology, São Paulo, SP,
Brazil

1. Introduction

Hematopoietic stem cells (HSCs) are multipotent stem cells defined by their ability to self-renewal, differentiation and maintenance of all blood cell types in the hematological system during the entire lifetime of the organism. This physiological process, called hematopoiesis, is controlled by several complex interactions between genetic processes in blood progenitor cells and bone marrow microenvironment. Hemostasis is maintained by a delicate balance between processes such as self-renewal, proliferation and differentiation versus apoptosis and cell-cycle arrest in HSCs. Over the last two decades, several studies have been made to understand possible mechanisms of cell malignancy and tumor growth, both in solid and hematological cancers. Leukemias are hematological malignancies that arise from cancer stem cells (CSCs). Neoplastic transformation of hematopoietic stem or progenitor cells occurs by unbalanced critical mechanisms. Blood cancers, as acute myeloid leukemia (AML), are sustained by leukemic stem cells (LSCs) which, like normal HSCs, present a range of biological characteristics that enable their long-term survival. AML is a well studied hematological cancer type characterized by an accumulation of clonal myeloid progenitor cells that do not differentiate normally. However, there is still no consensus about the mechanisms by which the HSCs transformation occurs. In this chapter, the hematopoietic stem cells and leukemic stem cells will be focused on leukemia development, mainly in AML.

2. Hematopoietic stem cells

Hematopoietic stem cells are a well characterized stem cell type which has been used in bone marrow transplantation for treatment of hematological malignancies as well as non-malignant disorders (Warner et al, 2004). In fact, bone marrow (BM) has been, for many years, transplanted as an unfractionated cell pool, until researchers discovered which cellular components were responsible for the engraftment of the donor hematopoietic and immune systems in marrow-ablated patients.

HSCs present self-renewal potential and differentiation capacity into blood lineages. The self-renewal concept means that when stem cells divide, 50% of the daughter cells, on average, is committed with a cell lineage; the remaining 50% do not differentiate; therefore the process maintains the same number of stem cells. This is accomplished by the so-called asymmetric cell division, so that each dividing stem cell originates one new stem cell and one differentiated cell (Gordon, 2005) (Figure 1). In the symmetric division, the stem cells originate 100% of identical stem cells.

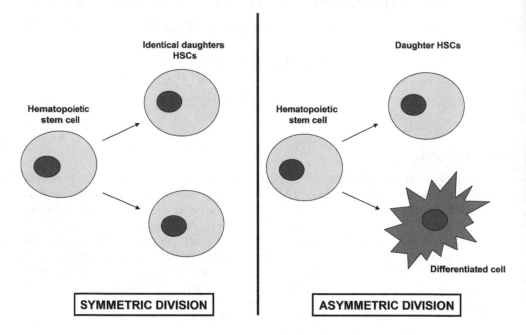

Fig. 1. Schematic illustration of two different types of HSCs division. On the left, the symmetric division in which mitosis originates two identical stem cell daughters. On the right, the characteristic stem cells asymmetric division where each dividing stem cell forms one new stem cell and one differentiated cell.

HSCs are classified as multipotent stem cells due to their ability to differentiate in lymphoid as well as myeloid cells types; however, some studies showed that transplanted bone marrow cells can contribute to the repair and regeneration of a spectrum of other tissue cell types including those from brain, muscle, lung and liver.

Lymphoid cell lineage includes T and B cells, while megakaryocytes, erythrocytes, granulocytes and macrophages belong to the myeloid lineage. These two lineages derive from different progenitor cells. Common lymphoid progenitors (CLPs) can differentiate into all types of lymphocytes without noticeable myeloid potential under physiological conditions. Similarly, common myeloid progenitors (CMPs) can give rise to all classes of myeloid cells with no or extensively low levels of B-cell potential (Kondo, 2010). It is likely that differences in the expression levels of transcription factors determine the lineage affiliation of a differentiating cell (Figure 2). The transcription factors PU.1 and GATA-1 have been implicated in myeloid and erythroid/megakaryocyte lineage differentiation, respectively (Gordon, 2005).

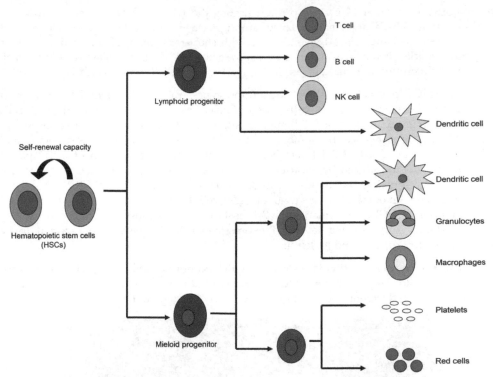

Fig. 2. HSCs differentiation pathways. HSCs could differentiate into specific lymphoid and myeloid cell types. Common lymphoid progenitors (CLPs) can differentiate into all types of lymphocytes and common myeloid progenitors (CMPs) can give rise to all classes of myeloid cells (megakaryocytes, erythrocytes, granulocytes and macrophages) (Adapted from Du et al., 2008).

2.1 Characterization

Morphologically, hematopoietic stem cells are undifferentiated and resemble small lymphocytes. Normally, a large fraction is quiescent, in the G_0 phase of the cell cycle, which protects them from the action of cell cycle-dependent drugs. The quiescent state of stem cells is maintained by transforming growth factor-β (TGF-β). The activity of TGF-β is mediated by p53, a tumor suppressor gene that regulates cell proliferation and targets the cyclin-dependent kinase inhibitor p21 (Gordon, 2005). Quiescence of HSCs is critical not only for protecting the stem cell compartment and sustaining stem cell pools during long periods of time, but also by minimizing the accumulation of replication-associated mutations.

Quiescence regulation in HSCs is also of great importance for understanding the pathophysiological origins of many related disorders. Interestingly, many of the intrinsic transcriptional factors that maintain HSCs quiescence are found to be associated with leukemias. For example, chromosomal translocations resulting in the fusion of FoxOs and myeloid/lymphoid or mixed lineage leukemia have been reported in acute myeloid leukemias.

The majority of normal HSCs are present among the CD34+/CD38− bone marrow cell fractions; some HSCs are also observed among CD34−/Lin− cells; CD34+/CD38+ cell fractions contain some HSCs but endowed with short-term repopulating activity. Other recognized marker is the tyrosine kinase receptor c-kit (CD117), concomitantly with the lack of terminal differentiation markers (as CD4 and CD8; Figure 3) (Rossi et al., 2011).

Primitive HSCs populations show low fluorescence ratios after Hoechst 33342 and Rhodamine 123 staining; these cells are described as side population (SP). SP cells demonstrate high expression of ATP binding cassette (ABC) transporters as P-glycoprotein (P-gp/ABCB1), breast cancer resistance protein (BCRP/ABCG2) and lung resistance protein (LRP) (Huls et al., 2009). MDR1 has been implicated in the protection of cells against apoptotic cell death induced by a variety of methods including growth factor deprivation, UV irradiation, ionizing radiation, or tumor necrosis factor-α treatment. BCRP is a half-transporter and characterized as a novel stem cell transporter. Like MDR1, enforced overexpression of BCRP in human MCF-7 breast cancer cells confers a broad spectrum of drug resistance, and elevated levels of expression of BCRP have been reported to be associated with acute myeloid leukemia.

Since ABC transporter function is associated with both normal and aberrant hematopoiesis, it is important to fully characterize the function of this class of transporter proteins in hematopoietic cell differentiation and to define the underlying mechanisms.

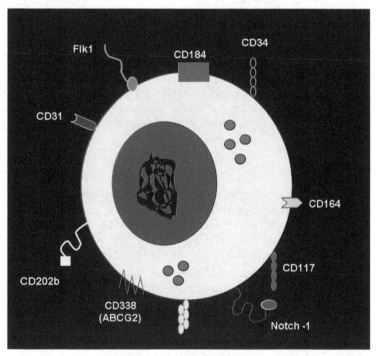

Fig. 3. HSCs main surface markers. HSCs express typical antigens as: CD34, CD117, CD164, CD202b, CD31, Flk-1, CD184, CD338 or ABCG2, Notch-1 concomitantly with the lack of terminal differentiation markers (CD4 and CD8).

2.2 Classification

According to its hematopoietic repopulation capacity, the hematopoietic stem cell pool can be subdivided into three main groups:

a. short-term HSCs, capable of generating clones of differentiating cells for only 4–6 weeks;
b. intermediate-term HSCs, capable of sustaining a differentiating cell progeny for 6–8 months before becoming extinct;
c. long-term HSCs, capable of maintaining hematopoiesis indefinitely (Testa, 2011).

2.3 HSC sources

HSCs can be harvested from healthy donors either by bone marrow aspiration, peripheral stem cell mobilization or from umbilical cord blood (Dick, 2003). HSCs located in the bone marrow present an estimated frequency of 0.01% of total nucleated cells and can be collected by iliac crest puncture and then separated from the other blood cells by magnetic beads or cell sorting.

Umbilical cord blood (UCB) is a source of the rare but precious primitive HSCs and progenitor cells that can reconstitute the hematopoietic system in patients with malignant and nonmalignant disorders treated with myeloablative therapy. UCB cells possess an enhanced progenitor cell proliferation capacity and self-renewal *in vitro*. UCB is usually discarded and it exists in almost limitless supply. The blood remaining in the delivered placenta is safely and easily collected and stored. The predominant collection procedure currently involves a relatively simple venipuncture, followed by gravity drainage into a standard sterile anti-coagulant-filled blood bag, using a closed system, similar to that utilized for whole blood collection (Bojanic & Golubic Cepulic, 2006).

Peripheral blood hematopoietic stem cells (PBSCs) have numerous advantages in comparison with traditionally used bone marrow. PBSCs collection by leukapheresis procedure is simple and better tolerated than bone marrow harvest. PBCSs are mobilized by myelosupressive chemotherapy or/and hematopoietic growth factors. Leukapheresis product contains PBSCs along with committed lineage of progenitors and precursors which contribute to faster hematopoietic recovery.

Unfortunately, the expansion of HSCs *in vitro* is difficult to achieve because the proliferation is accompanied by differentiation. This is presumably caused by a lack of appropriate cues that are provided *in vivo* by the microenvironment. The most excellent defined culture medium for HSCs expansion is supplemented with cytokines such as fetal liver tyrosine kinase-3 ligand (FLT3-L), stem cell factor (SCF), interleukin-3 (IL-3) and thrombopoietin (TPO). Interestingly, mesenchymal stem cells (MSCs), which are characterized by multi-differentiation potential, are important players of the bone marrow HSCs niche. In recent years, MSCs have been shown to support HSCs maintenance and engraftment (Jing et al., 2010).

3. Factors involved in hematopoiesis

Hematopoiesis is a highly coordinated process wherein HSCs differentiate into mature blood cells supported by a physical environment called **niche** (Figure 3). The bone marrow niche is the most important post-natal microenvironment in which HSCs proliferate, mature and give rise to myeloid and lymphoid progenitors. BM is present in the medullary cavities of all animal bones. Unlike secondary lymphoid organs such as spleen with distinct gross structures including red and white pulp, BM has no clear structural features, except for the endosteum that contains osteoblasts. The endosteum region comes in contact with calcified hard bones and provides a special microenvironment to HSCs, which is necessary for the maintenance of HSC activity (Kondo, 2010).

Within the niche, HSCs are believed to receive support and growth signals originating from several sources, including: fibroblasts, endothelial and reticular cells, adipocytes, osteoblasts and mesenchymal stem cells. The main function of the niche is to integrate local changes in nutrients, oxygen, paracrine and autocrine signals and to change HSCs quiescence, trafficking, and/or expansion in response to signals from the systemic circulation (Broner & Carson, 2009). Although the nature of true MSCs remains misunderstood, CXC chemokine ligand 12 (CXCL12) – expressing CD146 MSCs were recently reported to be self-renewing progenitors that reside on the sinusoidal surfaces and contribute to organization of the sinusoidal wall structure, produce angiopoietin-1 (Ang-1), and are capable of generating osteoblasts that form the endosteal niche (Konopleva & Jordan, 2011).

These CXCL12 reticular cells may serve as a transit pathway for shuttling HSCs between the osteoblastic and vascular niches where essential but different maintenance signals are provided. Cytokines and chemokines produced by bone marrow MSCs concentrate in particular niches secondary to varying local production and through the effects of cytokine-binding glycosaminoglycans. Of these, CXCL12/stromal cell–derived factor-1 alpha positively regulates HSCs homing, while transforming growth factors FMS-like tyrosine kinase 3 (Flt3) ligand and Ang-1 function act as quiescence factors.

CXCL12-CXCR4 signaling is involved in homing of HSCs into BM during ontogeny as well as survival and proliferation of colony-forming progenitor cells. The CXCR4-selective antagonist–induced mobilization of HSCs into the peripheral blood further indicates a role for CXCL12 in retaining HSCs in hematopoietic organs. BM engraftment involves subsequent cell-to-cell interactions through the BMSC-produced complex extracellular matrix. Thus, vascular cell adhesion molecule-1 (VCAM-1) or fibronectin is critical for adhesion to the BM derived MSCs.

In this way, the control of hematopoietic stem cell proliferation kinetics is critically important for the regulation of correct hematopoietic cells production. These control mechanisms could be classified in intrinsic or extrinsic to the stem cells, or a combination of both.

Extrinsic control means that self-renewal and differentiation can be controlled by external factors, such as cell–cell interactions in the hematopoietic microenvironment or cytokines as SCF (stem cell factor) and its receptor c-kit, Flt-3 ligand, TGF-β, TNF-α and others. Cytokines regulate a variety of hematopoietic cell functions through the activation of multiple signal transduction pathways. The major pathways relevant to cell proliferation and differentiation are the Janus kinase (Jak)/signal transducers and activators of transcription (STATs), the mitogen-activated protein (MAP) kinase and the phosphatidylinositol (PI) 3-kinase pathways.

Yet, in intrinsic control, the expression of other transcription factors has been shown to be essential for hematopoietic cell development from the earliest stages, as: SCL (stem cell leukaemia hematopoietic transcription factor); GATA-2; gene products involved in cell cycle control, such as the cyclin dependent kinase inhibitors (CKIs) p16, p21 and p27.

Notch-1–Jagged pathway may serve to integrate extracellular signals with intracellular signalling and cell cycle control. Notch-1 is a surface receptor on hematopoietic stem cell membranes that binds to its ligand, Jagged, on stromal cells. This results in cleavage of the cytoplasmic portion of Notch-1, which can then act as a transcription factor (Gordon, 2005).

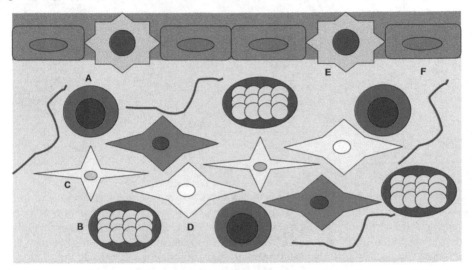

Fig. 4. Schematic representation of main bone marrow niche cells: A- hematopoietic stem cells, B- adipocytes, C- mesenchymal stem cells, D- reticular cells, E- osteoclasts, and F- osteoblasts.

4. Leukemia and leukemic development

Leukemia is the consequence of stepwise genetic alterations that confer both proliferative and survival advantage, as well as self-renewal capacity to the malignant cells (Lane et al., 2011). When the HSCs processes of self-renewal and differentiation become deregulated or uncoupled, leukemias can result, characterized by an accumulation of immature blast cells that fail to differentiate into functional cells. Two types of abnormal events can lead to leukemia. First, a normal stem cell acquires several mutations (from different types of genetic events) and, due to epigenetic changes that alter its growth control, the resistance to apoptosis is increased, interfering with the ability of its progeny to differentiate. Second, partially differentiated cells restore gene expression patterns that allow them to reacquire the unique self-renewal properties of stem cells while also interferes with their subsequent ability to differentiate (Testa, 2011).

Hanahan & Weinberg (2000) described the rules that govern the transformation of normal cells into a malignant cell. The six main properties that define malignant cells are: self-sufficiency in growth signals; insensitivity to growth inhibitory signals; evasion of programmed cell death (apoptosis); limitless replicative potential; sustained angiogenesis; and tissue invasion and metastasis.

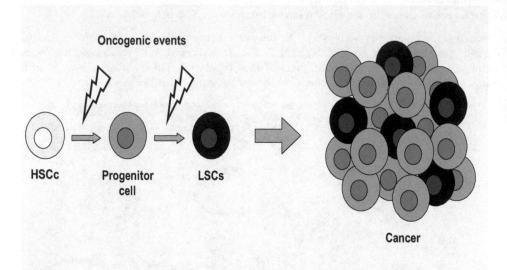

Fig. 5. Cancer stem cell hypothesis. A normal stem cell acquires several mutations and in consequence, by epigenetic changes that alter its growth control, its resistance to apoptosis increased and the ability of its progeny to differentiate is changed. Partially differentiated cells restore gene expression patterns that allow these cells to reacquire the unique self-renewal properties of stem cells while also interfere with their subsequent ability to differentiate.

The "cancer stem cell hypothesis" has gained considerable interest in recent years. This theory states that cells in a tumor are organized as a hierarchy similar to that of normal tissues, and are maintained by a small subset of tumor cells that are ultimately responsible for tumor formation and growth. These cells, defined as "cancer stem cells" (CSCs) or "tumor initiating cells" (TICs), possess several key properties of normal tissue stem cells including self-renewal, unlimited proliferative potential (i.e., the ability of a cell to renew itself indefinitely in an undifferentiated state), infrequent or slow replication, resistance to toxic xenobiotics, high DNA repair capacity, and the ability to give rise to daughter cells that differentiate. However, the major difference between cancer growth and normal tissue renewal is that whereas normal transit amplifying cells usually differentiate and die, at various levels of differentiation, the cancer transit-amplifying cells fail to differentiate normally and instead, accumulate (i.e. they undergo maturation arrest), resulting in cancer growth (Soltanian & Matin, 2011).

In the last years, studies have also clearly demonstrated that leukemia populations are highly heterogeneous and that the disease is propagated by a subpopulation of leukemia stem cells (LSC). LSCs, like normal hematopoietic stem cells, possess a range of biological characteristics that enable their long-term survival. Therefore, LSCs reside in a mostly quiescent state, and as a consequence, the overall activity of many chemotherapeutic agents that function by targeting cycling cells is likely diminished (Konopleva & Jordan, 2011).

LSCs infiltrate the bone marrow and interfere with the normal HSC-microenvironment homeostasis. Available data indicate that LSCs also interact with the hematopoietic microenvironment to maintain self-renewal and to mitigate the effects of cytotoxic chemotherapy (Lane et al., 2011)

4.1 Leukemia stem cells characterization

The immunophenotype and isolation of LSCs were first described by Lapidot et al.(1994) from primary human AML samples and, later, studies have shown that LSCs can be defined as expressing CD34, CD382, HLA-DR2, CD902, CD117 and CD123. Some of these markers are also detected in HSCs, but the expression of CD123 seems to be leukemic-specific (Blair et al., 1998).

Another LSC specific antigen is C-type lectin-like molecule-1, CLL-1. This antigen was demonstrated to be capable of identifying residual leukemic CD34+CD38− cells in clinical remission bone marrow samples. However, more recent data indicate that the phenotype of LSCs may be somewhat variable from patient to patient and that, in some cases, more than one phenotypically distinct subpopulation may possess LSC activity (Konopleva & Jordan, 2011).

Expression of Oct-4 is another similarity between normal and cancer stem cells. Oct-4, a member of the family of POU-domain transcription factors, is expressed in pluripotent embryonic stem and germ cells. Oct-4 mRNA is normally found in totipotent and pluripotent stem cells of pregastrulation embryos (Soltanian & Matin, 2011). Expression of this factor plays a crucial role in maintaining the self-renewing, cancer stem-cell-like, and chemoradioresistant properties in lung cancer-derived CD133+ cells (Chen et al., 2008).

Oct-4 gene product is expressed in several types of adult pluripotent stem cells including kidney, breast, epithelial, pancreatic, mesenchymal, gastric and liver, as well as in tumor cell lines derived from pancreas and liver (Tai et al., 2005). According to Marques et al. (2010) it is also possible that the resistance phenotype developed by leukemic cells is determined by ABC transporter expression which is probably activated by the induction of the Oct-4 transcription factor. The ABCB1, ABCG2 and ABCC1 transporters exhibit binding sites (octamer-ATGCAAAT) for the Oct-4 transcription factor. The presence of these binding sites in the gene promoter of these transport proteins suggests that the transporter regulation pathways may be initiated at the Oct-4 recognized binding sites. However, the presence of Oct-4 alone is not always sufficient for induction of transporter genes. Transporter expression levels are often dependent upon Oct-4 interactions with other transcription factors.

4.2 Genetic pathways of LSCs

4.2.1 Wnt/Catenin

The Wnt/Catenin signaling has been implicated in the self-renewal of LSCs. Wnt proteins are a large family of glycoproteins that bind to Frizzled receptors and LRP5/6 coreceptors. By stabilizing the mediator β-catenin, they start a complex signaling cascade that plays a significant role in regulating cell proliferation and differentiation. Wnt cascade has appeared as a critical regulator of stem cells self-renewal. Comparing the expression of normal hematopoietic stem cells to that of AML leukemic stem cells, evidences show that the Wnt signaling pathway is aberrantly regulated in leukemic stem cells.

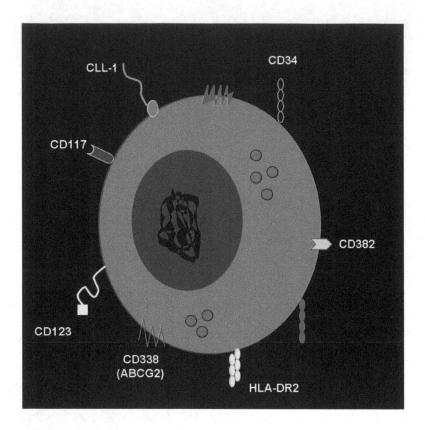

Fig. 6. LSCs main surface markers. LSCs can be defined as CD34, CD382, HLA-DR2, CD902, CD117 and CD123. The expression of CD123 seems to be leukemic-specific. Another LSC specific antigen is C-type lectin-like molecule-1, CLL-1.

4.2.2 PTEN (Akt/mTOR)

PTEN is a phosphatase that negatively regulates signaling through the PI3K pathway, attenuating proliferation and survival signals. PTEN deficiency causes an initial expansion of normal hematopoietic stem cells due to their cycling, followed by their exhaustion. In contrast to this requirement for PTEN in the maintenance of hematopoietic stem cells, leukemic stem cells arise and expand in numbers following PTEN deletion. The observation that PTEN deletion had opposite effects on normal hematopoietic stem cells compared to leukemic stem cells raised possibility for therapeutic targeting of this pathway to eliminate only the leukemic stem cells, without affecting normal hematopoietic stem cells. Since PTEN deletion causes increased AKT and mTOR activation, it seems logical that mTOR targeting by pharmacological agents, such as rapamycin, could represent an interesting option for AML treatment (Testa, 2011).

4.2.3 NF-kB

In addition to genes involved in the control of stem cell self-renewal, leukemic stem cells are expected to express, at high levels, genes involved in anti-apoptotic mechanisms. In this context, particular attention has been focused on the study of NF-kB. NF-kB plays a critical role in inflammation, anti-apoptotic responses, and carcinogenesis. High NF-kB expression was found in primitive AML blasts. In particular, the constitutive activation of NF-kB was observed in AML cell populations enriched in leukemic stem cells, but not in normal hematopoietic stem cells. According to these observations, it seemed clear that NF-kB could be a potential therapeutic target for attempting leukemia stem cell eradication (Guzman et al., 2001).

4.2.4 BMI1

BMI1 is a polycomb group protein which, together with Ring1 proteins, is part of PRC1 complex that has histone H2A-K119 ubiquitin E3 ligase activity. BMI1 has a role in HOX gene (HOXC13) silencing by H2A ubiquitylation (Cao et al, 2005). BMI1 is also known to be important in the regulation and maintenance of proliferative/self-renewal potential in both normal hematopoietic and leukemic stem cells (Park et al, 2003). Upon knockdown of BMI-1, cells lose their ability to engraft and reconstitute leukemia in mice (Bomken et al., 2010).

4.3 Xenotransplantation model of leukemia

A key component for understanding the biological mechanisms for tumor heterogeneity is the ability to functionally assess the capacity for limitless proliferative capacity for segregated populations of tumor cells. Unfortunately, for hematologic malignancies, *in vitro* culture assays are not entirely effective as a means of functionally assessing self-renewal capacity. Thus, transplantation assays in which candidate populations are assessed for their ability to establish long-term serial engraftment of recipient animals is the gold standard for assigning limitless proliferative capability, i.e. self-renewal. For murine studies, the availability of syngeneic transplantation models has been responsible in large part for our in depth understanding of the normal murine hematopoietic hierarchy.

Since the 70 s, there is ample evidence supporting the existence of a discrete compartment of slowly cycling leukemic cells that are resistant to standard chemotherapeutic agents. These cell populations were felt to represent the leukemic stem cells and though many observations were consistent with this hypothesis, there was no direct evidence that this was indeed the case. As the first direct evidence for the existence of cancer stem cells, the work of Lapidot et al. (1994) represented a milestone in the history of the leukemic stem cell model. This study identified an infrequent population of leukemic cells capable of recapitulating the human tumor in xenotransplants. A key finding was that the SCID mouse leukemia repopulating cell, SRC, possessed a phenotype that was similar to that of the normal hematopoietic stem cell (CD34+ and CD38−).

4.4 Acute myeloid leukemia

Acute myeloid leukemia (AML) is a clonal disorder characterized by arrest of differentiation in the myeloid lineage coupled with an accumulation of immature progenitors in the bone marrow, resulting in hematopoietic failure (Pollyea et al., 2011). AML is the most common acute leukemia in adults, affecting roughly three out of 100.000 people. AML patients are predominantly elderly, with a median age at diagnosis of 67 (National Cancer Institute 1975–2007).

In AML, there is wide patient-to-patient heterogeneity in the appearance of the leukemic blasts. Conventionally, AML is classified into seven French–American–British (FAB) subtypes corresponding to the maturation stage of the leukemia (Warner et al., 2004).

The discovery of leukemia-initiating cells in acute myeloid leukemias (AMLs) started with the discovery that the large majority of AML blasts do not proliferate and only a small minority is capable of forming new colonies (Testa, 2011).

A common feature to all AML cases is the arrested aberrant differentiation leading to an accumulation of more than 20% blast cells in the bone marrow (Gilliland & Tallman, 2002). More than 80% of myeloid leukemias are associated with at least one chromosomal rearrangement (Pandolfi, 2001), and over 100 different chromosomal translocations have been cloned (Gilliland & Tallman, 2002). Frequently, these translocations involve genes encoding transcription factors that have been shown to play an important role in hematopoietic lineage development. Thus, alteration of the transcriptional machinery appears to be a common mechanism leading to arrested differentiation (Pandolfi, 2001; Tenen, 2003).

Clinical investigation and experimental animal models suggest that at least two genetic alterations are required for the clinical manifestation of acute leukemia. According to the model proposed by Gilliland & Tallman (2002), cooperation between class I activating mutations and class II mutations that induce termination of differentiation give rise to AML. The class I mutations, such as mutations in the receptor tyrosine kinase genes FLT3 and KIT, RAS family members, and loss of function of neurofibromin 1, confer proliferative and/or survival advantage to hematopoietic progenitors, typically as a consequence of aberrant activation of signal transduction pathways. The class II mutations lead to a halt in differentiation via interference with transcription factors or co-activators (Frankfurt et al., 2009).

While the LSC appears to share many of the cell surface markers previously identified for HSC such as CD34, CD38, HLA-DR, and CD71, there have been several groups who have reported surface markers that are differentially expressed in the two populations. CD90 or Thy-1 is one marker that has been described to be potentially specific of the LSC compartment. Thy-1 is downregulated in normal hematopoiesis as the most primitive stem cells progress toward the progenitor stage. This finding of the lack of expression on LSC might suggest that the primitive stem cell does not contribute to the primary pathological event, or that Thy-1 expression is downregulated as a result of the leukemogenic events (Hope et al., 2003).

The interaction between CXCL12 (stromal cell–derived factor-1 alpha) and its receptor CXCR4 on leukemic progenitor cells contributes to their homing to the bone marrow microenvironment. CXCR4 levels are significantly elevated in leukemic cells from patients with AML and CXCR4 expression is associated with poor outcome (Konopleva & Jordan, 2011). Constitutive activation of the nuclear factor kappa B (NF-kB) pathway in primary human AML stem cells provided evidence that NF-kB plays a significant role in the overall survival of LSCs as well as AML cell types in general. This pathway is strongly implicated as a central target in developing LSC-specific therapies (Konopleva & Jordan, 2011).

FLT3, a member of the class III tyrosine kinase receptor family, is expressed in normal hematopoietic progenitors as well as in leukemic blasts, and it plays an important role in cell proliferation, differentiation, and survival. Activation of the FLT3 receptor by the FLT3 ligand leads to receptor dimerization and phosphorylation, and activation of downstream signaling pathways, including the Janus kinase (JAK) 2 signal transducer (JAK2), signal transducer and activator of transcription (STAT) 5, and mitogen-activated protein kinase (MAPK) pathways. Mutations in the FLT3 gene, found in approximately 40% of patients with AML, are believed to promote its autophosphorylation and constitutive activation, leading to ligand-independent proliferation (Frankfurt et al., 2009).

The adhesion receptor CD96 (TACTILE) is a transmembrane glycoprotein possessing three extracellular immunoglobulin-like domains. It is a member of the Ig gene superfamily and was first identified as a gene expressed in activated T cells. CD96 was described as a tumor marker AML stem cell (Konopleva & Jordan, 2011). Hosen et al. (2011) showed that AML-LSC can be distinguished from normal HSC by the presence of CD96 expression. This finding suggests that CD96 also may prove to be an excellent target for antibody therapy against LSC because hematopoietic progenitors are regenerated rapidly from HSC.

Another adhesion molecule, CD44, has been demonstrated to be a key regulator of AML LSCs homing to microenvironmental niches, maintaining a primitive state. CD44 mediates adhesive cell-cell and cell–complex extracellular matrix interactions through binding to its main ligand, hyaluronan, a glycosaminoglycan highly concentrated in the endosteal region. Other ligands include osteopontin, fibronectin, and selectin, all of which are involved in cell trafficking and lodgment. Beyond its adhesion function, CD44 can also transduce multiple intracellular signal transduction pathways when bound to hyaluronan or to specific function-activating monoclonal antibodies (Konopleva & Jordan, 2011).

5. Conclusions

Adult hematopoietic stem cells are undifferentiated cells capable of self-renewal and differentiation potential in several cell types that comprise the hematopoietic tissue. These cells have been used in bone marrow transplantation for treatment of hematological malignancies as well as non-hematological diseases. The HSC is the main component in the process of hematopoiesis which, together with the cells that make up the bone marrow stromal environment and other intrinsic and extrinsic factors, orchestrates the entire production of progenitors and terminally differentiated blood cells.

However, when this process of cell production is unbalanced, leading to an exacerbated and uncontrolled proliferation of blood progenitor cells, leukemia may develop.The ultimate challenge in coming years will be to understand the stem cell 'programme', particularly the control of self-renewal, in an attempt to develop novel, stem cell-directed therapies. An improved understanding of clonal evolution will be critical if we are to ensure that cancers are not able to evolve mechanisms to evade the new directed therapies. However, reducing the risk of relapse and minimizing long-term side effects should always remain the ultimate goal of understanding the CSCs.

With little doubt, the leukemia stem cell model has had the greatest clinical impact on our understanding and treatment of Philadelphia chromosome positive leukemias. Effective targeted agents and the ability to follow the impact of therapy on critical rare sub-populations of the malignant clone has greatly advanced our understanding of chronic myeloid leukemia.

For AML, the clinical impact of the leukemic stem cell model is less clear. The ability to isolate and characterize rare LSC populations has had a significant importance on our understanding of the biology of AML. In the past decade, we have gained considerable insight into the properties that distinguish leukemic stem cells from their normal counterparts and some of the rules that govern the leukemic hierarchy.

Despite the wide variance in techniques and to some degree expression profiles, common signaling pathways have been shown to play a role not only in AML stem cells, but also in cancer stem cells in general. These include BMI1, Wnt, Sonic Hedgehog, Notch, and NF-kB. These pathways are being evaluated for their role in LSC biology and agents targeting these pathways are making their way through the pre-clinical focus.

6. References

Becker, M. W. & Jordan, C. T. (2011). Leukemia stem cells in 2010: Current understanding and future directions. *Blood Reviews* Vol.25, No. 2, (March 2011), pp. 75–81.

Blair, A.;Hogge, D.E. & Sutherland, H.J. (1998). Most acute myeloid leukemia progenitor cells with long-term proliferative ability in vitro and in vivo have the phenotype CD34þ/CD71-/HLA-DR-. *Blood* Vol.92, No. 11, (December 1998), pp. 4325–4335.

Bojanić, I. & Golubić Cepulić, B. (2006).Umbilical cord blood as a source of stem cells. *Acta Medica Croatica* Vol.60, No. 3, (June 2006),pp. 215-225.

Bomken, S., Fiser, K., Heidenreich, O. (2010). Vormoor, J. Understanding the cancer stem cell. *British Journal of Cancer* Vol.103, No. 4, (August 2010), pp. 439 – 445.

Broner, F. & Carson, M C. *Topics in bone biology.* Springer. 2009; 4: pp. 2-4. New York, USA.

Buting, K. D. (2002). ABC transporters as phenotypic markers and functional regulators of stem cells. *Stem Cells* Vol.20, No. 12, (December 2002), pp. 11-20.

Cao, R., Tsukada, Y., Zhang, Y. (2005). Role of Bmi-1 and Ring1A in H2A ubiquitylation and Hox gene silencing. *Molecular Cell* Vol.22, No. 6, (December 2005),pp. 845-854.

Chen, Y.C., Hsu, H.S., Chen, Y.W., Tsai, T.H., How, C.K., Wang, C.Y., Hung,S.C.,Chang,Y.L.,Tsai,M.L.,Lee,Y.Y.,Ku,H.H.,Chiou,S.H.(2008).   Oct-4 expression maintained cancer stem-like properties in lung cancer-derived CD-133 positive cells. *PLoS ONE* Vol.3, No. 7, (July 2008), pp. 2637.

Dick, J.E. (2003). Stem cells: Self-renewal writ in blood. *Nature* Vol.423, No. 6937, (May 2003), pp. 231–233.

Du, W., Adam, Z., Rani, R., Zhang, X., Pang, Q. (2008). Oxidative stress in Fanconi anemia hematopoiesis and disease progression. *Antioxidants & Redox Signaling* Vol.10, No. 11 (November 2008), pp. 1909-1921.

Frankfurt, O., Licht, J.D., Tallman, M.S. (2007). Molecular characterization of acute myeloid leukemia and its impact on treatment. *Current Opinion in Oncology* Vol.19, No. 6, (November 2007), pp. 635–649.

Gilliland, D.G.& Tallman, M.S. (2002). Focus on acute leukemias. *Cancer Cell.* Vol.1, No. 5, (June 2002), pp. 417-420.

Gordon, M. *Stem cells and haemopoiesis*. In: Hoffbrand, V., Catovsky, D., Tuddenham, E.G., 5th ed. Blackwell Publishing, (2005): Differential niche and Wnt requirements during acute myeloid leukemia. pp. 1-12. New York.

Guzman ML, Neering SJ, Upchurch D, Grimes B, Howard DS, Rizzieri DA, Luger SM, Jordan CT (2001). Nuclear factor-KB is constitutively activated in primitive human acute myelogenous leukemia cells. *Blood*: 2301-2307.

Hanahan, D. & Weinberg, R.A. (2000). The hallmarks of cancer. *Cell* Vol.100, No. 1, (January 2000), 57-70.

Hope, K. J., Jin, L., Dick, JE. (2003). Human Acute Myeloid Leukemia Stem Cells. *Archives of Medical Research* Vol.34, No. 6, (November-December 2003), pp. 507–514.

Hosen, N., Park, C.Y., Tatsumi, N., Oji, Y., Sugiyama, H., Gramatzki, M., Krensky, A.M., Weissman, I.L. (2007). CD96 is a leukemic stem cell-specific marker in human acute myeloid leukemia. *Proceedings of National Academy of Science of U S A* Vol.104, No. 26, (June 2007), pp. 11008-11013.

Huls, M., Russel, F.G., Masereeuw, R. (2009). The role of ATP binding cassette transporters in tissue defense and organ regeneration. *Journal of Pharmacogycal Experimental Therapy* Vol.328, No. 1, (January 2009), pp. 3-9.

Jing, D., Fonseca, A.V., Alakel, N., Fierro, F.A., Muller, K., Bornhauser, M., Ehninger, G., Corbeil, D., Ordemann, R. (2010). Hematopoietic stem cells in co-culture with mesenchymal stromal cells-modeling the niche compartments in vitro. *Haematologica* Vol.95, No. 4, (April 2010), pp. 542550.

Kohler, B.A., Ward, E., McCarthy, B.J., Schymura, M.J., Ries, L.A., Eheman, C., Jemal, A., Anderson, R.N., Ajani, U.A., Edwards, B.K. (2011). Annual report to the nation on the status of cancer, 1975-2007, featuring tumors of the brain and other nervous system. *Journal of National Cancer Institute* Vol.103, No. 9, (May 2011), pp. 714-736.

Kondo, M. (2010). Lymphoid and myeloid lineage commitment in multipotent hematopoietic progenitors. *Immunology Reviews* Vol. 238, No. 1, (January 2010), pp. 37-46.

Konopleva, M.Y. & Jordan, CT. (2011). Leukemia Stem Cells and Microenvironment. *Biology and Therapeutic Targeting* Vol.29, No. 5, (May 2011), pp. 591-599.

Lane, S.W., Wang, Y.J., Lo Celso, C., Ragu, C., Bullinger, L., Sykes, S.M., Ferraro, F., Shterental, S., Lin, C.P., Gilliland, D.G., Scadden, D.T., Armstrong, S.A., Williams, D.A. (2011). Differential niche and Wnt requirements during acute myeloid leukemia progression. *Blood* (July 2011), *in press*.

Lapidot, T, Sirard, C., Vormoor, J., Murdoch, B., Hoang, T., Caceres-Cortes, J., Minden, M., Paterson, B., Caliguri, M.A., Dick, J.E. (1994). A cell initiating human acute myeloid leukaemia after transplantation into SCID mice. *Nature* Vol.367, No. 6464, (February 1994), pp. 645–648.

Marques, D.S., Sandrini, J.Z., Boyle, R.T., Marins, L.F., Trindade, G.S. (2010). Relationships between multidrug resistance (MDR) and stem cell markers in human chronic myeloid leukemia cell lines. *Leukemia Research* Vol.34, No. 6, (June 2010), pp. 757–762.

Pandolfi, P.P. (2001). In vivo analysis of the molecular genetics of acute promyelocytic leukemia. *Oncogene* Vol.20, No. 40, (September 2001), pp. 5726-5735.

Pollyea, D.A., Kohrt, H.E., Medeiros, B.C. (2011). Acute myeloid leukaemia in the elderly: a review. *British Journal of Haematology* Vol.152, No. 5, (March 2011), pp. 524-542.

Rossi, L., Challen, G.A., Sirin, O., Lin, K.K., Goodell, M.A. (2011). Hematopoietic Stem Cell Characterization and Isolation. *Methods in Molecular Biology*. Vol.750, No. 2, (2011), pp. 47-59.

Soltanian, S. & Matin, M. (2011). Cancer stem cells and cancer therapy. *Tumor Biology* Vol.32, No. 3, (June 2011), pp. 425–440.

Tai, M.H., Chang, C.C., Olson, L.K., Tosko, J.E. (2005). Oct-4 expression in adult human stem cells: evidence in support of the stem cell theory of carcinogenesis. *Carcinogenesis* Vol.26, No. 2, (February 2005),pp. 495–502.

Tenen, D.G. (2003). Disruption of differentiation in human cancer: AML shows the way. *Nature Reviews of Cancer* Vol.3, No. 2, (February 2003), pp. 89-101.

Testa, U. (2011). Leukemia stem cells. *Annals of Hematology* Vol.90, No. 3, (March 2011), pp. 245–271.

Warner, J., Wang, J.C., Hope, K.J., Jin, L., Dick, J.E. (2004). Concepts of human leukemic development. *Oncogene* Vol.23, No. 43, (September 2004), pp. 7164–7177.

4

Hematopoietic Derived Fibrocytes: Emerging Effector Cells in Fibrotic Disorders

Carolina García-de-Alba, Moisés Selman and Annie Pardo

Instituto Nacional de Enfermedades Respiratorias,
Universidad Nacional Autónoma de México
México

1. Introduction

Fibrocytes constitute a unique population of mesenchymal progenitor cells from hematopoietic origin. They display a unique spectrum of immune and molecular characteristics such as the simultaneous expression of mesenchymal (collagen types I and III, fibronectin), leukocyte (CD45), monocyte (CD14), and hematopoietic stem cell (CD34) markers. Fibrocytes were initially described in the context of wound repair and since their original description in 1994, our understanding and knowledge of this novel cell population has grown considerably. They have the potential to differentiate into fibroblasts and myofibroblasts among other mesenchymal cells such adipocytes, osteoblasts, and chondrocytes. Fibrocytes are a rich source of inflammatory cytokines, growth factors, and chemokines that provide important intercellular signals within the local tissue microenvironment. Moreover, fibrocytes possess the immunological features typical of an antigen-presenting cell (APC), and they have the capacity for the presentation of antigens to naïve T-cells.

The aim of this chapter is to present a comprehensive overview over the history and recent findings on the biology of fibrocytes as well as their putative participation in fibrotic disorders.

2. History

After an injury occurs, a number of extracellular and intercellular responses are initiated and coordinated in order to restore the tissue integrity and homeostasis. Wound healing is a dynamic, interactive process in which cellular components of the immune system, the blood coagulation cascade and the inflammatory pathways are activated. The cells involved including neutrophils, monocytes, lymphocytes, dendritic cells, endothelial cells, keratinocytes and fibroblasts undergo marked changes in gene expression and phenotype, leading to cell proliferation, differentiation and migration (Singer & Clark 1999; Arabi et al., 2007; Gurtner et al., 2008)

Tissue fibroblasts play a key role not only in normal reparative processes, but also in pathological fibrotic processes. In the past decade it has been established that fibroblasts/myofibroblasts, which participate in repair and fibrosis have their origin not only in the fibroblasts already present in the injured tissues, but also may derive from other sources such as mesenchymal and hematopoietic stem cells (Hinz et al., 2007). The notion of a monocytic fibroblast precursor was first proposed more than a hundred years ago by James Paget, and probably represents the first observations of cells with the molecular features of circulating fibrocytes (Herzog & Bucala 2010). Afterward in the early 1960´s the hypothesis of the blood borne origin of fibroblast appeared again in the literature; of particular significance are the observations of Petrakis and co-workers who reported the in vivo differentiation of human leukocytes into fibroblasts, histiocytes and adipocytes in subcutaneous diffusion chambers (Petrakis et al., 1961). More recently, it was demonstrated that bone-marrow (BM) contributes to the expansion of the fibroblast population in multiple organs and tissues, including skin, stomach and esophagus using mouse transplantation models, and in human liver fibrosis (Direkze et al 2003, 2004 and Forbes et al 2004). Regarding the lung, a pioneer work published in 2004 described that the collagen-producing fibroblasts in experimental pulmonary fibrosis are derived from BM progenitor cells (Hashimoto et al., 2004). While these studies documented the BM origin of at least part of the tissue fibroblasts during injury, they did not resolve whether these BM derived fibroblasts were from hematopoietic stem cells (HSCs) or mesenchymal stem cells. Later, through a model of transplantation of clones of cells derived from a single HSC from transgenic enhanced green fluorescent protein (EGFP) mice, it was clearly demonstrated that fibrocytes are derived from HSCs (Ebihara et al., 2006).

The circulating fibrocyte was first described in 1994 by Bucala, in a model of wound healing response, with the surgical implantation of wound chambers into the subcutaneous tissues of mice. The implantation resulted in a rapid influx of peripheral blood cells such as neutrophils, monocytes, and lymphocyte subpopulations within 24 hr. They noticed that 10% of the cells present in the wound chamber, were spindle shaped cells and expressed collagen I, and CD34, (Bucala et al., 1994). The idea that these cells were of circulating origin arose from the observation that their arrival in to the wound chamber was much faster than would be expected by entry of fibroblasts from the surrounding tissue, since the fibroblasts would have to migrate across the permeable plastic layer, enter the wound chamber, and begin matrix deposition, (Bucala, 2008). Hence, the entrance of large numbers of fibroblast-like cells simultaneously with circulating inflammatory cells suggested that this cell population was from peripheral blood origin and not exclusively by slow migration from adjacent connective tissue (Bucala et al., 1994). This new leukocyte sub-population was termed "fibrocytes", which combines the greek "kytos" referring to cell, and "fibro", which is from the latin denoting fiber. This nomenclature may lead to some overlap as the term "fibrocyte" is also used in histopathologic literature as a synonym for "mature" fibroblasts, and to name a cell constituent of the inner ear spiral ligament, (Quan et al., 2004).

Now it is known that fibrocytes are a hematopoietic stem cell source of fibroblasts/myofibroblasts that participate in the mechanisms of wound healing and fibrosis in many organs (Schmidt et al., 2003; Mori et al., 2005; Ebihara et al., 2006; Andersson-Sjöland et al., 2008; El-Asrar et al., 2008; Strieter et al., 2009).

3. Purification and culture

The current methods and techniques employed for the isolation and characterization of peripheral blood fibrocytes are based mainly in the derivation of these cells from the buffy coat of peripheral blood obtained from human or animal sources. Circulating fibrocytes comprise the ~0.1-0.5% of the non-erythrocytic cells in the peripheral blood and they can be quantified and analyzed by flow cytometry (Bucala et al., 1994, Moeller et al., 2009).

Fibrocytes can be obtained and/or differentiated in vitro from the complete peripheral blood mononuclear cell (PBMC) population as well as from an enriched CD14+ population (Abe et al., 2001, Pilling et al., 2009, García-de-Alba et al., 2010). Accordingly, fibrocytes represent one of the variety of cell types that can differentiate from monocytes, including macrophages, osteoclasts and dendritic cells (Wu & Madri 2010; Seta et al., 2010; Castiello et al., 2011).

The fibrocytes obtained from human or mouse blood, either from PBMCs or CD14+ enriched cells, are grown commonly in Dubelcco´s Modified Eagle Medium (DMEM) supplemented with 20% human AB serum (HAB) or fetal calf or bovine serum without the addition of any other growth factors. Some authors have reported the use of RPMI instead of DMEM with good results (Curnow et al., 2010). The resulting fibrocyte population (≥95% pure) is then characterized based on the combined expression of extracellular surface markers including cluster of differentiation (CD) antigens, major histocompatibility complex (MHC)-like molecules, extracellular matrix protein (ECM) markers, and chemokines receptors expression patterns (Metz, 2003) (table 1).

Marker type	Function
Extracellular matrix proteins	
Collagen I and III	Extracellular matrix
Type I pro-collagen	Collagen I precursor
Prolyl -4-hydroxilase	Collagen hydroxiproline
α-smooth muscle actin	Contractile element
Vimentin	Intermediate Filament
CD markers	
CD11a (LFA-1)	L subunit of integrin LFA-1, adhesion molecule
CD11b (Mac 1)	M subunit of integrin CR3, adhesion molecule
CD13	Pan-myeloyd antigen
CD34	Hematopoietic stem cell antigen, endothelial cell
CD45	Leukocyte common antigen
CD54 (ICAM)	Intracellular adhesion molecule binds LFA-1 and Mac-1
CD58 (LFA-3)	Adhesion molecule, binds CD2
CD80 (B7-1)	Co-stimulatory molecule binds CD28
CD86 (B7-2)	Co-stimulatory molecule binds CD28 and CTLA-4
MHC-related markers	
MHC class II	
HLA-DP	Major histocompatability molecule for antigen
HLA-DQ	presentation
HLA-DR	
Chemokine receptors	
CCR3	Receptor for secondary lymphoid chemokine (SLC)
CCR5 (CD195)	Receptor for RANTES (CCL5), MIP-1α and MIP-1β
CCR7 (CD197)	Receptor for CCL19 and CCL21
CXCR4	Receptor for CXCL12 (SDF-1α)

Table 1. Human fibrocytes surface and intracellular phenotype. Reviewed in Bucala et al., 1994, Chesney et al., 1998, Abe et al., 2001, Hartlapp et al., 2001

It was previously reported that the differentiation of fibrocytes is inhibited by serum amyloid P (SAP), a major constituent of serum, (Pilling et al., 2003) and more recently it was described that in the absence of serum the process of differentiation of fibrocytes can be accelerated with cells with the spindle-shaped morphology appearing in culture after only ~2-5 days, compared to ~8-14 days when fibrocytes are cultured with serum supplemented medium (Curnow et al., 2010). They also reported a difference in the ability of serum free and serum complemented fibrocytes to differentiate from PBMC and CD14+ peripheral blood cells, with more efficient generation of fibrocytes from PBMC cultured without serum, and from CD14+ cells when these were cultured in the presence of serum complemented medium (Curnow et al., 2010).

Cell population obtained regardless of the initial method for enrichment (PBMC or CD14+ enriched cell culture) are cells expressing a combination of CD45 or other haematopoietic markers (CD34, CD11b), as well as collagen I and III, with an elongated spindle-shaped morphology, making clear that the cells differentiated under both conditions can be classified as fibrocytes, based on the current definition: spindle-shaped cell that expresses both haematopoietic and mesenchymal cell markers, (Bucalla et al., 1994, C. Metz 2003),

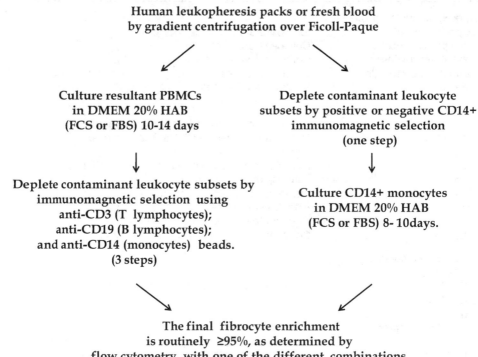

Fig. 1. Schematic description of the two most common methods for fibrocytes culture and enrichment.

3.1 Flow cytometry analysis

Flow cytometry is a critical technique for the characterization and quantification of circulating fibrocytes after their enrichment and in vitro differentiation as well as for fibrocytes obtained directly from fresh blood samples.

Cell preparation. Flow analysis requires a single cells suspension. Ice cold 0.05% EDTA in PBS or trypsin-EDTA 0.05% are recommended to detach the cells from the plastic surface, just covering it for 1-2 min at 37° C. Since trypsin is toxic for the cells, they must be observed closely to adjust and change the timing of the trypsin digestion. Immediately, media complemented with 10% serum is added to neutralize the enzymatic activity of the trypsin present in the buffer (normal human AB serum, FCS or FBS). Horizontal shear force can be applied, or cells can be gently scraped if needed for harvesting and they are immediately washed in cold PBS. The number of dead cells should be estimated by trypan blue exclusion.

Number of cells required for staining. Approximately 2.5-5 x 10^5 cells with a minimum volume of 300ul of staining buffer (1% BSA-PBS) in polystrene tubes 12X75 are needed for the analysis of the in vitro cultured fibrocytes; fewer cells mean longer collection time and potentially more background noise. For the analysis of circulating fibrocytes from fresh blood samples, ~ 0.5- 1 × 10^6 cells in 300ul of staining buffer (1% BSA-PBS) in polystrene tubes 12X75 are needed, since the normal percentage of this cells in the circulation is 0.1-0.5% of the total leukocytes it is better to analyze at least 50,000 events, the use of high performance flow cytometers is recommended.

Protocol for staining cell surface and intracellular antigens for fibrocytes analysis. The following steps are the same for both cell types (fresh PBMC´s or cultured cells).

Cells are centrifuged and resuspended in staining buffer (1% BSA-PBS). The optimum amount of buffer to incubate depends on the protocol suggested by the antibody´s manufacturer technical data sheet, commonly 100μl is an adequate volume. Cells are incubated with the corresponding fluorochrome-labeled antibodies for surface markers (i. e., CD45, CD34, CD11b, and CXCR4) and then fixed and permeabilized with a commercial kit recommended for this purpose (i.e., BD Cytofix/Cytoperm™ Fixation/Permeabilization Solution Kit, BD Biosciences) prior to staining with the anti-collagen antibody or its corresponding isotype control. It is important to consider that isotype controls are critical in the analysis of these cells, since they have to be permeabilized and fixed and a high percentage of nonspecific binding can occur. Also non-stained cells treated with the same process are required as control to discriminate collagen fibers autofluorescence. The number of markers that can be analyzed depend on the capacity (i.e., lasers, filters) of the cytometer to be used, at least 2- 3 fibrocyte markers (i.e., CD45+/Collagen I or CD45+/CXCR4+/Collagen I) are needed to meet the minimum criteria of the fibrocytes definition.

3.2 Fibrocyte to myofibroblast differentiation

Fibrocytes increase the expression of α-smooth muscle actin (α-SMA) spontaneously in culture, and gradually loose the expression of CD34 and CD45 over time, which likely reflects terminal differentiation or other phenomena related specifically to a particular tissue microenviroment (Schmidt et al., 2003, Mori et al., 2005, Bucala, 2008). The differentiation of fibrocytes into myofibroblasts can be enhanced by transforming growth factor (TGF)-β or endothelin-1, which results in an increment in the synthesis of collagen and the myofibroblast marker α–SMA (Schmidt et al., 2003; Bucala, 2008).

For myofibroblast differentiation as described in the literature (Hong et al., 2007): a population of enriched fibrocytes has to be previously obtained with one of the techniques described above. The percentage of enrichment needs to be verified by flow cytometry in each culture to ensure reproducibility of the results.

Fibrocytes are treated with serum-free DMEM with 10 ng/ml TGF-β1 for 3 weeks, refreshing TGF-β1 supplemented medium every 48-72hs. If the objective is to analyze changes in the pattern of gene and protein expression, time curves should be performed previously since these effects might be different depending on the gene or protein of interest.

The signaling pathways that are activated by TGF-β1 to induce α-SMA transcription and thus fibrocyte differentiation to myofibroblast-like cells include Smad2/3 and stress-activated protein kinase (SAPK)/c-Jun N-terminal kinase (JNK) - mitogen-activated protein kinase (MAPK). Interestingly, it was reported that treatment with troglitazone (TGZ, a synthetic agonist of peroxisome proliferator-activated receptor gamma: PPARγ), inhibits TGF-β1 induced α-SMA expression and this effect is modulated through attenuation of the SAPK/JNK activity leading to decreased Smad2/3 levels and transactivation activity, (Hong et al., 2007).

3.3 Adipocyte differentiation

Hong et al., demonstrated in a model of differentiation of human circulating adipogenic progenitors to adipocytes in SCID mice, that fibrocytes, in the presence of specific environmental characteristics can give rise to adipocytes. By gene microarray analysis they found a significant up-regulation of specific mature adipocyte genes and proteins after fibrocyte differentiation to adipocyte, including fatty acid binding protein 4 (FABP4), leptin, and PPARγ; remarkably certain genes, such as those involved in cell motility, chemotaxis, or metalloproteinase activity where also upregulated in the process of differentiation to adipocytes. These findings indicate that fibrocytes may retain unique functions for motility and chemoattractive activity that might allow them to participate in migration and trafficking despite their differentiation into adipocytes (Hong et al., 2005). Differentiation of fibrocytes into adipocytes appears to be mediated by PPARγ that leads to lipid accumulation and induction of aP2 gene expression (Rival et al., 2004). By contrast, this process is inhibited by TGF-β through SAPK/JNK pathway activation (Hong et al., 2007).

For adipocyte differentiation: fibrocytes are treated with PBM culture media (Cambrex Bio Science) supplemented with 10 M troglitazone. Culture media has to be changed every 48 h for 21 days. Following 21 days in culture, the cells accumulate lipids in intracellular vacuoles. Oil Red O Staining can be used to confirm fibrocytes differentiation to adipocytes (Hong et al., 2007).

3.4 Osteoblast and chondrocyte differentiation

Osteoblasts and chondrocytes, which are derived from a common mesenchymal precursor cell, are critical in bone and cartilage formation respectively (Knothe et al., 2010). It has recently been reported that fibrocytes possess the ability to differentiate into chondrocytes and osteoblasts in vitro when the appropriate combination of cytokines and growth factors are used (Choi et al., 2010). These findings, taken together with their capacity to differentiate into myofibroblasts and adipocytes, indicate that fibrocyte may differentiate toward several types of mesenchymal cell types and that this process is influenced by a complex profile of cytokines within the local microenvironment of the host tissue or tissue injury.

Induction of the differentiation of fibrocytes to osteoblasts: Purified fibrocytes are seeded at a concentration of 1×10^5 cells/well in a fibronectin-coated 12 well plate, they are treated with osteogenic basal media (this media is commercially available) supplemented with dexamethasone, ascorbate, mesenchymal cell growth supplement (MCGS), l-glutamine, 1× Penicillin/Streptomycin, and β-glycerophosphate. β-glycerophosphate is critical to stimulate calcified matrix formation in combination with the effects of dexamethasone and ascorbate. Cells are cultured during 21 days with media replacement every 3 days (Choi et al., 2010).

Induction of the differentiation of fibrocytes to chondrocytes: Purified fibrocytes are seeded at the concentration of 5×10^4 cells/tube in 15ml sterile polypropylene tubes, followed by centrifugation at ~300×g for 10min to form pellets. Supernatant has to be carefully removed in order not to disrupt the fibrocyte micromass pellet. Fibrocytes are additioned with chondrogenic differentiation cocktail: basal chondrogenic media (also commercially available) supplemented with 1×10^{-7}M dexamethasone, 0.1 M ascorbate, l-glutamine, Penicillin/Streptomycin, 1 M sodium pyruvate, proline and 10 ng/ml of TGF-β3. Cells are cultured for 21 days with media replacement every 2 - 3 days (Barry et al., 2001; Choi et al., 2010). Fig. 2.

4. Fibrocytes participation in repair processes

Wound repair is a complex process that results from the coordinated release of cytokines, chemokines, and growth factors, leading successively to the recruitment and activation of different cells into the injured site from the very initial phases of repair (Gurtner GC et al., 2008). Fibrocytes have been postulated as important players of the tissue repair process since they have the ability to rapidly home to sites of tissue together with the infiltrating inflammatory cells that act to prevent infection and degrade damaged connective tissue components (Bucala et al., 1994).

Fibrocytes secrete proinflammatory cytokines such as tumor necrosis factor alpha (TNFα), interleukin (IL)-6, IL-8, IL-10, macrophage inflammatory protein-1α/β (MIP-1α/β) CC-chemokine ligands (CCL) -3 and -4 in response to IL-1β which is an important mediator of wound healing response (Chesney et al., 1998). The fibrocyte products MIP-1α , MIP-1β, and monocyte chemotactic protein-1 (MCP-1) are potent T cell chemoattractants and may act to specifically recruit CD4+ T cells into the tissue repair microenvironment; moreover, the fibrocytes increase the cell surface expression of leukocyte adhesion molecules, such as intercellular adhesion molecule 1 (ICAM1), which would enhance leukocyte trafficking (Chesney et al., 1998). Interestingly, in addition to these functions, fibrocytes may play an early and important role in the initiation of antigen-specific immunity. Thus, it has been demonstrated that peripheral blood fibrocytes: express the surface proteins required for antigen presentation, including class II major histocompatability complex molecules: HLA-

DP, -DQ, and -DR; the costimulatory molecules CD80 and CD86, and the adhesion molecules CD11a, CD54, and CD58. Fibrocytes are potent stimulators of antigen-specific T cells in vitro, and migrate to lymph nodes and sensitize naïve T cells in situ (Chesney et al., 1997). Likewise, fibrocytes may also participate in the development of the innate immune response; in porcine models, specific in vitro stimulation of fibrocytes for TLR 2, 4, 7 or TLR3 leads rapidly to the translocation of the NF-kB transcription factor and the production of high levels of IL-6 (Balmelli et al., 2007); on the other hand, exposure to innate immune stimulation in the form of TLR agonists induces an increased expression of MHC class I and II molecules and of the co-stimulatory proteins CD80 and CD86 on fibrocytes, which enables these cells to function as antigen-presenting cells for the activation of cytotoxic CD8+ T cells. All these findings indicate that fibrocytes may recognize a large variety of pathogens such as viruses or bacteria and could be part of the initiation of innate immune responses (Balmelli et al., 2005 and 2007).

Blood vessel formation during normal physiological processes, such as wound healing, is highly regulated by a delicate balance between pro- and antiangiogenic factors. As mentioned, circulating fibrocytes have been shown to migrate to early wound sites where angiogenesis occurs, fibrocytes produce and secrete active matrix metalloproteinase 9 and 2 (MMP-9: gelatinase B; MMP-2: gelatinase A) (Hartlapp I et al., 2001, García-de-Alba et al., 2010), which are implicated in the proteolysis of the basement membrane early during the invasion stage of angiogenesis. In addition, cultured fibrocytes constitutively secrete vascular endothelial growth factor (VEGF), basic fibroblast growth factor (bFGF), platelet derived growth factor (PDGF), insulin growth factor (IGF-I) and hematopoietic factors as granulocyte monocyte-colony stimulating factor (GM-CSF) that induce endothelial cell migration, proliferation, and alignment of endothelial cells into tubular-like structures in vitro. In like manner cultured fibrocytes (and fibrocyte-conditioned media) showed the ability to promote angiogenesis in vivo using a Matrigel implant model, (Hartlapp I et al., 2001).

Interestingly, it has been reported that Th2 cytokines (IL-4 and IL-13) induce, whereas Th1 cytokines (IFN-γ and IL-12) inhibit the CD14+ monocyte to fibrocyte differentiation. When added together the profibrocyte activities of IL-4 and IL-13 and the fibrocyte-inhibitory activities of IFN-γ and IL-12 counteract each other in a concentration-dependent form. By contrast, the fibrocyte-inhibitory activity of the plasma protein serum amyloid P (SAP) dominates over the profibrocyte activities of IL-4 and IL-13. These results might indicate that the complex mix of cytokines and plasma proteins present in inflammatory lesions, wounds, and fibrosis will influence fibrocyte differentiation (Shao et al., 2008). Consistent with this data, it was recently reported that CD14+ monocytes can differentiate in vitro into two different subtypes of fibrocytes depending on the presence or absence of serum in the culture media, which could resemble the changes in serum protein concentrations that occur during tissue repair, inflammation and its resolution (Curnow et al., 2010).

Fibrocytes also contribute to normal wound healing by serving as the contractile force of wound closure via α-smooth muscle actin expression (Abe et al., 2001; Metz, 2003), and secreting components of the extracellular matrix (collagen I, collagen III, fibronectin) (Abe et al., 2001; Bucala et al., 1994). Interestingly, it has been reported that the capacity to produce collagen of fibrocytes from normal subjects or from burn patients is less than that of fibroblasts (dermal and lung fibroblasts) (Wang et al., 2007; García-de-Alba et al., 2010), which raises the question if fibrocytes main contribution to the process of tissue repair is only a direct participation in the production of ECM components. In this context, it is important to emphasize that fibrocytes secrete paracrine growth factors such as connective tissue growth factor (CTGF), PDGF, FGF and TGF-β1 that induce proliferation, migration and differentiation of fibroblasts to myofibroblasts in culture (Chesney et al., 1998, Wang et al., 2007). These findings suggest that the predominant role of fibrocytes in scarring could be the regulation of the functions of local fibroblasts.

Proteins secreted by fibrocytes	Pattern of Expression
Growth factors	
Platelet-Derived Growth Factor A (PDGF-α)	
Fibroblast Growth Factor basic (bFGF)	
Granulocyte-Monocyte Colony Stimulating Factor (GM-CSF)	
Insulin Growth Factor 1 (IGF1)	Constitutive
Vascular Endothelial Cell Growth Factor (VEGF)	
Transforming Growth Factor-beta1 (TGF-β1)	
Connective Tissue Growth Factor (CTGF)	
Hepatocyte Growth Factor (HGF)	
Cytokines	
Tumoral Necrosis Factor-alpha (TNF-α)	Induced by IL-1β stimulation
IL-6	Induced by IL-1β or TNF-α stimulation
IL-10	Induced by IL-1β or TNF-α stimulation
IL-1α	Constitutive
Chemokines	
IL-8	
GROα	
MIP-1α	Constitutive; ↑ with TGF-β1 or IL-1β
MIP-1β	
MCP-1	
MMPs	
MMP-2 MMP-9	Constitutive; ↑ with TGF-β1
MMP-7 MMP-8	Constitutive; ↓ with TGF-β1

Table 2. Fibrocytes pattern of expression for diverse proteins.

4.1 Migration and homing

Fibrocytes trafficking from the bone marrow and circulation to the organs or site of lesion is given through several chemokines. Human fibrocytes express diverse chemokine receptors, including CCR3, CCR5, CCR7, and CXCR4; whereas mouse fibrocytes express CXCR4, CCR7, and CCR2 (Abe et al., 2001; Phillips et al., 2004; Moore et al., 2005; Mehrad et al., 2009). Secondary lymphoid tissue chemokine (SLC/CCL21) and its receptor CCR7 was the first chemokine-chemokine receptor system described to induce the recruitment of fibrocytes as a mechanism of migration to wound sites (Abe et al., 2001). In humans as in mice CCL21 is constitutively abundant in lymphoid tissues, particularly in the lymph nodes and spleen but it is also expressed at lower levels in some non-lymphoid tissues, including the kidneys and lungs (Gunn et al., 1998; Abe et al., 2001; Sakai N et al., 2006).

CXCR4 is an important chemokine receptor for stem and immune cell migration, high levels of CXCL12, which is the only known ligand for CXCR4, were found in the lungs and plasma of patients with IPF and these levels correlated with circulating fibrocyte concentrations (Mehrad B et al., 2007; Andersson-Sjöland A et al., 2008).

Recently (Mehrad et al., 2009) reported that most (but not all) freshly isolated human fibrocytes expressed CXCR4, whereas 46% expressed CCR2 and 9% expressed CCR7. Approximately 30% were CCR2/CXCR4+ and most CCR7+ cells also expressed CCR2, but there was no overlap between CXCR4+ and CCR7+ receptors.

It has been reported an association between serum concentration of MCP-1 and high levels of CD45/pro-Col-I+ fibrocytes in the circulation of scleroderma patients with interstitial lung disease (ILD) or in healthy aging subjects, suggesting that MCP-1 may be also involved in mobilization of fibrocytes into the peripheral blood. (S. Mathai et al., as cited in Herzog & Bucala , 2010),

Thus, fibrocytes can use different chemokine–chemokine receptor axis for tissue homing and this might be related to the type of process (acute or chronic) or to the organs involved; however, the mechanisms implicated in the migration through basement membranes and extracellular matrix and subsequent tissue homing remain unclear. In this context, it was recently reported that fibrocytes express several MMP's (MMP- 2, 7, 8 and 9) (Fig 3) that may facilitate the process of migration of fibrocytes from the circulation to the tissues in response to chemokine gradients (Garcia-de-Alba et al., 2010). In this work it was showed that fibrocytes transmigration towards CXCL12 or PDGF through collagen I coated migration chambers, was highly associated with the collagenase MMP8, while migration through a combination of proteins of basal membrane was facilitated by gelatinases MMP2 and MMP9. Thus, these MMPs may ease cell migration by breaking down matrix barriers or affecting the state of cell-matrix interactions and also may play an important role in the remodelling of ECM. Interestingly, PDGF showed to be a more potent chemotactic agent when migration was given through collagen I coated chambers, possibly indicating that when fibrocytes have arrived to lung interstitium, PDGF plays an important role as a chemoattractant through lung parenchyma.

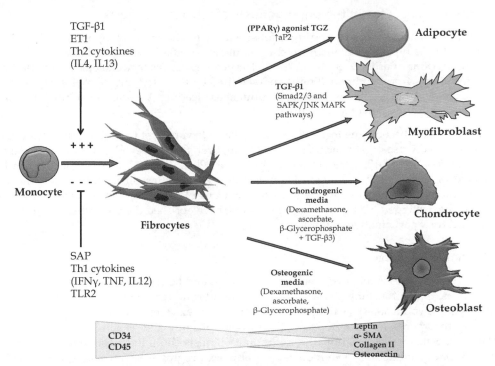

Fig. 2. Schematic summary of the mediators and inhibitors of CD14+monocyte to fibrocyte differentiation, and fibrocytes differentiation to other mesenchymal cells. TGZ: trogliotazone. A crosstalk between PPARγ and TGF-β1 exists, where they can strongly inhibit each other signaling, making clear that a complex and critical balance exists between both of them. It is noteworthy that the expression of hematopoietic markers decrease as fibrocytes differentiate into other mesenchymal cells, while specific markers for that given cell increase their expression during differentiation.

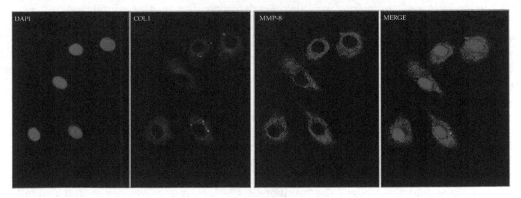

Fig. 3. Fluorescent immunocytochemistry showing a group of fibrocytes positive for collagen I and MMP-8 staining.

5. Role of fibrocytes in the pathogenesis of fibrotic disorders

In contrast to acute inflammatory reactions, which are characterized by rapidly resolving events; fibrosis typically results from chronic unsolved inflammation or aberrant epithelial activation (King, Pardo & Selman, 2011). Despite having distinct etiological and clinical manifestations, fibrotic remodelling is characterized by fibroblast/myofibroblast activation, and excessive extracellular matrix accumulation leading to scarring formation and progressive dysfunction of a given organ.

Fibrocytes have become the focus of research of a wide variety of focal and diffuse fibrosing disorders in diverse organs including lung, heart, liver, and kidney (Barth et al., 2005; Sakai et al., 2006, 2008, 2010; Andersson-Sjöland et al., 2008; Scholten et al., 2011); primarily because of their ability to home into tissues and secret extracellular matrix components. More recently however, a large and varied amount of new knowledge about fibrocytes biology has emerged, rising new hypothesis that have enriched the understanding of these cells and their participation in fibrotic diseases.

5.1 Pulmonary fibrosis

Pulmonary fibrosis is the final result of a numerous and heterogeneous group of disorders known as interstitial lung diseases (ILD). Lung fibrotic remodeling is characterized by fibroblast/myofibroblast activation, and excessive extracellular matrix accumulation leading to progressive destruction of the lung architecture and usually terminal outcome (Pardo & Selman, 2002). Idiopathic pulmonary fibrosis (IPF), the most common form of the idiopathic interstitial pneumonias, is a chronic, progressive, irreversible, and usually lethal lung disease of unknown cause (King, Pardo & Selman 2011). IPF is characterized by the presence of clusters of fibroblasts and myofibroblasts circumscribed from surrounding cells (fibroblastic foci), which represent sites of active fibrogenesis (Selman, King & Pardo, 2001).

During a long time, proliferation of local (resident) fibroblasts and differentiation to myofibroblasts were considered the main source of extracellular matrix deposition in pulmonary fibrosis. The first report of the possible participation of mesenchymal stem cells in the pathogenesis of pulmonary fibrosis, described that collagen-producing cells with fibroblast characteristics were derived from BM progenitor cells, in a model of bleomycin induced pulmonary fibrosis (Hashimoto et al., 2004). The mice in this model were engrafted with BM from GFP transgenic mice that allow to easily follow the fate of these BM-derived cells. Though this group did not prove that these cells were actually fibrocytes, they recognize the possibility of this premise. Not much later, a work that showed that human CD45+Col I+CXCR4+ circulating fibrocytes were able to migrate to the lung of mice treated with bleomycin was published (Phillips et al., 2004). These authors also described that maximal intrapulmonary recruitment of CD45+Col I+CXCR4+ fibrocytes directly correlated with increased collagen deposition in the lungs. Likewise, they identified a second fibrocyte population that is CD45+Col I+CCR7+ and also traffics to the lungs of bleomycin-treated mice; interestingly the absolute number of CCR7+ fibrocytes found in the fibrotic lung was two to three fold lower than the number of CXCR4+ fibrocytes present under similar conditions, indicating that CXCR4 predominates for the recruitment of fibrocytes to injured lungs (Phillips et al., 2004).

Fibrocyte recruitment to damaged lungs has been proved to be mediated by several chemokine/chemokine receptor interactions. Thus, in a model of fluorescein isothiocyanate (FITC)-induced lung fibrosis, it was demonstrated that significantly higher numbers of fibrocytes are present in the airspaces of fluorescein isothiocyanate-injured CCR2$^+$/$^+$ mice compared to CCR2$^-$/$^-$ mice (Moore et al., 2005; 2006). Fibrocytes isolated from the lung expressed CCR2 and migrated toward CCL2 and CCL12 ligands. Interestingly, CCL2 stimulated collagen secretion by lung fibrocytes, which differentiated towards a myofibroblast phenotype, transition that was associated with loss of CCR2 expression (Moore et al 2005).

Importantly, interruption of the chemokine axis attenuated both fibrocyte accumulation and pulmonary fibrosis (Phillips et al., 2004; Moore et al., 2006), strengthening the notion that these chemokine/chemokine receptor axis are the main responsible of fibrocytes trafficking to the lungs; however, under which biological/pathological conditions one or other chemokine/chemokine receptor system is activated, or if they represent redundant mechanisms, yet remains to be elucidated.

Recently several independent research groups have identified fibrocytes in different forms of fibrotic human lung disease. In an initial study, it was reported that circulating fibrocytes expressing CXCR4 and both lung and plasma levels of CXCL12 were elevated in IPF patients (Mehrad 2007). CXCL12 levels showed a positive correlation with higher number of circulating fibrocytes in the peripheral blood of these patients. Later, Andersson-Sjöland et al., evaluated the presence of fibrocytes in the lung of patients with idiopathic pulmonary fibrosis by immunofluorescence and confocal microscopy. Fibrocytes were identified with different combinations of markers in most fibrotic lungs; interestingly, no fibrocytes were identified in normal lungs. They also found a positive correlation between the abundance of fibroblastic foci and the amount of lung fibrocytes and a negative correlation between plasma levels of CXCL12 with lung function tests (lung diffusing capacity for carbon monoxide and oxygen saturation on exercise) (Andersson-Sjöland et al., 2008). These findings indicate that circulating fibrocytes may contribute to the expansion of the fibroblast/myofibroblast population in idiopathic pulmonary fibrosis.

On the other hand, as mentioned earlier in this chapter, fibrocytes constitutively synthesize and release to the medium important amounts of MMP-2, MMP-7, MMP-8, and MMP-9 (García-de-Alba et al., 2010).

MMPs consist of a large family of zinc endoproteases, collectively capable of degrading all ECM components (Pardo et al., 2006). However, ECM represents only a fraction of their proteolytic targets, and moreover, a given MMP can act on various proteins and, in turn, affect a variety of processes. Gelatinases (MMP-2 and MMP-9) have been found up-regulated in human pulmonary fibrosis and animal models of lung fibrosis (Swiderski et al., 1998; Selman et al., 2000; Oikonomidi et al., 2009). The overexpression of MMP-2 and MMP-9 has been mainly associated with their capacity to provoke disruption of alveolar epithelial basement membrane and enhanced fibroblast invasion into the alveolar spaces (Ruiz et al., 2003; Pardo et al., 2006). In the case of fibrocytes, these MMPs may facilitate the process of migration from the circulation to the interstitial and alveolar spaces in response to SDF-1/CXCL12 synthesized by alveolar epithelial cells (Andersson-Sjöland et al., 2008; García-de-Alba et al., 2010). TGF-β1–stimulated fibrocytes significantly increase gene and protein expression of both MMP-2 and MMP-9 in vitro. Another putative pathogenic role of these two enzymes is that cell surface localized MMP-2 and MMP-9 can activate latent TGF-β, and this constitutes a mechanism that may operate in normal tissue remodeling as well as in fibrosis, tumor growth, and invasion (Yu et al., 2000). Fibrocytes also synthesize MMP-7 and MMP-8; the presence of MMP-7 is interesting because this metalloproteinase has been associated with pulmonary fibrosis since is one of the most up-regulated genes in IPF and display several profibrotic activities (Zuo et al., 2002, Pardo et al., 2005). Moreover, MMP-7 and MMP-1 have been related to alveolar and bronchiolar cell migration over different matrices during IPF lung remodeling (Oikonomidi, 2009). In addition, MMP-7 cleave E-cadherin, which may influence several aspects of cell behavior, such as epithelial-to-mesenchymal transition, which is a well-recognized event that recently has gained importance as a mechanism in the pathogenesis of fibrosis (Lochter et al.,1997; Noe et al., 2001; Hinz et al., 2007). MMP-8 or collagenase-2 specifically degrades fibrillar collagen types I, II and III, and is known to play an important regulatory role in both acute and chronic inflammation (Prikk et al., 2001). In the context of fibrocytes it seems to have an important role in the transmigration of these cells through collagen I (García-de-Alba et al., 2010).

Recently it has been suggested that circulating fibrocytes could have a role as biomarkers for disease severity in IPF; Moeller and coworkers quantified circulating fibrocytes from patients with IPF and found that high percentages of these cells in blood were predictive of poor clinical outcomes; they compared fibrocyte levels in peripheral blood from patients with idiopathic pulmonary fibrosis (stable and during an exacerbation), patients with acute respiratory distress syndrome, and normal controls. Fibrocytes were significantly elevated in patients with stable idiopathic pulmonary fibrosis compared with normal controls, but showed a prominent increase during acute exacerbations of the disease. The number of fibrocytes in patients with acute respiratory distress syndrome was not significantly different from patients with stable idiopathic pulmonary fibrosis or normal controls (Moeller et al., 2009). These data suggest that serial measurements of fibrocyte percentages may predict acute exacerbations (Moore, 2009). This work was the first to bring up the notion that fibrocytes measurements may be a useful biomarker in this disease but larger studies are needed to confirm this hypothesis.

Finally, a recently published work exploring senescence-accelerated prone mice found increased levels of CXCR4 expressing fibrocytes in the blood of these mice when compared to wild type controls. The senescence-prone mice also displayed increased lung fibrosis when exposed to intratracheal bleomycin, suggesting the possibility that the increased number of fibrocytes contributed to disease. This is an interesting observation since IPF is considered an age related disease (Selman M et al., 2010). Actually, unpublished data from Mathai et al (Mathai et al., as cited in Herzog & Bucala 2010) indicates that the blood of healthy aged individuals contain increased concentrations of CD45+/Col-1+ fibrocytes and high circulating levels of MCP-1 and IL-13, suggesting that fibrocytes may be associated with certain aging processes.

5.2 Asthma

Asthma is an inflammatory disorder of the conducting airways which undergo distinct structural and functional changes, leading to non-specific bronchial hyper-responsiveness

(BHR) and airflow obstruction. It is among the commonest chronic conditions in Western countries affecting 1 from 7 children and 1 from 12 adults (Holgate et al., 2009).

It has long been known that architectural and structural remodeling occur in the airways of asthmatic patients. These changes include increased collagen (type III and IV) and fibronectin deposition, increased thickness of subepithelial basement membrane, angiogenesis, and fibrosis. All these processes collectively contribute to severe alterations of the normal bronchial architecture in response to the inflammatory tissue injury, leading to progressive airway obstruction and a permanent impairment in respiratory function (Holgate et al., 2009, Hamid & Tulic 2009). Pathologic examination of these tissues demonstrates subepithelial fibrosis and myofibroblast accumulation. Fibrocytes have been identified in the airways of patients with asthma, and it has been reported that allergen exposure induced an increment of fibrocyte-like cells in the bronchial mucosa of patients with allergic asthma (Shmidt et al., 2003). In a mouse model of allergic asthma, fibrocytes were recruited into the bronchial tissue following allergen exposure and differentiated into myofibroblasts providing evidence for the first time that these cells might be a source of myofibroblasts in allergic asthma (Shmidt et al., 2003). Nihlberg and his group showed that fibrocytes in patients with mild asthma were primarily localized, either individually or in clusters, close to the epithelium and to blood vessels. Fibrocyte numbers correlated to the thickness of the basement membrane, supporting that these cells may participate in airway wall remodeling. The increase number of fibrocytes expressing α-SMA seen in patients with increment in the basement membrane thickness may indicate a more differentiated phenotype (Nihilberg et al., 2006). More recently, in two different works, fibrocytes percentages in peripheral blood were shown to be increased in patients with asthma with chronic airway obstruction and severe refractory asthma (Saunders et al., 2008; Chun-Hua et al., 2009). Additionally, a yearly decline in lung function has been significantly associated with the percentage of circulating fibrocytes in patients with chronic obstructive asthma (Saunders et al., 2008).

5.3 Renal fibrosis

Renal tubulo-interstitial fibrosis is a non-specific process, representing the common end-stage for kidney diseases, regardless of their etiology. The histological characteristics include the presence of tubular atrophy and dilation, interstitial leukocyte infiltration, accumulation of fibroblasts, and increased interstitial matrix deposition (Strutz et al., 2006). Fibrocytes have also been implicated in the pathogenesis of renal fibrosis in diverse models. For example, in an experimental model of unilateral ureteral obstruction, fibrocytes appeared in injured parenchyma in a time dependent fashion. Thus, a remarkable number of fibrocytes dual-positive for CD45 or CD34 and type I collagen infiltrated the interstitium, reaching a peak at day 7. Morphological interstitial fibrosis and collagen content were reduced by almost 50% in mice treated with anti-CCL21 antibodies 7 days after ureteral ligation. A similar reduction was observed in CCR7-null mice (Sakai et al., 2006). Interestingly, most fibrocytes were positive for CCR7 and CCL21, and the blockade of CCR7 reduced the number of infiltrating fibrocytes indicating that for this organ, CCR7/CCL21 might be the main recruitment axis. The same investigators showed later that fibrocytes might contribute to fibrosis by an angiotensin II dependent pathway (Sakai et al., 2008). Using two models of renal fibrosis (unilateral ureteral obstruction and chronic angiotensin II infusion), angiotensin II type 2 receptor (AT2R)-deficient mice developed increased renal fibrosis and fibrocyte infiltration and a concomitant upregulation of procollagen type I compared with wild-type mice. Pharmacologic inhibition of angiotensin II type 1 receptor (AT1R) with valsartan reduced the degree of renal fibrosis and the number of fibrocytes in both the kidney and the bone marrow. In isolated human fibrocytes, inhibition of AT2R signalling increased the angiotensin II-stimulated expression of type I collagen, whereas inhibition of AT1R decreased collagen synthesis. These results suggest that AT1R/AT2R signalling may contribute to the pathogenesis of renal fibrosis by at least two fibrocytes-related mechanisms: by regulating the number of fibrocytes in the bone marrow, and by activation of these cells in the tissues (Sakai et al. 2008).

More recently, the presence of fibrocytes was investigated by immunohistochemistry in kidney biopsy specimens from 100 patients with chronic disease; in addition 6 patients with thin basement membrane disease were studied as a disease control. In patients with chronic kidney disease, the infiltration of fibrocytes was observed mainly in the interstitium and their numbers were higher than that in patients with thin basement membrane disease. Moreover, there was an inverse correlation between the number of interstitial fibrocytes and kidney function at the time of biopsy (Sakai et al., 2010). These results suggest that fibrocytes may be involved in the pathogenesis of human chronic kidney disease though the mechanisms involved in their participation are yet to be studied.

CD34+spindle-shaped cells have also been detected in tubulointerstitial lesions in patients with renal interstitial fibrosis. Although in this work the complete phenotype corresponding to fibrocytes was not documented, it is possible that the described CD34+ cells were actually fibrocytes (Okona et al., 2003).

5.4 Liver fibrosis

Hepatic fibrogenesis represents a wound-healing response of liver to a variety of insults. The net accumulation of extracellular matrix (ECM) in liver injury arises from increased synthesis by activated hepatic stellate cells and other hepatic fibrogenic cell types, as well as from bone marrow and circulating fibrocytes (Guo & Friedman, 2007).

Fibrocytes participation in liver fibrosis is a growing field of research and has been assessed in different models. In a murine model of bile duct ligation-induced liver fibrosis, investigators found bone marrow derived collagen-expressing GFP+ cells in the liver of chimeric mice (Kisseleva et al., 2006). The majority of these bone marrow derived cells co-expressed collagen-GFP+ and CD45+, suggesting that collagen-producing fibrocytes were recruited from the bone marrow to the damaged liver (Kisseleva et al., 2006). Later, fibrocyte migration in response to liver injury was investigated using bone marrow (BM) from chimeric mice expressing luciferase (Col-Luc-wt) or green fluorescent protein (Col-GFP-wt) under control of the α1(I) collagen promoter and enhancer, respectively. Migration of CD45+Col I+ fibrocytes was regulated by chemokine receptors CCR2 and CCR1. In addition to CCR2 and CCR1, egress of BM CD45+Col I+ cells was regulated by TGF-β and liposaccharide in vitro and in vivo. Interestingly, development of liver fibrosis was also increased in aged mice and correlated with high numbers of liver fibrocytes (Kisseleva et al., 2011). However, it is unknown what proportion of tissue myofibroblasts/fibrocytes are derived from bone marrow or circulating fibrocytes, whether myofibroblasts of these origins transition through a stellate cell phenotype, and what happens to activated myofibroblasts from various sources when liver injury resolves (Guo & Friedman, 2007).

5.5 Cardiovascular disease

Deposition and remodeling of connective tissue in the heart plays a critical role in cardiac repair and response to injury. Fibrosis also occurs on a reactive basis around coronary vessels (perivascular fibrosis) and in the interstitial space (Haudek et al., 2006). It is generally considered that both reactive and reparative fibrosis may contribute to adverse remodeling. A number of studies have supported the contribution of bone marrow progenitor cells or fibrocytes to remodeling in diverse areas of the cardiovascular system where fibrotic response seems to be a common feature.

In a mouse model of fibrotic ischemia/reperfusion cardiomyopathy (I/RC) it was observed a prolonged elevation of MCP-1, and concomitantly a population of small spindle-shaped fibroblasts with a distinct phenotype appeared in the sites of lesion. These cells were highly proliferative and expressed collagen I and α-smooth muscle actin as well as CD34, and CD45; these cells represented 3% of all non myocyte live cells. Haudek and coworkers confirmed the bone marrow origin of these cells creating a chimeric mice expressing lacZ; I/RC injury resulted in a large population of spindle-shaped fibroblasts containing lacZ. Interestingly, the administration of SAP in vivo markedly reduced the number of proliferative spindle-shaped fibroblasts and completely prevented I/RC-induced fibrosis and global ventricular dysfunction (Haudek et al., 2006). Similar results were reported later, in a model induced by Ang-II. Ang-II infusion resulted in the appearance of bone marrow-derived CD34+/CD45+ fibroblasts that expressed collagen type I and the cardiac fibroblast marker DDR2 while local fibroblasts were CD34−/CD45−. Genetic deletion of MCP-1 (MCP-1-deficient mice) prevented the Ang-II-induced cardiac fibrosis and the appearance of CD34+/CD45+ fibroblasts. Interestingly, Ang-II-treated hearts showed induction of types I and III collagens, TGF-β1, and TNF mRNA expression. Apparently the differentiation of a CD34+/CD45+ fibroblast precursor population in the heart is induced by Ang-II and mediated by MCP-1 (Haudek et al., 2010).

Neointimal hyperplasia is a common feature of various cardiovascular diseases such as atherosclerosis, postangioplasty restenosis and transplant arteriopathy. Neointima usually consists of smooth muscle cells and deposited extracellular matrix. In an in vivo ovine model of carotid artery synthetic patch graft, circulating leukocytes were shown to express collagen and α-SMA. Importantly, these cells also expressed markers unique to fibrocytes (CD34, CD45, vimentin; Varcoe et al., 2006), suggesting an association between intimal hyperplasia and fibrocyte migration. In other work performed in a rat model of transplant vasculopathy, accelerated transplant vasculopathy was associated with increased levels of host-endothelial chimerism and increased neointimal smooth muscle cell proliferation; moreover, accelerated transplant vasculopathy was associated with increased frequency of circulating CD45+vimentin+ fibrocytes (Onauta et al., 2009).

CD34+ fibrocyte-like cells are detectable in normal mitral valves. In cases of myxomatous degeneration CD34+ fibrocytes make up the majority of mitral valve stromal cells (Barth et al., 2005). Since major factors in the development of myxomatous valve degeneration are the MMP-9 and collagen I and III, which are secreted by CD34+ fibrocytes, they propose that these cells might be involved in the pathogenesis of myxomatous mitral valve (Barth et al., 2005).

5.6 Skin disease

Fibrocytes are thought to play a role in skin repair by several mechanisms such as the secretion of ECM, antigen presentation, cytokine production, angiogenesis, and wound closure (Metz, 2003). After the original work by Bucala, several groups examined the participation of fibrocytes in the wound healing process. Mori and coworkers examined the phenotype of fibrocytes and myofibroblasts present in the wounded skin of BALB/c mice and observed that during wound healing, between 4 and 7 days post-wounding, more than 50% of the cells present at the site of injury were CD13+/collagen I+ fibrocytes that could be isolated at an early stage of the healing process from digested fragments of wounded tissue by fluorescence-activated cell sorting (Mori et al., 2005). Fibrocytes have been identified in postburn hypertrophic scar tissue but were absent from normal skin, moreover, the number of fibrocytes was higher in hypertrophic than in mature scar tissue (Yang et al., 2005). It is noteworthy that over time the expression of CD34 on fibrocytes present in these wounds decreases, whereas the expression of proline-4-hydroxylase (an enzyme involved in collagen synthesis) increases in both hypertrophic or keloid scars (Aiba and Tagami, 1997). This finding has been corroborated by other authors (Abe et al., 2001; Phillips et al., 2004) and it's an important feature to be considered for the analysis of these cells in organ fibrosis. In other words, it seems that fibrocytes, once in the tissues, progressively lose their typical markers and can be difficult to identify.

Also, the participation of fibrocytes in wound healing of human skin has been postulated as a useful marker for wound age determination in the legal pathology area. In an interesting study (Ishida et al., 2009) a double-color immunofluorescence analysis was carried out using anti-CD45 and anti-collagen type I antibodies to examine the time-dependent appearance of fibrocytes in 53 human skin wounds with different wound ages. Fibrocytes were initially observed in wounds aged 4 days, and their number increased in lesions proportionally with advances in wound age. These findings imply that human skin wounds containing fibrocytes are at least 4 days old. Moreover, a fibrocyte number of over 10 indicates a wound age between 9 and 14 days. Fibrocytes numbers, evaluated with these markers (CD45+/Col I+) showed a marked decrease from day 17 to 21 which was the longest time of evaluation, exposing the need to use other parameters to confirm the wound ages since fibrocytes numbers in day 4 were similar to numbers in day 17-21.

Yang and his group reported high percentages of fibrocytes present in the cultures of peripheral blood mononuclear cells obtained from burn patients compared with controls (89.7 +/- 7.9% versus 69.9 +/- 14.7%, p < 0.001) and this percentages were consistently higher in patients with more than 30% extent of burn; moreover, they found a positive correlation between the levels of serum TGF-β1 and the percentage of fibrocytes developed in the cultures of PBMC derived from these patients (Yang et al., 2002). Interestingly, it has been postulated that the principal role of fibrocytes in burn injury as well as in hypertrophic scars is the regulation of the function of local fibroblasts. Thus, dermal fibroblasts treated with conditioned medium obtained from burn patient fibrocytes, but not by those derived from normal subjects, showed an increase in cell proliferation and migration (Wang et al., 2007). Furthemore, it has been suggested that fibrocytes can be reprogrammed by changes in the culture media, and that this reprogrammed fibrocytes have the ability to increase cell proliferation and MMP-1 expression in dermal fibroblasts (Medina, A & Ghahar, A. 2010). These findings have opened a new research line worthy of follow up.

5.7 Nephrogenic systemic fibrosis

Fibrocytes have been also identified in the skin of patients with cutaneous fibrosing diseases, such as nephrogenic systemic fibrosis. Nephrogenic systemic fibrosis (NSF) is a recently described cutaneous fibrosing disorder that exhibits pathologic similarities with scleroderma but occurs exclusively in patients with renal insufficiency who have received gadolinium containing magnetic resonance contrast agents. The onset of the disease varies from days to several months following exposure to gadolinium-based contrast. It is a debilitating disease characterized by the development of discolored plaques on the skin of the extremities and trunk. Over time, contractures develop and complete loss of range of motion can occur (Cowper & Bucala, 2003; Cowper et al., 2008). Skin biopsies from patients with this disease have revealed an important accumulation of CD34, pro-Col-I+ fibrocytes in the dermis with abundant connective tissue matrix production; it is noteworthy that in vitro studies revealed that gadolinium may decrease the ability of endogenous mediators, such as SAP and IL-12, to inhibit fibrocyte outgrowth (Vakil et al., 2009). The reason for why fibrocytes are present in high numbers and are such a prominent feature of the dermatopathology of NSF remains unclear, but may be due to the acute and abrupt development of skin fibrosis (Bucala, 2008).

6. Opportunities for research and therapeutic targets

The study of fibrocytes and their participation in the pathogenesis of chronic inflammation and fibroproliferative diseases presents both important challenges and opportunities for researchers. To advance this field, detailed molecular characterization of these cells and establishment of defined experimental strategies in animals and humans will be necessary to catalyze progress in this area of investigation. Recent studies and emerging concepts have significantly improved our understanding of the participation of fibrocytes in health and disease and so have opened the door to new hypotheses and approaches aimed at therapeutic targets and strategies.

One of the main therapeutic targets, suggested since the initial works on fibrocyte biology research, was the serum amyloid P (SAP), a member of the pentraxin family of proteins. In this context, it was first demonstrated that SAP could inhibit the differentiation of monocytes into fibrocytes (Pilling et al., 2003). SAP binds to Fcγ receptors through which apparently mediates its anti-fibrotic activities affecting peripheral blood monocyte differentiation and activation states (Lu et al., 2008). In a rat model of bleomycin-induced lung injury it was shown that purified rat SAP could suppress development of lung fibrosis which correlated with reduced fibrocyte numbers within the lung tissue (Pilling et al., 2007). More recently, SAP ability to reduce fibrosis was tested in models of renal and lung fibrosis where this therapeutic potential was confirmed. In both models, the mechanisms through which SAP exerts its antifibrotic effect seemed to be independent of monocyte to fibrocyte differentiation (Casraño et al., 2009; Murray 2010). Further analysis of this molecule and its potential as antifibrogenic therapy is needed to identify all the mechanisms involved in its effect as well as the feasibility of its use in human disease.

Several chemokines are abundantly expressed in experimental models of fibrosis and in the human disease (Agostini & Gurrieri 2006). Regarding fibrocytes, several studies have focused on the role of chemokines in recruiting these cells to the injured lung. In human IPF, the

CXCL12/CXCR4 axis may be of particular significance (Andersson-Sjoland et al., 2008). As mentioned human circulating fibrocytes express CXCR4 and α-SMA, and can traffic toward the unique CXCR4 ligand, CXCL12 (Mehrad et al., 2007; Andersson-Sjoland et al., 2008). Supporting a major role of this axis in the lung disease, it was demonstrated that the administration of neutralizing anti-CXCL12 antibodies to bleomycin-treated mice resulted in a significant reduction of fibrocyte lung homing and collagen deposition, but interestingly without affecting the numbers of other leukocyte populations in the lungs (Phillips et al., 2004). These data suggest that blocking or interfering with chemokine/chemokine receptor networks may help to diminish or stop fibrocyte recruitment in fibrotic lung disorders. Recently, two groups have explored this hypothesis. Xu et al., 2007 used an antagonist of the receptor CXCR4 (TN14003) in a model of bleomycin-induced pulmonary fibrosis. Intraperitoneal treatment of mice with TN14003 attenuated the development of lung fibrosis and blocked in vitro migration of bone marrow derived stem cells towards CXCL12 or lung homogenates of bleomycin treated mice. Likewise, Song and coworkers showed that intraperitoneal treatment of mice with AMD3100 (Plerixafor, which is a small synthetic specific inhibitor of CXCR4), resulted in decreased levels of CXCL12 in the bronchoalveolar fluid and decreased numbers of fibrocytes in the lungs of mice treated with bleomycin (Song et al 2010). Collagen deposition and pulmonary fibrosis were also attenuated by treatment with AMD3100 (Song et al., 2010). Though the initial results seem to be optimistic, this is still an area of active research, and further studies are needed to elucidate whether pharmacologic inhibition of the CXCR4/CXCL12 axis could modify the lung fibrotic process in human disease.

The potential use of circulating fibrocytes as biomarkers in fibrosing diseases is a window of opportunity that has to be explored; diverse groups have reported differences in the percentages of circulating fibrocytes between healthy controls and patients (Mehard et al., 2007; Moeller et al., 2008; Chun-Hua et al., 2008). An increase in the percentages of circulating fibrocytes was demonstrated in a cohort of 51 patients with stable IPF, compared to healthy controls, but more important, a huge increase was observed during an acute exacerbation, a highly lethal process in IPF. Moreover, the number of fibrocytes returned to the values of stable IPF in the few patients that recovered. In general, fibrocyte numbers were an independent predictor of early mortality (Moeller et al., 2008).

However, higher number of patients should be evaluated and larger longitudinal studies should be done in order to establish if differences in percentages of circulating fibrocytes as well as changes in the percentages of circulating fibrocytes in a given patient with a given disease may predict outcome. The possibility of using differences in the percentages of circulating fibrocytes as biomarkers for disease diagnostic, outcome, or therapeutic response is an important biomedical area of research that needs attention.

Fibrocytes are progenitor cells capable to differentiate not only into myofibroblasts but also in other mesenchymal cells (Hong et al., 2005 and 2007; Choi et al., 2010). The ability of fibrocytes to undergo differentiation to osteoblasts and chondrocytes like cells when treated with specific cytokines and defined media raises the opportunity of their use for regenerative therapy related to bone or articular cartilage repair. Hypothetically, circulating fibrocytes could be isolated from the patient's own blood, processed for differentiation into osteoblasts or chondrocytes, followed by transplantation into the damaged tissue. Tissue engineering is a growing field in the biomedical sciences, and the role of fibrocytes in regenerative therapy has to be assessed with future studies in the area.

7. References

Aarabi, S; Longaker, MT & Gurtner, GC. (2007). Hypertrophic scar formation following burns and trauma: new approaches to treatment. *PLoS Medicine*, Vol 4, pp: e234 (1464-1470).

Abe, R; Donnelly, S. C.; Peng, T; Bucala, R. and Metz, C. N. (2001). Peripheral blood fibrocytes: differentiation pathway and migration to wound sites. *Journal of Immunology*. 166: 7556–7562

Agostini, C & Gurrieri, C. (2006). Chemokine/cytokine cocktail in idiopathic pulmonary fibrosis. *Proccedings of the American Thoracic Society*, Vol. 3, pp:357–363

Andersson-Sjöland, A; Garcia-de Alba, C; Nihlberg, K; Becerril, C; Ramirez, R; Pardo, A; Westergren-Thorsson, G and Selman M. (2008). Fibrocytes are a potential source of lung fibroblasts in idiopathic pulmonary fibrosis. *The International Journal of Biochemistry & Cell Biology*, Vol. 40, pp: 2129–2140

Balmelli, C, Ruggli N, McCullough, K. & Summerfield, A. (2005). Fibrocytes are potent stimulators of anti-virus cytotoxic T cells. *Journal of Leukocyte Biology*, Vol. 77, pp: 923–933

Balmelli, C; Alves, MP; Steiner, E; Zingg, D; Peduto, N; Ruggli, N; Gerber, H; McCullogh, K and Summerfield, A. (2007). Responsiveness of fibrocytes to Toll-like receptor danger signals. *Immunobiology, Vol.* 212, pp: 693–699

Barry, F; Boynton, RE; Liu, B and Murphy, JM. (2001). Chondrogenic differentiation of mesenchymal stem cells from bone marrow: differentiation-dependent gene expression of matrix components. *Experimental Cell Research*, Vol. 268, No. 2, pp: 189-200.

Barth, PJ; Köster, H & Moosdorf R. (2005). CD34+ fibrocytes in normal mitral valves and myxomatous mitral valve degeneration. *Pathology, Research & Practice.* Vol. 201, No. 4, pp: 301-304.

Broekema, M; Harmsen, MC; van Luyn, MJ; Koerts, JA; Petersen, AH; van Kooten, TG; van Goor, H; Navis, G & Popa ER.(2007). Bone marrow-derived myofibroblasts contribute to the renal interstitial myofibroblast population and produce procollagen I after ischemia/reperfusion in rats. *Journal of the American Society of Nephrology*, Vol. 18, pp: 165–175.

Bucala, R; Spiegel, L. A; Chesney, J; Hogan, M. & Cerami, A. (1994) Circulating fibrocytes define a new leukocyte subpopulation that mediates tissue repair. *Molecular Medicine, Vol.* 1, pp: 71–81

Bucala, R. (2008). Circulating fibrocytes: cellular basis for NSF. *Journal American College of Radiology*; Vol. 5, pp: 36–39

Bujak, M; Dobaczewski, M; Gonzalez-Quesada, C; Xia, Y; Leucker, T; Zymek, P; Veeranna, V; Tager, AM; Luster, AD; & Frangogiannis. NG. (2009). Induction of the CXC chemokine interferon-gamma-inducible protein 10 regulates the reparative response following myocardial infarction. *Circulatory Research*, Vol. 105, pp: 973-983.

Castaño, AP; Lin, SL; Surowy, T; Nowlin, BT; Turlapati, SA; Patel, T; Singh, A; Li, S; Lupher, ML Jr & Duffield, JS. (2009). Serum amyloid P inhibits fibrosis through Fc gamma R-dependent monocyte-macrophage regulation in vivo. *Science Translational Medicine*, Vol.1, Num. 5, pp: 5ra13.

Castielo, L; Sabatino, M; Jin, P; Clayberger, C; Marincola, FM; Krensky, AM & Stroncek, DF. (2011). Monocyte-derived DC maturation strategies and related pathways: a transcriptional view. *Cancer Immunology and Immunotherapy*, Vol. 60, No. 4, pp: 457-466.

Chesney, J; Bacher, M; Bender, A & Bucala, R. (1997) The peripheral blood fibrocyte is a potent antigen-presenting cell capable of priming naive T cells in situ. *Proceedings of the National Academy Sciences USA* Vol. 94, pp. 6307–6312.

Chesney, J; Metz, C; Stavitsky, A. B; Bacher, M & Bucala, R. (1998) Regulated production of type I collagen and inflammatory cytokines by peripheral blood fibrocytes. *Journal of Immunology*, Vol. 160, pp: 419–425

Choi, ES; Pierce, EM; Jakubzick, C; Carpenter, KJ; Kunkel, SL; Evanoff, ;, Martinez, FJ; Flaherty, KR; Moore, BB; Toews, GB; Colby, TV; Kazerooni, EA; Gross, BH; Travis, WD & Hogaboam, CM. (2007) Focal interstitial CC chemokine receptor 7 (CCR7) expression in idiopathic interstitial pneumonia. *Journal of Clinical Pathology*. Vol.59, No. 1, pp: 28-39

Choi, YH; Burdick, MD & Strieter, RM . (2010) Human circulating fibrocytes have the capacity to differentiate osteoblasts and chondrocytes. *The International Journal of Biochemistry & Cell Biology* Vol 42, pp: 662–671.

Chu, PY; Mariani, J; Finch, S; McMullen, JR; Sadoshima, J; Marshall, T & Kaye, DM. (2010). Bone marrow-derived cells contribute to fibrosis in the chronically failing heart. *American Journal of Pathology*, Vol. 176, pp: 1735-1742.

Cowper, SE & Bucala, R. (2003). Nephrogenic fibrosing dermopathy: suspect identified, motive unclear. *American Journal of Dermatopathology*. Vol.25, pp: 358

Cowper, SE; Rabach, M & Girardi, M. (2008) Clinical and histological findings in nephrogenic systemic fibrosis. *European Journal of Radiology*, Vol. 66, pp: 191–199.

Curnow, SJ; Fairclough, M; Schmutz, C; Kissane, S; Denniston, A;, Nash, K; Buckley, CD; Lord, JM & Salmon M.. (2010) Distinct Types of Fibrocyte Can Differentiate from Mononuclear Cells in the Presence and Absence of Serum. *PLoS ONE*, Vol. 5, No. 3, pp: e9730. doi:10.1371/journal.pone.0009730

Direkze, NC; Forbes, SJ; Brittan, M; Hunt, T; Jeffery, R; Preston, SL; Poulsom, R; Hodivala-Dilke, K; Alison, M & Wright, NA. (2003) Multiple organ engraftment by bone-marrow-derived myofibroblasts and fibroblasts in bone-marrow-transplanted mice. *Stem Cells, Vol* 21, No. 5, pp: 514-20.

Direkze, NC; Hodivala-Dilke, K; Jeffery, R; Hunt, T; Poulsom, R; Oukrif, D; Alison, MR & Wright, NA. (2004). Bone marrow contribution to tumor-associated myofibroblasts and fibroblasts. *Cancer Research*. Vol. 64, No.23, pp: 8492-8495.

Ebihara, Y; Masuya, M; Larue, AC; Fleming, PA; Visconti, RP; Minamiguchi, H; Drake, CJ & Ogawa, M: (2006) Hematopoietic origins of fibroblasts: II. In vitro studies of fibroblasts, CFU-F, and fibrocytes. *Experimental Hematology*, Vol 34, No. 2, pp: 219-229

El-Asrar, AM; Struyf, S; Van Damme, J & Geboes K. (2008). Circulating fibrocytes contribute to the myofibroblast population in proliferative vitreoretinopathy epiretinal membranes. *Brithish Journal Ophthalmology*, Vol. 92, pp:699-704

Forbes, SJ; Russo, FP; Rey, V; Burra, P; Rugge, M; Wright, NA & Alison MR. (2004) A significant proportion of myofibroblasts are of bone marrow origin in human liver fibrosis. *Gastroenterology, Vol.* 126, No. 4, pp: 955-963

García-de-Alba, C,; Becerril, C; Ruiz, V; González, Y; Reyes, S; García-Alvarez, J; Selman, M & Pardo A. (2010) Expression of matrix metalloproteases by fibrocytes: possible role in migration and homing. *American Journal of Respiratory and Critical Care Medicine.* Vol. 182, No. 9, pp: 1144-1152.

Gunn, MD; Tangemann, DK; Tam, C; Cyster, JG; Rosen, SD & Williams LT. (1998). A chemokine expressed in lymphoid high endothelial venules promotes the adhesion and chemotaxis of naïve T lymphocytes. *Proceedings of the National Academy Sciences USA,* Vol. 95, pp: 258–263.

Gurtner, GC; Werner, S; Barrandon, Y & Longaker, MT. (2008) Wound repair and regeneration. *Nature,* Vol 453, pp: 314-321.

Hamid, Q & Tulic, M. (2009). Immunobiology of Asthma. *The Annual Review of Physiology,* Vol. 71, pp: 489–507

Hartlapp, I; Abe, R; Saeed, R. W; Peng, T; Voelter, W; Bucala R. & Metz, CN. (2001). Fibrocytes induce an angiogenic phenotype in cultured endothelial cells and promote angiogenesis in vivo. *FASEB J.* 15: 2215–2224

Hashimoto, N; Jin, H; Liu, T; Chensue, SW & Phan SH.(2004) Bone marrow-derived progenitor cells in pulmonary fibrosis. *Journal of Clinical Investigation, Vol.* 113, pp: 243–252.

Haudek, SB; Xia, Y; Huebener, P; Lee, JM; Carlson, S; Crawford, JR; Pilling, D; Gomer, RH; Trial, J; Frangogiannis, NG & Entman, ML. (2006). Bone marrow-derived fibroblast precursors mediate ischemic cardiomyopathy in mice. *Proccedings of the National Academy of Sciences USA,* Vol. 103, pp:18284-18289.

Haudek, SB; Cheng, J; Du, J; Wang, Y; Hermosillo-Rodriguez, J; Trial, J; Taffet, GE & Entman ML. (2010) Monocytic fibroblast precursors mediate fibrosis in angiotensin-II-induced cardiac hypertrophy. *Journal of Molecular Cell Cardiology,* Vol. 49, No. 3, pp:499-507.

Herzog, EL; Chai, L & Krause, DS.(2003). Plasticity of marrow-derived stem cells. *Blood,* Vol. 102, pp: 3483–3493.

Herzog, EL & Bucala, R. (2010) Fibrocytes in health and disease. *Experimental Hematology.* Vol.38, No. 7, pp: 548-556.

Hinz, B; Phan, SH; Thannickal, VJ; Galli, A; Bochaton-Piallat, ML & Gabbiani G. (2007) The myofibroblast: one function, multiple origins. *American Journal of Pathology ,* Vol. 170, No. 6, pp: 1807-1816.

Holgate, ST; Arshad, HS; Roberts, GC; Howarth, PH; Thurner, P & Davies DE. (2009) A new look at the pathogenesis of asthma. *Clinical Science.* Vol.118, No.7, pp:439-50.

Hong, KM; Belperio, JA; Keane, MP; Burdick, MD & Strieter RM. (2007). Differentiation of Human Circulating Fibrocytes as Mediated by Transforming Growth Factor-β1 and Peroxisome Proliferator-activated Receptor γ. *The Journal of Biological Chemistry* Vol. 282, No. 31, pp. 22910–22920.

Hong, KM; Burdick, MD; Phillips, RJ; Heber, D & Strieter RM. (2005). Characterization of human fibrocytes as circulating adipocyte progenitors and the formation of human adipose tissue in SCID mice. *FASEB Journal.* Vol. 14, pp:2029-2031

Ishida, Y; Kimura, A; Takayasu, T; Eisenmenger, W & Kondo T. (2009). Detection of fibrocytes in human skin wounds and its application for wound age determination. *International Journal of Legal Medicine,* Vol. 123, pp: 299–304

Kisseleva, T; Uchinami, H; Feirt, N; Quintana-Bustamante, O; Segovia, JC; Schwabe, RF & Brenner, DA. (2006). Bone marrow-derived fibrocytes participate in pathogenesis of liver fibrosis. *Journal of Hepatology*; Vol. 45, pp: 429–438

King, TE Jr; Pardo, A & Selman M. (2011). Idiopathic Pulmonry Fibrosis. *The Lancet. PMID: 21719092*

Knothe Tate, ML; Falls, TD; McBride, SH; Atit, R & Knothe UR. (2008) Mechanical modulation of osteochondroprogenitor cell fate. *International Journal of Biochemistry and Cell Biology.* Vol 40, No.12, pp: 2720-2738.

Lochter, A; Galosy, S; Muschler, J; Freedman, N; Werb, Z & Bissell, MJ. (1997). Matrix metalloproteinase stromelysin-1 triggers a cascade of molecular alterations that leads to stable epithelial-to-mesenchymal conversion and a premalignant phenotype in mammary epithelial cells. *Journal of Cell Biology, Vol.* 139, pp:1861–1872.

Lu, J; Marnell, LL; Marjon, KD; Mold, C; Du Clos, TW & Sun P. (2008). Structural recognition and functional activation of FcgammaR by innate pentraxins. *Nature,* Vol. 456, No. 7224, pp: 989-92

Medina, A & Ghahar, A. (2010) Fibrocytes can be reprogrammed to promote tissue remodeling capacity of dermal fibroblasts. *Mollecular Cell Biochemistry,* Vol. 344, pp:11–21.

Mehrad, B; Burdick, MD; Zisman, DA; Keane, MP; Belperio, JA & Strieter RM. (2007). Circulating peripheral blood fibrocytes in human fibrotic interstitial lung disease. *Biochemestry Biophysics Research Community*; Vol. 353, pp:104–108

Mehrad, B; Burdick, MD & Strieter RM. (2009). Fibrocyte CXCR4 regulation as a therapeutic target in pulmonary fibrosis. *International Journal of Biochemistry and Cell Biology,* Vol. 41, pp: 1708-1718.

Metz, C.. (2003). Fibrocytes: a unique cell population implicated in wound healing. *Cellular and Molecular Life Sciences,* Vol. 60, pp: 1342–1350.

Moeller, A; Gilpin, S; Ask, K; Cox, G; Cook, D; Gauldie, J; Margetts, P; Farkas, L; Dobranowski, J; Boylan, C; O'Byrne, P; Strieter, R & Kolb M. (2009) Circulating Fibrocytes Are an Indicator of Poor Prognosis in Idiopathic Pulmonary Fibrosis. *American Journal of Respiratory and Critical Care Medicine,* Vol. 179, pp: 588–594,

Moore, BB; Kolodsick, JE; Thannickal, VJ; Cooke, K; Moore, TA; Hogaboam, C; Wilke, CA & Toews GB. (2005). CCR2-mediated recruitment of fibrocytes to the alveolar space after fibrotic injury. *American Journal of Pathology,* Vol. 166, pp: 675–684.

Moore, BB; Murray, L; Das, A; Wilke, CA; Herrygers, AB & Toews, GB.(2006). The role of CCL12 in the recruitment of fibrocytes and lung fibrosis. *American Journal of Respiratory Cell and Molecular Biology.* Vol. 35 No. 2, pp: 175-181

Moore, B. (2009). Fibrocytes as Potential Biomarkers in Idiopathic Pulmonary Fibrosis. *International Journal of Respiratory and Critical Care Medicine.* Vol 179, pp: 524-525

Mori, L; Bellini, A; Stacey, MA; Schmidt, M & Mattoli S. (2005) Fibrocytes contribute to the myofibroblast population in wounded skin and originate from the bone marrow. *Experimental Cell Research,* Vol 304, pp: 81–90

Murray, LA; Rosada, R; Moreira, AP; Joshi, A; Kramer, MS, Hesson, DP; Argentieri, RL; Mathai, S; Gulati, M; Herzog, EL & Hogaboam CM. (2010) Serum Amyloid P Therapeutically Attenuates Murine Bleomycin-Induced Pulmonary ia Its Effects on

Macrophages. *PLoS ONE*, Vol. 5, No. 3, pp: e9683. doi:10.1371/journal.pone. 0009683

Nihlberg, K; Larsen, K; Hultgårdh-Nilsson, A; Malmström, A; Bjermer, L & Westergren-Thorsson G. (2007) Tissue fibrocytes in patients with mild asthma: a possible link to thickness of reticular basement membrane? *Respiratory Research*. Vol.7, pp:50

Noe, V; Fingleton, B; Jacobs, K; Crawford, HC; Vermeulen, S; Steelant, W; Bruyneel, E; Matrisian, LM & Mareel M. (2001). Release of an invasion promoter E-cadherin fragment by matrilysin and stromelysin-1. *Journal of Cell Sciences* Vol. 114, pp:111–118.

Oikonomidi, S; Kostikas, K; Tsilioni, I; Tanou, ;, Gourgoulianis, KI & Kiropoulos, TS.(2009). Matrix metalloproteinases in respiratory diseases: from pathogenesis to potential clinical implications. *Current Medical Chemestry, Vol.* 16, pp: 1214–1228.

Okona, K; Szumera, A; & Kuzniewski M. (2003). Are CD34+ cells found in renal interstitial fibrosis? *American Journal of Nephrology*, Vol. 23, pp: 409–414.

Onuta, G; van Ark, J; Rienstra, H; Boer, MW; Klatter, FA; Bruggeman, CA; Zeebregts, CJ; Rozing, J & Hillebrands JL. (2010). Development of transplant vasculopathy in aortic allografts correlates with neointimal smoothmuscle cell proliferative capacity and fibrocyte frequency. *Atherosclerosis*, Vol. 209, pp: 393-402

Pardo, A & Selman, M. (2002). Molecular mechanisms of pulmonary fibrosis. *Frontiers in Biosciences*. Vol. 7, pp: d1743-1761

Pardo, A& Selman, M. (2006) Matrix metalloproteases in aberrant fibrotic tissue remodeling. *Proceedings of the American Thoracic Society*; Vol. 3, No. 4, pp: 383-388

Petrakis, NL; Davis, M & Lucia, SP. (1961) The in vivo differentiation of human leukocytes into histiocytes, fibroblasts and fat cells in subcutaneous diffusion chambers. *Blood*, Vol 17, pp: 109-18.

Pilling, D; Buckley, CD; Salmon, M & Gomer, RH. (2003). Inhibition of fibrocyte differentiation by serum amyloid P. *Journal of Immunology*, Vol. 171, No. 10, pp: 5537-5546

Pilling, D; Roife, D; Wang, M; Ronkainen, SD; Crawford, JR; Travis, EL & Gomer RH. (2007). Reduction of bleomycin-induced pulmonary fibrosis by serum amyloid P. *Journal of Immunology, Vol.* 179, pp: 4035–4044

Pilling, D; Vakil, V & Gomer RH. (2009). Improved serum-free culture conditions for the differentiation of human and murine fibrocytes. *Journal Immunology Methods, Vol.* 351, pp: 62-70

Phillips, RJ; Burdick, MD; Hong, K; Lutz, MA; Murray, LA; Xue, YY, Belperio, JA; Keane, MP & Strieter RM.(2004). Circulating fibrocytes traffic to the lungs in response to CXCL12 and mediate fibrosis. *Journal of Clinical Investigation*, Vol. 114, pp: 438–46.

Prikk, K; Maisi, P; Pirila, E; Sepper, R; Salo, T; Wahlgren, J & Sorsa T. (2001). In vivo collagenase-2 (MMP-8) expression by human bronchial epithelial cells and monocytes/macrophages in bronchiectasis. *Journal of Pathology*, Vol. 194, pp: 232–238

Rabkin, E; Aikawa, M; Stone, JR; Fukumoto, Y; Libby, P & Schoen, FJ. (2001). Activated interstitial myofibroblasts express catabolic enzymes and mediate matrix remodeling in myxomatous heart valves. *Circulation*, Vol. 104, pp: 2525-2532.

Rival Y, Stennevin A, Puech L, Rouquette A, Cathala C, Lestienne F, Dupont-Passelaigue E, Patoiseau JF, Wurch T, Junquéro D. (2004) Human adipocyte fatty acid-binding protein (aP2) gene promoter-driven reporter assay discriminates nonlipogenic peroxisome proliferator-activated receptor gamma ligands. *Journal of Pharmacology and Experimental Therapy.* Vol 311, No. 2, pp:467-475

Roufosse, C; Bou-Gharios, G; Prodromidi, E; Alexakis, C; Jeffery, R; Khan, S; Otto, WR; Alter, J; Poulsom, R & Cook HT. (2006). Bone marrow-derived cells do not contribute significantly to collagen I synthesis in a murine model of renal fibrosis. *Journal of the American Society of Nephrology.* Vol.17, pp: 775–782.

Ruiz, V; Ordoñez, RM; Berumen, J; Ramírez, R; Uhal, B; Becerril, C; Pardo, A & Selman, M. (2003). Unbalanced collagenases/TIMP-1 expression and epithelial apoptosis in experimental lung fibrosis. *American Journal of Physiology Lung Cell Molecular Physiology,* Vol. 285, pp: L1026–L1036.

Sakai, N; Wada, T; Yokoyama, ; Lipp, M; Ueha, S; Matsushima, K & Kaneko S. (2006) Secondary lymphoid tissue chemokine (SLC/CCL21)/CCR7 signaling regulates fibrocytes in renal fibrosis. *Proceedings of the National Academy Sciences USA;* Vol 103, No. 38, pp:14098-14103.

Sakai, N; Wada, T; Matsushima, K; Bucala, R; Iwai, M; Horiuchi, M & Kaneko S. (2008) The renin-angiotensin system contributes to renal fibrosis through regulation of fibrocytes. *Journal of Hypertens*ion. Vol.26, No.4, pp:780-90.

Sakai, N; Furuichi, K; Shinozaki, Y; Yamauchi, H; Toyama, T; Kitajima, S; Okumura, T; Kokubo, S; Kobayashi, M; Takasawa, K; Takeda, S; Yoshimura, M; Kaneko, S & Wada, T. (2010). Fibrocytes are involved in the pathogenesis of human chronic kidney disease. *Human Pathology.* Vol; 41, No. 5, pp:672-67

Selman, M; Ruiz, V; Cabrera, S; Segura, L; Ramirez, R; Barrios, R & Pardo A. (2000). TIMP-1, -2, -3 and -4 in idiopathic pulmonary fibrosis. A prevailing non degradative lung microenvironment? *American Journal of Physiology* Vol. 279, pp: L562–L574.

Selman, M; King, TE & Pardo A. (2001) Idiopathic pulmonary fibrosis: prevailing and evolving hypotheses about its pathogenesis and implications for therapy. *Annals of Internal Medicine,* Vol. 134, No. 2, pp: 136-51

Selman, M; Rojas, M; Mora, AL & Pardo A. (2010). Aging and interstitial lung diseases: unraveling an old forgotten player in the pathogenesis of lung fibrosis. *Seminars in Respiratory and Critical Care Medicine,* Vol. 31, pp: 607-17

Seta, N & Kuwana, M (2010). Derivation of multipotent progenitors from human circulating CD14+ monocytes. *Experimental Hematology,* Vol. 38, No. 7, pp: 557-563.

Singer, AJ & Clark RA. (1999) Cutaneous wound healing. *New England Journal of Medicine,* Vol 341, pp 738–746

Shao, DD; Suresh, R; Vakil, V; Gomer, RH & Pilling D. (2008) Pivotal Advance: Th-1 cytokines inhibit, and Th-2 cytokines promote fibrocyte differentiation influence fibrocyte differentiation. *Journal of Leukocyte Biology, Vol.* 83, pp: 1323–1333

Schmidt, M; Sun, G; Stacey, MA; Mori, L & Mattoli S. (2003). Identification of Circulating Fibrocytes as Precursors of Bronchial Myofibroblasts in Asthma. *Journal of Immunology,* Vol. 170, pp: 380–389.

Scholten, D; Reichart, D; Paik, YH; Lindert, J; Bhattacharya, J; Glass, CK; Brenner,DA & Kisseleva T. (2011) Migration of Fibrocytes in Fibrogenic Liver Injury. *American Journal of Pathology,* Vol. 179, pp: 189–198

Song, JS; Kang, CM; Kang, HH; Yoon, HK; Kim, YK; Kim, KH; Moon, HS & Park SH. (2010). Inhibitory effect of CXC chemokine receptor 4 antagonist AMD3100 on bleomycin induced murine pulmonary fibrosis. *Experimental Mollecular Medicine,* Vol.42, pp: 465-472

Strieter, RM; Keeley, EC; Hughes, MA; Burdick, MD & Mehrad B. (2009) The role of circulating mesenchymal progenitor cells (fibrocytes) in the pathogenesis of pulmonary fibrosis. *Journal of Leukocyte Biology, Vol* 86, No. 5, pp: 1111-1118.

Strutz, F & Zeisberg, M. (2006). Renal fibroblasts and myofibroblasts in chronic kidney disease. Journal of the American Society of Nephrology, Vol. 17, pp:2992–2998.

Swiderski, RE; Dencoff, JE; Floerchinger, CS; Shapiro, SD & Hunninghake, GW. (1998). Differential expression of extracellular matrix remodeling genes in a murine model of bleomycin-induced pulmonary fibrosis. *American Journal of Pathology,* Vol. 152, pp: 821–828

Varcoe, RL; Mikhail, M; Guiffre, A;, Pennings, G; Vicaretti, M; Hawthorne, WJ; Fletcher, JP & Medbury, HJ. (2006). The role of the fibrocyte in intimal hyperplasia. *Journal of Thrombosis and Haemostasis,*Vol. 4, pp:1125-1133.

Vakil, V; Sung, JJ; Piecychna, M; Crawford, JR; Kuo, P; Abu-Alfa, AK; Cowper, SE; Bucala, R & Gomer RH. (2009). Gadolinium-containing magnetic resonance image contrast agent promotes fibrocyte differentiation. *Journal of Magnetic Resonance and Imaging.* Vol. 30, No. 6, pp: 1284-8.

Wang, JF; Jiao, H; Stewart, TL; Shankowsky, HA; Scott, PG & Tredget EE.(2007) Fibrocytes from burn patients regulate the activities of fibroblasts. *Wound Repair and Regeneration, Vol.* 15, pp: 113–121

Wang, J; Jiao, H; Stewart, TL; Shankowsky, HA; Scott, PG, & Tredget EE. (2007). Improvement in postburn hypertrophic scar after treatment with IFN-alpha2b is associated with decreased fibrocytes. *Journal of Interferon Cytokine Research.* Vol. 11, pp: 921-930.

Wu, Y & Madri J. (2010). Insights into monocyte-driven osteoclastogenesis and its link with hematopoiesis: regulatory roles of PECAM-1 (CD31) and SHP-1. *Critical Review in Immunology,* Vol. 30, No. 5, pp: 423-33.

Xu, J; Mora, A; Shim, H; Stecenko, A; Brigham, KL & Rojas M. (2007) Role of the SDF-1/CXCR4 axis in the pathogenesis of lung injury and fibrosis. *Am J Respir Cell Mol Biol.,* Vol. 37, No. 3, pp:291-299.

Xu, J; Gonzalez, ET; Iyer, SS; Mac, V; Mora, AL; Sutliff, RL; Reed, A,; Brigham, KL; Kelly, P & Rojas M. (2009) Use of senescence-accelerated mouse model in bleomycin-induced lung injury suggests that bone marrow-derived cells can alter the outcome of lung injury in aged mice. *Journal of Gerontology A Biological Science Medical Science.* Vol. 64, No. 7, pp: 731–739

Yang, L,; Scott, PG; Giuffre, J; Shankowsky, HA; Ghahary, A & Tredget, EE. (2002). Peripheral blood fibrocytes from burn patients: identification and quantification of fibrocytes in adherent cells cultured from peripheral blood mononuclear cells. *Laboratory Investigation.* Vol. 82, No. 9, pp: 1183-1192.

Yang, L; Scott, PG; Dodd, C; Medina, A; Jiao, H; Shankowsky, HA; Ghahary, A & Tredget, EE. (2005). Identification of fibrocytes in postburn hypertrophic scar. *Wound Repair And Regeneration.* Vol.4, pp:398-404.

Yu, Q & Stamenkovic I. (2000). Cell surface-localized matrix metalloproteinase-9 proteolytically activates TGF-b and promotes tumor invasion and angiogenesis. *Genes Development, Vol.* 14, pp: 163–176.

Zulli, A; Buxton, BF; Black, MJ & Hare, DL.. (2005). CD34 Class III positive cells are present in atherosclerotic plaques of the rabbit model of atherosclerosis. *Histochemestry and Cell Biology*, Vol. 124, pp: 517-522.

Zuo, F; Kaminski , N; Eugui, E; Allard, J; Yakhini, Z; Ben-Dor, A; Lollini, L; Morris, D; Kim, Y; DeLustro, B ; Sheppard D; Pardo, A; Selman, M & Heller, RA. (2002). Gene expression analysis reveals matrilysin as a key regulator of pulmonary fibrosis in mice and humans. *Proccedings of the National Academy of Sciences USA*, Vol.99, pp: 6292–6297.

5

Distribution of SDF1-3'A, GNB3 C825T and MMP-9 C-1562T Polymorphisms in HSC CD34+ from Peripheral Blood of Patients with Hematological Malignancies

Ben Nasr Moufida[2] and Jenhani Faouzi[1,2]
[1]Cellular Immunology and Cytometry and Cellular Therapy Laboratory,
National Blood Transfusion Center,
[2]Immunology Unit research, Faculty of Pharmacy, Monastir
Tunisia

1. Introduction

Mobilized peripheral blood stem cells (MPBSC) have nearly replaced bone marrow (BM). So, they become the primary source of hematopoietic grafts especially for patients with hematological malignancies undergoing aggressive myelosuppressive or myeloablative chemotherapy. It allows faster engraftment and equivalent disease-free survival compared with bone marrow cells [Siena S et al, 2000; To LB et al, 1997; Roberto M. Lemoli and Alessandra D'Addio, 2008].

Some reports suggested that hematopoietic stem cell mobilization involves a complex interplay between adhesion molecules, cytokines, proteolytic enzymes such as MMP-9 and MMP-2, stromal cells and chemokines among them (e.g.; SDF-1/CXCR4) play a central role [Roberto M. Lemoli and Alessandra D'Addio, 2008; Tsevee Lapidot and Isabelle Petit, 2002]. It has been reported that increased secretion of SDF-1 downmodulates CXCR4 on CD34+ cells, thus preventing the homing of hematopoietic progenitors to the bone marrow [Signoret N et al, 1997]. Moreover, Dlubek D et al, have observed a negative correlation between mobilization capacity and a reduced expression of CXCR4 on mobilized HPC CD34+ in the leukapheresis product [Dlubek D et al, 2006].

These data suggested a central role for CXCR4 and SDF-1 on mobilization of hematopoietic stem cell as well as their homing to the bone marrow [Dlubek D et al, 2006].

The reason for poor mobilization of hematopoietic stem cells that occur in many donors or patients is fully recognized and patients' characteristics (age, BMI, mobilization regimen, diagnosis and clinical status or ulterior therapy) did not explain the whole thing.

Benboubker and his colleagues identified an association of a polymorphism in the SDF-1 gene, designated as SDF1-3'A, with the rate of mobilization of HPCs CD34+ into peripheral blood [Benboubker L et al, 2001]. Hence, we hypothesized that individual genetic factors might explain, at least in part, this variability and that polymorphism analysis can be used to anticipate CD34+ cells mobilization.

So, identifying SNPs predictive of poor or good response to G-CSF or any mobilization regimen, in terms of number of CD34+ cells mobilized, might be useful in discussing the possibility of using a different mobilizing agent or a different source of CD34+ cells for auto-HSCT and allo-HSCT.

In this issue, we proposed to study the distribution of three genetic polymorphisms: SDF1-3'A, MMP-9 C-1562T and GNB3 C825T in Tunisian patients with malignant hematological diseases who underwent stem cell mobilization for autologous transplantation compared to a group of healthy allogenic PBPC donors.

2. Materials and methods

2.1 Study population

250 subjects (144 men, 106 women) admitted to the Cellular Immunology and Cytometry and Cellular Therapy Laboratory of National Blood Transfusion Center of Tunis –Tunisia, for autologous PBPC mobilization were enrolled.

Our patients can be divided in 4 subgroups distributed as follows: Group 1: 85 Non-Hodgkin's Lymphoma (57 men, 28 women) which comprises 80 Diffuse B Cell Lymphoma, 4 Mantle Cell Lymphoma and a patient with Follicular Lymphoma.

Group 2: 87 Multiple Myeloma (48 men, 39 women).

Group 3: 63 Hodgkin's disease (31 men, 32 women).

Group 4: composed of 15 patients with Acute Myeloid Leukemia (9 men, 6 women).

Besides, a group composed of 41 subjects (24 men, 17 women) with mean age of 32 years (range 12-63 years) designated for peripheral blood stem cells (PBSC) mobilization. They were visiting the Cellular Immunology and Cytometry and Cellular therapy Laboratory of National Blood Transfusion Center of Tunis–Tunisia as allogenic donors for stem cell transplantation.

Then, a group of 165 healthy blood donors visiting the Blood Transfusion Service of National Blood Transfusion Center of Tunis -Tunisia served as a control group was enrolled in the study. Whole details concerning the subjects will be resumed in Table 1.

Written informed consent was obtained from all subjects according to a protocol approved by the ethical committee for scientific and medical research of the National Blood Transfusion Center and National Bone marrow transplantation center of Tunis (Tunisia) in accordance with the Declaration of Helsinki.

Circulating hematopoietic progenitors CD34+ were evaluated daily by flow cytometry and PBSC collections or apheresis were begun when peripheral CD34+ cells were ~20 cells/µl. Apheresis was usually performed daily using continuous flow blood cell separators COBE SPECTRA and MCS+.

2.2 DNA extraction and genotyping

Genomic DNA was prepared from EDTA anticoagulated peripheral blood by using a common salting-out procedure [Miller SA et al, 1988].

Distribution of SDF1-3'A, GNB3 C825T and MMP-9 C-1562T Polymorphisms in HSC CD34+ from Peripheral
Blood of Patients with Hematological Malignancies

85

	PATIENTS				PBSC DONORS		
	Total	<2x10e6 CD34+/kg	>2x10e6 CD34+/kg	p	Total	<3x10^6 CD34/kg	≥3x10^6 CD34/kg
Age (years) Median	40.58				33.25 (12-63)	32.25 (15-57)	33.5 (12-63)
Range	12-64						
Male	144	27	117	NS	24	6	11
Female	106	26	80		17	6	6	18
Diagnosis							
NHL (non Hodgkin's lymphoma)		25	60				
Diffuse large Cell Lymphoma	80						
FL(follicular lymphoma)	1						
ML (mantle Cell lymphoma)	4						
Hodgkin's Disease	63	14	49				
Multiple Myeloma	87	12	77				
AML (acute myeloid leukemia)	15	7	8				
Prior radiotherapy	62	19	23				
Prior chemotherapy	250						
time from last chemotherapy to mobilization							
< 1 month	121	-					
1 to 2 months	20						
2 to 3 months	4						
> 3 months	5						
Chemomobilization							
Rituximab ESHAP/ rituximab DSHAP	59	-					
rituximab CHOP	2						
ICE/ RICE	21						
Others	168						
Mobilization regimen growth factor only							
Lenograstim (Granocyte®)	80	-					
filgrastim (Neupogen®)	75	-					
G/C [endoxan+ G-CSF]	95	-					

Table 1. patients and healthy allogenic PBPC donors charachteristics Abbreviations: G-CSF, granulocyte colony-stimulating factor; G/C, G-CSF- chemotherapy; ICE, ifosfamide, carboplatin, etoposide; ESHAP/DHAP, etoposide, cytarabine, methylprednisolone,

2.3 Genotyping

The reaction mixture consisted of 1µl PCR buffer 10x, 2 mM of MgSo4, 0.2 mM of each dNTP, 400mM of each primer, and 0,5units/reaction Taq DNA polymerase (Bio Basic Inc).

The reaction conditions were: For SDF1–3'A an initial denaturation at 95°C for five minutes, then 35 cycles at 94°C for 30 seconds, at 58°C for 30 seconds, at 72°C for 1min, and finally extension at 72°C for 7 minutes.

All specimens were examined for the presence of amplifiable DNA. PCR products were digested with 10units HpaII/reaction (Fermentas) at 37°C for overnight [Benboubker L et al, 2001] (figure 1).

For, MMP-9 C-1562T, PCR conditions as above, with annealing temperature at 67°C. PCR products were digested with 10units Hin1II/reaction (Fermentas) at 37°C for overnight [Zhang B et al, 1999; Toru Ogata et al, 2005] (figure 2).

For GNB3 C825T, the PCR-reaction began with denaturation at 95°C for 5 min, followed by 35 cycles of denaturation at 94°C (for 30 seconds), annealing at 55°C (30 s), extension at 72°C (1min), and a final extension at 72°C (7 min). PCR products were digested with BseDI at 60°C (4 h), separated on 2% agarose gels, and visualized under UV illumination [Cheng-Ho Tsai MD et al, 2000] (figure 3)

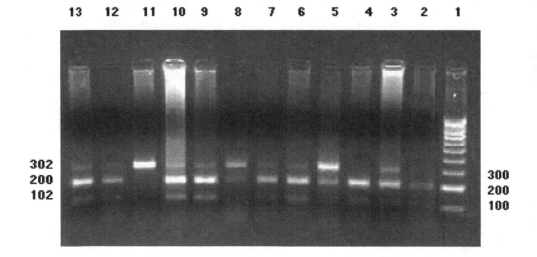

Fig. 1. SDF-1 genotyping by PCR-RFLP analysis followed by separation on 2% agarose gel as described in text. Lane 1, 100pb ladder; lanes 2 and 4, G/G; lanes 3 and 5, G/A; lane 11, A/A

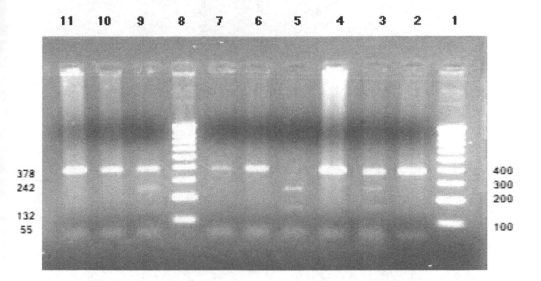

Fig. 2. MMP-9 genotyping by PCR-RFLP analysis followed by separation on 2% agarose gel as described in text. Lanes 1 and 8, 100 pb ladder; lanes 2 and 6, C/C; lanes 3 and 9, C/T; lane 5, T/T.

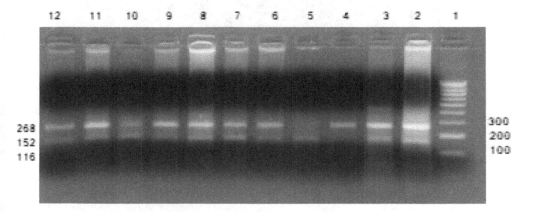

Fig. 3. GNB3 C825T genotyping by PCR-RFLP analysis followed by separation on 2% agarose gel as described in text. Lane 1, 100 pb ladder; lanes 2 and 3, C/T; lane 4, T/T; lane 5, C/C.

Gene	Variant	rs #	Forward and Reverse PCR Primer Sequences 5'–3'	PCR Product lenght, pb	Restriction enzyme	Restriction Fragments Generated, bp
SDF-1	SDF-1-3'A	rs1801157	5'-CAGTCAACCTGGGCAAAGCC-3' 5'-AGCTTTGGTCCTGAGAGTCC-3'	302	HpaII	G allele: 102 and 200 bp A allele: 302 bp
MMP-9	C-1562T	rs3918242	5'-ATGCTCATGCCCGTAATCCT-3' 5'-TGGGAAAAACCTGCTAACAACT-3'	435	Hin1II	C allele: 378- and 55-bp T allele: 242, 132 and 55pb
GNB3	C825T	rs5443	5'-TGACCCACTTGCCACCCGTGC-3' 5'-GCAGCAGCCAGGGCTGGC-3'	268	BseDI	C allele: 153- and 116-bp T allele: 268pb

Table 2. All genotyping Details, corresponding to each polymorphism studied are provided.

Distribution of SDF1-3'A, GNB3 C825T and MMP-9 C-1562T Polymorphisms in HSC CD34+ from Peripheral
Blood of Patients with Hematological Malignancies

89

2.4 Statistical analysis

Allele and genotype frequencies of the studied polymorphisms in patients and healthy controls were formulated by direct counting. Statistical analysis was performed using SPSS software (SPSS 16.0 for windows; SPSS Inc., Chicago, IL.).

The allele frequencies of SDF1-3'A, GNB3 C825T and MMP-9C-1562T polymorphisms were tested for the Hardy–Weinberg equilibrium of the whole group or subgroups of patients and were compared to the respective frequencies of the control group using the Pearson chi-square test or Fisher's exact test when appropriate. The same test was applied to compare the genotype frequency between patients and controls. Association of the allelic frequencies with the clinico-pathologic parameters was evaluated by $\chi 2$ test. The odds ratios (OR) and 95% confidence intervals (CI) were calculated too. P<0.05 was required for statistical significance.

3. Results

3.1 Patient's distributions according to their CD34+ cell yield and failure rates

Overall 83% of patients included in this study collected $\geq 2x10^6$ CD34+ cells/kg after a maximum of 4 aphereses, among them 20% collected 2-5x10^6 CD34cells/kg, and 63% collected $\geq 5x10^6$ CD34 cells/kg. Beside, 10% are remobilizers as they did not achieve the threshold of CD34+ cell yield of 2x10^6 CD34/kg within 4 apheresis days and are subjects to another mobilization protocol. Among them, the group of NHL represented the highest rate (40%), the lower ones, the group of MM and AML, which represented respectively 19% and 13%. By contrast, others are designed as first mobilizers (90%) since they have already collected $\geq 2x10^6$CD34+ cells/kg after a maximum of 4 aphereses days. Amongst them the group of multiple myeloma was the most frequent (40%), thereafter the group of Non-Hodgkin's lymphoma (34%) and Hodgkin's disease with 26%. For the patients included in this study, mobilization failure was defined as <2x10^6 CD34+ cells/kg obtained within 4 apheresis days. So, especially MM patients collected $\geq 5x10^6$CD34+ cells/kg and contained the highest CD34+ cell yield (8,89x10^6 CD34/kg for MM, and 5,51x10^6 CD34/kg for the others patients). Furthermore, the fact that MM patients had higher yield of CD34+ cells compared to NHL and HD is likely since that NHL and HL patients are frequently more heavily pretreated with cytotoxic chemotherapy than patients with MM [Iskra Pusic et al, 2008] (figure 4).

3.2 Analysis of the studied polymorphisms in the 4 subgroups of patients according to disease: A comparison between healthy donors of PBSC and patients

According to this study, SDF1-3'A and MMP-9 C-1562 T polymorphisms were significantly different between the patients and healthy controls (table 3). Particularly, we found significant differences in all the allelic and genotypic frequencies of the SDF1-3'A polymorphism in the MM group (p<0.05; OR=3.245 CI (95%) [1.830-5.753] for A allele; p= 0.017; OR= 3.324 CI (95%) [1.182-9.348]; p= 0.009; OR= 2.072 CI (95%) [1.200-3.580] for AA and GA genotypes, respectively).

Concerning the MMP-9 C-1562 T polymorphism its distribution was significantly different in the same MM group of patients compared to the control group, significant differences were observed exclusively for the T allele (p=0.041; OR=2.295 CI (95%) [1.020-5.168]) and also for the CC and CT genotypes (p= 0.039; p= 0.004; Table 3).

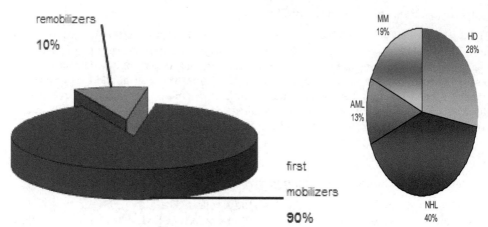

A number of first mobilization and remobilization in database

Distribution of remobilizers in the 4 subgroup of patients

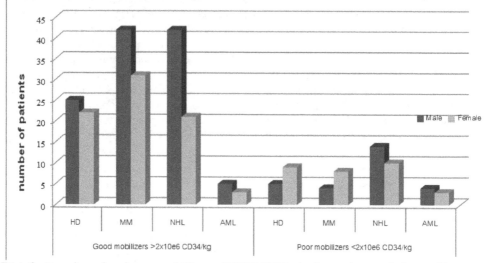

Distribution of good and poor mobilizers of PBPC CD34+ in the study population and by sex

Fig. 4. Overview of autologous stem cell transplantation database by disease as well as the distribution of good/poor mobilizers of PBSC CD34+ within the study population and by sex is already represented

Distribution of SDF1-3'A, GNB3 C825T and MMP-9 C-1562T Polymorphisms in HSC CD34+ from Peripheral Blood of Patients with Hematological Malignancies

91

	MM					NHL					HD					AML				
SDF-1	N	af	P	OR	CI	N	af	P	OR	CI	N	af	P	OR	CI	N	af	P	OR	CI
Alleles																				
A	75	0.436	<0.05	3.24	[1.830-5.753]	60	0.34	0.019	1.88	[1.104-3.209]	40	0.345	NS			9	0.3	NS		
G	97	0.464	0.013	0.30	[0.113-0.810]	114	0.65	NS			76	0.665	0.027§	0.27	[0.096-0.802]	21	0.7	NS		
Genotypes	N	gf				N	gf				N	gf				N	gf			
GG	22	0.256	<0.05	0.31	[0.176-0.567]	32	0.36	0.029	0.54	[0.315-0.941]	26	0.449	NS			7	0.467	NS		
GA	53	0.616	0.009	2.07	[1.200-3.580]	50	0.57	NS			24	0.413	NS			7	0.467	NS		
AA	11	0.128	0.017	3.32	[1.182-9.348]	5	0.05	NS			8	0.138	0.028§	3.62	[1.199-10.972]	1	0.066	NS		
MMP-9	N'	af				N'	af				N'	af				N'	af			
Alleles																				
T	14	0.16	0.041	2.29	[1.020-5.168]	21	0.22	<0.05	4.05	[1.901-8.646]	14	0.16	0.041	2.29	[1.020-5.168]	21	0.223	<0.05	4.05	[1.901-8.646]
C	74	0.84	NS			73	0.77	NS			74	0.84	NS			73	0.777	NS		
Genotypes	N'	gf				N'	gf				N'	gf				N'	gf			
CC	31	0.705	0.039	0.43	[0.192-0.971]	27	0.57	<0.05	0.24	[0.115-0.521]	31	0.705	0.039	0.43	[0.192-0.971]	27	0.574	<0.05	0.24	[0.115-0.521]
CT	12	0.272	0.004	3.5	[1.435-8.535]	19	0.40	<0.05	6.33	[2.754-14.567]	12	0.272	0.004	3.5	[1.435-8.535]	19	0.404	<0.05	6.33	[2.754-14.567]
TT	1	0.023	NS			1	0.02	NS			1	0.023	NS			1	0.021	NS		
GNB3	N''	af				N''	af				N''	af				N''	af			
Alleles																				
A	42	0.72	NS			30	0.45	NS			20	0.52	NS			6	0.6	NS		
G	25	0.084	NS			36	0.55	NS			18	0.48	NS			4	0.4	NS		
Genotypes	N''	gf				N''	gf				N''	gf				N''	gf			
GG	2	0.069	NS			8	0.24	NS			1	0.052	NS			0	0	NS		
GA	21	0.72	NS			20	0.6	NS			16	0.84	NS			4	0.8	NS		
AA	6	0.206	NS			5	0.15	NS			2	0.1057	NS			1	0.2	NS		

Table 3. Allele and genotype frequencies of *SDF-1, GNB3* and *MMP-9 polymorphisms* in the groups of patients with MM, NHL, Hodgkin's' Disease and AML

In table 3 are provided: all genotypic and allelic frequencies according to each polymorphism studied and corresponding to all patients. Distribution of genotypic and allelic frequencies by each disease included in this study. Then, all frequencies are calculated by statistical software SPSS 16.0 as well as p value and odd ratios (OR) are provided.

For the group of NHL, the distribution of the SDF1-3'A polymorphism was significantly different between patients and healthy controls especially for the A allele which seemed to be associated to this disease (p=0,019). Moreover, a decrease in GG genotype frequency compared to the control group was observed too reaching a statistically significance (p=0.029).

Concerning the MMP-9 C-1562T polymorphism, like the MM group, high significant differences were seen especially for the T allele (P<0.05; OR=4.055; CI (95%) [1.901-8.646]) and CT genotypes (P<0.05; OR=6.333; CI (95%) [2.754-14.567]). Similar results were obtained concerning the distribution of the MMP-9 C-1562T polymorphism in the group of Hodgkin's disease where significant differences were found in the T allele and CT genotype frequencies (p<0.05; Table 3).

While, the distribution of the SDF1-3'A polymorphism was not significantly different between the group of patients with AML and the control group, MMP-9 C-1562T distribution was significantly different essentially for the T allele (p=0.019, OR= 7.298, CI (95%) [1.511-35.249]) and the CT genotypes (p=0.004, OR= 12.444, CI (95%) [2.485-62.319]) Table 3.

So the presence of the MMP-9 C-1562T might be associated with this disease.

When considering the GNB3 C825T polymorphism, we observed that the TT genotype was more frequent in patient with MM and NHL with respectively 20.69% and 15.15% compared to the Hodgkin's disease group (only 10.52%). Whereas, the CC genotype was more frequent in the NHL group (24.24%) (Table 3).

3.3 Association of the SDF1-3'A allele with a good mobilizing capacity

As the clinicians have defined mobilization failure as <2x106 CD34+ cells/kg obtained within 4 apheresis days, two mainly group of patients emerged: the subjects with a good capacity of mobilization who collected ≥2x106 CD34+ cells/kg obtained within 4 apheresis days. Others with a poor mobilizing capacity and didn't collect 2x106 CD34+ cells/kg within 4 apheresis days. For the healthy allogenic PBSC donors, the mobilization failure was defined as <3x106 CD34+ cells/kg obtained within 4 apheresis days.

When considering the SDF1-3'A polymorphism, significant difference was observed in the SDF1-3'A allele carriers and GG carriers (p=0.023). A higher concentration of CD34+ cells in the leukapheresis products was detected in SDF1-3'A positive patients compared to GG homozygous subjects

Besides, a lower increase in the GG genotypes was observed in the "poor" mobilizer group compared to the "good" ones reaching a statistical significance (p=0.023; OR =0.494; CI (95%) [0.268-0.912]) (Table 4).

Thus, the SDF1-3'A allele carriers, especially the SDF1-3'AA homozygous individuals in the group of healthy allogenic PBSC donors had a better mobilization potential (table 4).

Distribution of SDF1-3'A, GNB3 C825T and MMP-9 C-1562T Polymorphisms in HSC CD34+ from Peripheral Blood of Patients with Hematological Malignancies

93

	Patients (285*, 161**)		Healthy controls (165*, 124**)		P	OR	CI	Good mobilizers (219*, 126**)		Poor mobilizers (66*, 35**)		P	OR	CI
SDF-1														
Alleles	N	af	N	af				N	af	N	af			
A	218	0.383	80	0.24	<0.05	2.185	[1.477-3.232]	177	0.404	41	0.31	0.009	0.451	[0.252-0.807]
G	352	0.617	250	0.76	0.029	0.38	[0.163-0.885]	261	0.596	91	0.69	NS		
Genotypes	N	gf	N	gf				N	gf	N	gf			
GG	97	0.34	90	0.545	<0.05	0.425	[0.287-0.630]	67	0.306	30	0.4	0.007	2.161	[1.208-3.868]
GA	158	0.555	70	0.424	0.008	1.686	[1.145-2.482]	127	0.58	31	0.47	NS		
AA	30	0.105	5	0.031	0.003	3.875	[1.476-10.171]	25	0.114	5	0.076	NS		
MMP-9														
Alleles	N'	af	N'	af				N'	af	N'	af			
T	66	0.205	26	0.105	<0.05	3.428	[1.914-6.141]	49	0.195	17	0.243	NS		
C	256	0.795	222	0.895	NS			203	0.805	53	0.757	NS		
Genotypes	N'	gf	N'	gf				N'	gf	N'	gf			
CC	99	0.615	105	0.847	<0.05	0.286	[0.160-0.512]	81	0.643	18	0.514	NS		
CT	58	0.36	12	0.097	<0.05	5.307	[2.697-10.444]	41	0.325	17	0.486	0.038	0.438	[0.198-0.968]
TT	4	0.025	7	0.056	NS			4	0.032	0	0	NS		

Abbreviations: OR, odds ratio; af, allele frequency; gf, genotype frequency; CI, confidence interval (CI=95%); Corrected p value; NS, not significant; *, for SDF-1 polymorphism; ** for MMP-9 polymorphism, Good mobilizers (>2X10^6 CD34/kg), Poor mobilizers (<2x10^6CD34/kg)

Table 4. Allele and genotype frequencies of *SDF-1,* and *MMP*-9 polymorphisms in mobilized peripheral blood patients and healthy controls

In this table are provided:

All genotypic Allelic frequencies designed as "gf" and allelic frequencies designed as "af" of SDF1-3'A and MMP-9 C-1562T polymorphisms in all the study populations (all patients), then in a group of healthy blood donors (as control group)

Then when, dividing the whole patients according to their mobilization capacity into: good mobilizers (>2X10^6 CD34/kg), and poor mobilizers (<2x10^6CD34/kg).

OR designed as odd radio and p value of all genotypic and allelic frequencies are provided in the table by using statistical software (SPSS 16.0) as it was mentioned above in section materials and methods-statistical analysis.

However, when considering the group of remobilizers in our study population we have observed that 48% of subjects were GG, 12% were AA and 40% were GA. This led us to consider a probable association of the GG genotypes to mobilization failure.

For the MMP-9 C-1562T polymorphism, significant difference was obtained with CT genotypes between the two groups (p=0.004; OR= 0.297; CI (95%) [0.125-0.703]).

For the GNB3 C825T polymorphism, we didn't observe any difference between the 2 groups of poor and good mobilizers.

This let us consider that there's no association between GNB3 C825T polymorphism and the capacity of mobilization of hematopoietic stem cells.

For the group of healthy PBSC donors, and with respect to our classification according to mobilization failure (<3x106 CD34/kg within 4 apheresis days), we have found an important association of SDF1-3'A distribution with higher mobilization yield of hematopoietic stem cells CD34+ reaching a higher statistical significance (p=0.001; OR=12.6; table 5).

Besides, we have observed a similar increase in the SDF1-3'G allele in the intermediate to poor mobilizers' subgroup reaching a statistical significance (p=0.035; OR=1.25; table 4). Similarly, the association was already observed when comparing the genotypic frequencies between the two subgroups.

The AA genotype was absent in the poor mobilizer subgroup, then was highly increased in the other subgroup reaching a statistical significance (p=0.035; OR=1.25).

While, the GG genotype was more represented in the poor mobilizers and the differences were significant too (p=0.001; OR=0.079; table 4).

Healthy allogenic PBSC Donors						
Good mobilizers		Poor mobilizers		P	OR	CI
N	af	N	af			
32	0,55	5	0,208	0,001§	12,6	[2,407-65,953]
26	0,45	19	0,792	0,035§	1,25	[1,045-1,495]
N	gf	N	gf			
3	0,10	7	0,583	0,001§	0,079	[0,015-0,415]
20	0,69	5	0,417	NS		
6	0,20	0	0	0,035§	1,25	[1,045-1,495]
N'	af	N'	af			
7	0,17	6	0,23	0,633 (NS)		
33	0,82	20	0,77	NS		
N'	gf	N'	gf			
13	0,65	7	0,54	NS		
7	0,35	6	0,46	NS		
0	0	0	0	NS		

Abbreviations: OR, odds ratio; af, allele frequency; gf, genotype frequency; CI, confidence interval (CI=95%); Corrected p value; NS, not significant; *, for SDF-1 polymorphism; ** for MMP-9 polymorphism, for healthy allogenic PBPC donors: Good mobilizers (>3X106 CD34/kg), Poor mobilizers (<3x106CD34/kg)

Table 5. Allele and genotype frequencies of *SDF-1*, and *MMP-9* polymorphisms in mobilized peripheral blood of healthy allogenic PBSC donors

Distribution of SDF1-3'A, GNB3 C825T and MMP-9 C-1562T Polymorphisms in HSC CD34+ from Peripheral
Blood of Patients with Hematological Malignancies

95

4. Discussion

In the present study, we investigated the effect of polymorphisms in the genes SDF-1, GNB3 and MMP-9 on the outcome of mobilization of peripheral blood stem cells for autologous transplantation by using a PCR-RFLP analysis.

We observed a significant association for SDF-1 and MMP-9 polymorphisms exclusively in patients with MM, NHL and Hodgkin's disease suggesting that these polymorphisms are fair candidate gene variants to these 3 hematological diseases.

In fact, Association of these polymorphisms to cancer has been previously reported by many investigators [De Oliveira KB et al, 2009; Rabkin CS et al, 1999].

Our results were in agreement with other studies suggesting that SDF1-3'A polymorphism is a genetic determinant of NHL [Gabriela Gonçavales de Olivera Cavassin et al, 2004]. Furthermore; as the SDF1-3'A polymorphism is situated in the mRNAs of 3'UTR region (untranslated region) which has been identified as an important regulator of the mRNA transcript, as well as the translated product [Catia Andreassi and Antonella Riccio, 2004; Marilyn Kozak, 2004; Gavin S. Wilkie et al, 2003].

The second polymorphism studied encoded for MMP-9, J. Arai et al, have reported that SDF-1 mRNAs abundantly expressed in stromal cells from the lymph nodes of patients with malignant lymphoma, so that 3'A carriers NHL are good candidates for presenting proliferation of neoplasic cells in the lymph nodes since that SDF-1 variant is associated with an increase of SDF-1 levels [J. Arai et al, 2000; Gabriela Gonçavales de Olivera Cavassin et al, 2004].

De Oliveira KB et al, when studying distribution of SDF1-3'A polymorphism have reported also a significant difference in genotype distribution between NHL patients (GG: 51.4%; GA: 47.1%; AA: 1.5%) compared to healthy controls (GG: 65.6%; GA: 28.9%; AA: 5.5%). Whereas, they didn't find any significant differences in genotypes distributions with breast cancer and Hodgkin's lymphoma [De Oliveira KB et al, 2009].

Moreover, previous reports on AIDS related non-Hodgkin's lymphoma (NHL) demonstrated that the CXCL12-3'A chemokine variant was associated with approximate doubling of the NHL risk in heterozygotes and an approximately fourfold increase in homozygotes [Rabkin CS et al, 1999; A Zafiropoulos et al, 2004]. Hence, this might let us suggest the possible role of such variant in the pathogenesis of NHL.

In this present work, we did not find a significant association between SDF1-3'A polymorphism and our group of patients with AML, this could be due to the lower number of patients (15 patients).

However, Dommange et al, have reported the implication of SDF1-3'A polymorphism in the clinical representation of acute myeloid leukemia in 86 patients with AML, as an association between this polymorphism and the risk of tissue infiltration by malignant cell was established by an increased release of the blast from the bone marrow in the blood in the SDF1-3'A carriers suggesting that this SDF-1 variant is associated with clinical representation of AML [A Zafiropoulos et al, 2004].

MMP-9 is a zinc-dependent proteinase, which is involved in numerous physiological and pathological processes. In the present study, we reported the distribution of the functional

MMP-9 polymorphism -1567 C/T in the promoter region of the MMP-9 gene in group of patients with some haematological malignancies as well as in patients undergoing stem cell mobilization.

Then, we observed that the T allele was highly associated to the susceptibility to the four diseases studied (table 3). We have to investigate either this variant have major influence on the circulating levels of MMP-9.

Concerning the group of MM, we observed a significant association in all allelic and genotypic frequencies of SDF1-3'A polymorphism with statistical differences when compared to control. Hence, as increased angiogenesis was related to the pathogenesis of MM, and because SDF-1 chemokine induces increased VEGF production, which is responsible for an angiogenic activity [Florence Dommange et al, 2006], we hypothesize that the SDF1-3'A polymorphism might increase SDF-1 protein which would have a role in developing angiogenesis and in the pathogenesis of the disease.

On the other hand, frequent distribution of the SDF-1 3'A allele in multiple myeloma patients confirms the implication of SDF-1 in hematopoietic stem cells. This logical consequence of the widely distribution of SDF-1 3'A allele proving that multiple myeloma patient's could be considered as good mobilizers.

For the GNB3 polymorphism we've observed that the TT genotype and the T allele frequencies are more frequent especially in patients with MM (0.72 for Tallele frequency) and NHL (0.45 for Tallele frequency) compared to healthy donors of PBSC (peripheral blood stem cells) (Table 3) which is far from the others populations [Maggie C.Y et al, 2004] . Then, suggesting the possible relation with these diseases.

Maggie et al when studying the ethnic differences in the linkage disequilibrium and distribution of single-nucleotide polymorphisms in 35 candidate genes for cardiovascular diseases have reported that the frequency of the T allele of GNB3 polymorphism in Chinese population is about 0.545. Then, such frequency is far from those of the French and of the Spanish population (0.329 and 0.359) and more closer to our result in Tunisian population [Yair Gazitt & Cagla Akai, 2004].

When interesting to the capacity of mobilization which was largely demonstrated to vary from a subject to another, several studies have focused on such phenomena and have reported that 10–30% of patients with hematological malignances fail to mobilize PBSC [Ingrid G. Winkler & Jean-Pierre Levesque, 2006] and either a small proportion of normal donors (1-5%) fail to mobilize sufficient CD34+ cells.

Besides, many reports suggest that numerous factors are related to poorer mobilization including age, gender, type of growth factor, dose of the growth factor and in the autologous setting patient's diagnosis, chemotherapy regimen and number of previous chemotherapy cycles or radiation [Sugrue MW et al, 2001].

In our study we were interested in the possible implication of some genetic factors in mobilization and as we've found an association with the SDF-1 3'A variant only, then we supposed that this polymorphism is the only predictor of mobilization capacity of PBSC CD34+.

Distribution of SDF1-3'A, GNB3 C825T and MMP-9 C-1562T Polymorphisms in HSC CD34+ from Peripheral
Blood of Patients with Hematological Malignancies

97

In fact, when analyzing the distribution of the two functional polymorphisms SDF-1 G801A and MMP-9 C-1562T considering the two groups of "good" and "poor" mobilizers, we've found an association only with SDF1-3'A polymorphism. While no association with capacity of mobilization was observed with GNB3 C825T and MMP-9 C-1562T polymorphisms.

When observing the distribution of the two polymorphisms not only when considering the mobilization capacity but also in relation to each studied disease enrolled in this work we've found that the good mobilizer group was mainly composed of MM patients. Whereas the poor mobilizer group contains Hodgkin's disease who are considered in previous studies as hard-to-mobilize patients [Benboubker L et al, 2001; Patrick J Stiff, 1999].

The fact that multiple myeloma patients mobilized better PBSC CD34+ (peripheral blood stem cells) than the others groups seem to be related to their ulterior chemotherapy (dexamethasone + thalidomide) and didn't receive any radiation therapy unlike the HD and NHL groups.

In the good mobilizer group composed of patients needing fewer apheresis than the other group, genotypes frequencies for the GG,GA, AA represented respectively 30.6%, 58% and 11.4%, and corresponded respectively to 45.5%, 47% and 7.6% in the poor mobilizer's group, and significant differences were found for GG genotype (p=0.007) and for A allele (p=0.009).

This confirms on the one hand that the SDF1-3'A allele was associated with good mobilizing capacity not only in the group of patients but for instance in the group of healthy allogenic PBSC donors (see table 5). Thus, our results regarding patients undergoing autologous transplantation of haematopoietic stem cells concur with those reported by Benboubker et al [Bogunia-Kubik K et al, 2009].

Moreover this deduction is already found in the group of healthy allogenic transplantation donors as it was reported in the present study and by Bogunia-Kubik K et al who have suggested that the SDF1-3'A allele was associated with a higher yield of CD34+ cells from healthy donors of PBPC for allogeneic haematopoietic SCT (stem cell transplantation) compared to GG homozygotes [Patrick J Stiff, 1999].

Recent studies by the same group underlined an association of the SDF1-3'A allele with faster granulocyte and platelet recovery after transplantation. Therefore they suggested that the SDF-1 gene polymorphism could be a useful tool of prognostic value for recipients of autologous haematopoietic stem cells [A. Gieryng et al, 2010]. The allelic variant SDF1-3'A is a result of the SNP rs1801157, which is located in a highly demethylated area of the 3'UTR region. This SNP confers a G to A transition in the nucleotide position 801, resulting in a loss of a methylation site, which could affect the methylating effect of G-CSF [Nagler A et al, 2004], and leading to a more decreased SDF-1 expression in healthy individuals carrying the polymorphism.

So, it's of interest to investigate either this variant have major influence on the circulating levels of SDF-1 and its mRNA expression, one of our future's interests.

Further studies examining how these three polymorphisms interact with disease risk factors are needed.

Interestingly, the possible implication of others genes involved of homing and migration process of CD34+ cells and for instance VCAM-1 to higher or lower mobilization yield of PBPC might emphasize new strategies for poor mobilizers subjects and lead to the identification of new biomarkers and/or therapeutic targets.

5. Conclusion

In the present study, we observed a significant association for CXCL12 and MMP-9 polymorphisms exclusively in patients with MM, NHL and Hodgkin's disease suggesting that these polymorphisms are fair candidate gene variants to these 3 hematological diseases.

Furthermore we've confirmed that the SDF1-3'A allele was highly associated to a good mobilizing capacity especially in the group of healthy allogenic PBSC donors where the analysis not biased by background disease or chemotherapy.

Besides, we suggested a possible association of GG genotypes to poorer mobilization is already deduced.

6. Acknowledgment

We thank all participant and all patients in this work

7. References

Catia Andreassi and Antonella Riccio. (2004). To localize or not to localize: mRNA fate is in 3'UTR ends. Trends in Cell Biology; Vol.19 No.9

J. Arai, M Yasukawa, Y. Yakushijin, T. Miyazaki, S. Fujita. (2000). Stromal cells in lymph nodes attract B-lymphoma cells via production of stromal cell-derived factor-1. Eur. J. Haematol; 64:323-32.

Benboubker L, Watier H, Carion A, Georget MT, Desbois I, Colombat P, et al. (2001). Association between the SDF1-3_A allele and high levels of CD34+ progenitor cells mobilized into peripheral blood in humans. Br J Haematol; 113:247–50.

Belvisi MG and Bottomley KM. (2003). The role of matrix metalloproteinases (MMPs) in the pathophysiology of chronic obstructive pulmonary disease (COPD): a therapeutic role for inhibitors of MMPs? Inflamm. Res. 52: 95-100.

Bogunia-Kubik K, Gieryng A, Dlubek D, Lange A. (2009). The CXCL12-3'A allele is associated with a higher mobilization yield of CD34 progenitors to the peripheral blood of healthy donors for allogeneic transplantation. Bone Marrow Transplant:273-8.

Dlubek D, Drabczak-Skrzypek D, Lange A. (2006). Low CXCR4 membrane expression on CD34+ cells characterizes cells mobilized to blood. Bone Marrow Transplant 37:19.

Florence Dommange,* Guillaume Cartron, Claire Espanel, Nathalie Gallay, Jorge Domenech, Lotfi Benboubker, et al for the GOELAMS Study Group. (2006). CXCL12polymorphism and malignant cell dissemination/tissue infiltration in acute myeloid leukemia. FASEB J; 20: 1296–1300

De Oliveira KB, Oda JM, Voltarelli JC, Nasser TF, Ono MA, Fujita TC, et al. (2009). CXCL12 rs1801157 polymorphism in patients with breast cancer, Hodgkin's lymphoma, and non-Hodgkin's lymphoma. J Clin Lab Anal, 23(6):387-93.

Distribution of SDF1-3'A, GNB3 C825T and MMP-9 C-1562T Polymorphisms in HSC CD34+ from Peripheral
Blood of Patients with Hematological Malignancies

99

Gabriela Gonçavales de Olivera Cavassin, Fernando Luiz De Luca, Nayara Delgado André, Dimas Tadeu Covas, Maria Helena Pelegrinelli Fungaro, Júlio César Voltarelli, and Maria Angelica Ehara Watanabe. (2004). Molecular investigation of the stromal cell-derived factor-1 chemokine in lymphoid leukemia and lymphoma patients from Brazil. Blood Cells, Molecules, and Disease; 33: 90-93.

Yair Gazitt, Cagla Akai. (2004). Mobilization of myeloma cells involves SDF-1/CXCR4 signaling and downregulation of VLA-4. Stem Cells; 22:65-73.

A. Gieryng, K. Bogunia-Kubik, and A. Lange. (2010). CXCL12 Gene Polymorphism and Hematologic Recovery After Transplantation of Peripheral Blood Progenitor Cells. Transplantation Proceedings, 42, 3280–3283

Marilyn Kozak. (2004). How strong is the case for regulation of the initiation step of translation by elements at the 3' end of eukaryotic mRNAs? Gene; 343: 41–54

Tsevee Lapidot and Isabelle Petit. (2002). Current understanding of stem cell mobilization: the roles of chemokines, proteolytic enzymes, adhesion molecules, cytokines and stromal cells. Experimental Hematology; 30: 973-81.

Roberto M. Lemoli and Alessandra D'Addio. (2008). Hematopoietic stem cell mobilization. Haematologica; 93(3): 321.

Maggie C.Y., Ng Ying Wang, Wing-Yee So, Suzanne Cheng, Sophie Visvikis, Robert Y.L. Zee et al. (2004). Ethnic differences in the linkage disequilibrium and distribution of single-nucleotide polymorphisms in 35 candidate genes for cardiovascular diseases. Genomics, 83; 559–65.

Miller SA, Dykes DD, Polesky HF. (1988). A simple salting out procedure for extracting DNA from human nucleated cells. Nucleic Acids Res; 16:1215.

Nagler A, kollenstein-Ilan A, Amiel A, Avivi L. (2004). Granulocyte-colony stimulating factor generates epigenetic and genetic alterations in lymphocytes of normal volunteers donors of stem cells. Exp Hematol, 32 (1): 122-30.

Iskra Pusic, Shi Yuan Jiang, Scott Landua, Geoffrey L. Uy, Michael P. Rettig, Amanda F. Cashen, et al. (2008). Impact of Mobilization and Remobilization Strategies on Achieving Sufficient Stem Cell Yields for Autologous Transplantation. Biology of Blood and Marrow Transplantation; 14:1045-56.

Rabkin CS, Yang Q, Goedert JJ, et al. (1999). Chemokine and chemokine receptor gene variants and risk of non-Hodgkin's lymphoma in human immunodeficiency virus-1-infected individuals. Blood; 93(6):1838–42.

Siena S, Schiavo R, Pedrazzoli P, Carlo-Stella C. (2000). Therapeutic relevance of CD34+ cell dose in blood cell transplantation for cancer therapy. J Clin Oncol. 18:1360–77.

Signoret N, Oldridge J, Pelchen-Matthews A, et al. (1997). Phorbol esters and SDF-1 induce rapid endocytosis and down modulation of the chemokine receptor CXCR4. J Cell Biol 139:651

Stetler-Stevenson WG. (2001). The role of matrix metalloproteinases in tumour invasion, metastasis, and angiogenesis. Surg Oncol Clin N Am; 10:383–92.

Patrick J Stiff. (1999). Management strategies for the hard-to-mobilize patient. Bone Marrow Transplantation; (23), Suppl. 2: 29-33

Sugrue MW, Willians K, Pollok BH, et al. (2001). Characterization and outcome of "hard to mobilize" lymphoma patient sundergoing autologous stem cell transplantation. Leukemia Lymphoma; 39:509–19

To LB, Haylock DN, Simmons PJ, Juttner CA. (1997). The biology and clinical uses of blood stem cells. Blood; 89:2233–58.

Toru Ogata, Hidenori Shibamura, Gerard Tromp, Moumita Sinha, MStat, Katrina A. B. Goddard et al. (2005). Genetic analysis of polymorphisms in biologically relevant candidate genes in patients with abdominal aortic aneurysms. J Vasc Surg; 41: 1036–42.

Cheng-Ho Tsai, Hung-I Yeh, Yusan Chou, Hsin-Fu Liu, Tzu-Yao Yang , Jyh-Chwan Wang et al. (2000). G protein b3 subunit variant and essential hypertension in Taiwan – a case–control study. International Journal of Cardiology; 73 :191–95.

Gavin S. Wilkie, Kirsten S. Dickson and Nicola K. Gray. (2003). Regulation of mRNA translation by 5'- and 3'-UTR-binding factors .TRENDS in Biochemical Sciences; 28:182-88.

Ingrid G. Winkler and Jean-Pierre Levesque. (2006). Mechanisms of hematopoietic stem cell mobilization:When innate immunity assails the cells that make blood and bone. Experimental Hematology; 34:996–1009.

A Zafiropoulos, N Crikas, A M Passam and D A Spandidos. (2004). CXCL12-3'A in the development of sporadic breast cancer. J. Med. Genet; 41; e59

Zhang B, Ye S., Herrmann SM, Eriksson P, de Maat M, Evans A, et al. (1999). Functional polymorphism in the regulatory region of gelatinase B gene in relation to severity of coronary atherosclerosis. Circulation; 99:1788– 94.

Part 2

Hematopoietic Stem Cell Therapy

6

Hematopoietic Stem Cells Therapeutic Applications

Carla McCrave

Children's Mercy Hospital in Kansas City, MO,
USA

1. Introduction

Hematopoietic stem cell transplantation (HSCT) has become an established treatment for malignant hematological diseases, solid malignancies and non-malignant diseases (figure 1). Newer indications for HSCT have emerged because of better understanding of human immunology, tumor biology and immunotherapy (table 1). Novel approaches have resulted in increase number of transplants as well as significant reductions in the morbidity and mortality associated with HSCT. These include more suitable donors with the addition of unrelated cord blood units (single & double) and partially matched family members; and novel conditioning regimens (reduced & non-myeloablative) that allow patients with significant co-morbidities to undergo transplantation. On the other hand, the introduction of alternative therapies, such as imatinib (tyrosine kinase inhibitor) for chronic myelogenous leukemia (CML), has challenged well established indications. This chapter summarizes the current indications for HSCT in pediatrics and address recent clinical developments in the field of HSCT.

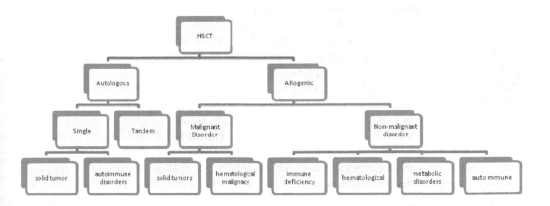

Fig. 1. Indications for HSCT

ALL	Immunodeficiency with hyper IgM
• In CR 1[a]	Leukocyte adhesion deficiency
• In CR 2	Omenn syndrome
• In CR 3 or further	Chediak-Higashi syndrome
AML in CR I or further	X-linked lymphoproliferative disease
CML	Kostmann syndrome
Myelodysplastic syndromes	Chronic granulomatosis disease
Hodgkin and non-Hodgkin lymphoma	Glanzmann thromboasthenia
Selected types of solid tumors[b]	Bernard-Soulier syndrome
Bone marrow failure syndromes (acquired & congenital)	Familial hemophagocytic lymphohistiocytosis
	Selected types of mucopolysaccharidoses,
Thalassemia major	Selected types of peroxisomal and lysosomal
Sickle cell disease	disorders
Infantile malignant osteopetrosis	Selected types of life-threatening autoimmune
SCID	disorders resistant to conventional treatments

Abbreviations: ALL= acute lymphoblastic leukemia; AML= acute myeloblastic leukemia; CML= chronic myeloid leukemia; CR1, 2, 3= first, second and third complete remission; SCID= severe combined immunodeficiency.

[a]Patients at high risk of recurrence (that is, t (9; 22) or t (4; 11); T-ALL with poor prednisone response, high levels of minimal residual disease).

[b]Stage IV neuroblastoma, renal cell carcinoma, very high risk Ewing sarcoma.

Table 1. Main Indications to allogeneic hematopoietic SCT in childhood

2. Indications for hematopoietic stem cell transplantation (HSCT) in pediatrics

There are two types of HSCT: autologous and allogeneic. Autologous HSCT consists of removal, storage and reinfusion of patients own hematopoietic stem cells as a way to restore the patient's depleted bone marrow after high dose myeloablative therapy (figure 2). Allogeneic HSCT consists of transferring both immature and mature blood cells to a patient from the bone marrow, peripheral blood or umbilical cord blood of a sibling, relative or an unrelated donor (figure 2) as a way to restore the patients bone marrow with a new immune system after a conditioning regimen (non-myeloablative or myeloablative chemotherapy). The success of an allo-HSCT is limited by the toxicity associated with the conditioning regimens, graft versus host disease (GVHD) and the development of opportunistic infections. New concepts and interventions over the last two decades have resulted in reduction of the morbidity and mortality associated with allo-HSCT. These include the utilization of reduced intensity regimens, more effective GVHD prophylaxis, new sources of progenitor hematopoietic stem cells, donor lymphocyte infusions and better prophylaxis and treatment for infectious diseases.

The decision to transplant or not to transplant should be determined on individual basis and several factors should be considered including the disease status, age, prior treatments and responses, donor availability and evolving alternative therapies.

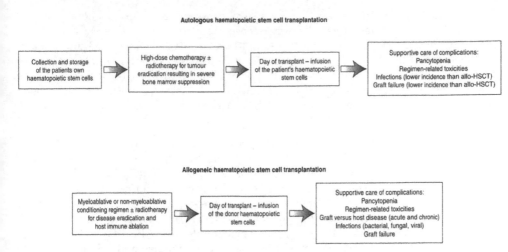

Fig. 2. Major Key Steps of HSCT.

2.1 Leukemias

2.1.1 Acute myeloid leukemia (AML)

Despite intensive chemotherapy, less than half of all patients with AML will survive in the long term (Creutzin, 2005; Gibson, 2005). Treatment outcome of pediatric AML is not as favorable as in ALL. AML treatment failure is due primarily to disease recurrence, although treatment-related mortality remains an important cause of treatment failure. Improvement in AML outcomes have been due primarily to intensification of therapy and improved supportive care guidelines. In AML, treatment intensity is an important determinator of outcome, and many studies have focused on the role of HSCT as post-remission intensification, utilizing both autologous as well as allogeneic HSCT. Allogeneic HSCT may provide a graft versus leukemia effect in pediatric AML. This is supported by a study from Bader et al that showed that preemptive immunotherapy following HSCT in patients with increasing (mixed chimerism) may lead to improved outcome. In another study Neudorf et al reported that children treated with allogeneic-HSCT in the children's cancer group 2891 study who developed acute graft versus host disease (GVHD) had fewer relapses (Bader, 2004; Neudorf et al., 2004).

The American society of bone marrow transplant position statement for the treatment of AML in children indicates that allogeneic HSCT should be recommended in the first complete remission because transplant has better overall survival and leukemia-free survival compared with chemotherapy alone (ASBMT, 2007; Oliansky, 2007). However, the role of allogeneic-HSCT in complete remission one (CR1) is declining because of the better outcome with modern multiagent chemotherapy and better methods of identifying patients that have low risk features at diagnosis and therefore are more likely to be cured with conventional chemotherapy. Recent AML trials (MRC-AML-12 & AML 0531) have shown that prognostic factors like cytogenetic and response to induction therapy are highly predictive of determining patients that are high risk at diagnosis and therefore would benefit from allogeneic-HSCT in CR1, while sparing lower risk patients the potential toxicities associated with an allogeneic-

HSCT (Ljungman, 2009). Recent analysis by several cooperative groups has now identified relapse risk group parameters based on cytogenetics abnormalities and early response to treatment : Low risk is defined as inversion (16)/t(16;16) or t(8,21). Down syndrome patients are also included in this low risk group; High risk is defined as monosomy 7, monosomy 5,5q deletions, or greater than 15% blasts at the end of induction I but who achieve complete remission after induction II, or high FLT3-ITD alleic ratio; Intermediate risk includes all other patients with no cytogenetic information available. This risk group is used to determine which patients should receive a HSCT in CR1.

Currently, HSCT is not recommended as frontline therapy for low-risk patients with AML in CR1, as they have an overall survival of 60% with conventional chemotherapy and HSCT has not been demonstrated to improve outcome for patients in CR1 (Gibson, 2005). HSCT is also not indicated for Myeloid Leukemia of Down Syndrome because HSCT is associated with excess toxicity with or without therapeutic gain (Lange et al., 1998). In addition, HSCT is also not indicated for acute promyelocytic leukemia (APL) due to excellent cure rates with conventional chemotherapy. However, for the few patients with APL who relapse or have persistent minimal residual disease, the prognosis is less favorable and HSCT might be a recommended choice (Oliansky et al., 2007). Allogeneic-HSCT from an HLA-identical sibling is an option for patients defined as intermediate risk. Allogeneic-HSCT from an HLA-identical sibling or an unrelated donor in CR1 is indicated for children with high risk AML including infant AML, therapy-related AML and children with M0 or M7 as it was proven to be more efficient than chemotherapy in some comparative studies with an event free survival ranging from 55 to 72% (Gibson, 2005). Regarding the use of haploidentical HSCT for AML, results in children with AML undergoing haploidentical HSCT have shown some effect of natural killer alloreactivity, suggesting that haploidentical HSCT may have a role in early phase very high AML patients (Marks et al., 2006).

HSCT also has an important role in the treatment of relapsed AML because outcome is poor with chemotherapy alone. Marrow transplantation in early first untreated relapse or CR2 results in a two-year EFS rate of 30-40%(Besinger,1995; Schimitz, 1998). Analyzes that attempt to compare outcome based on treatment have shown a survival advantage for patients who receive marrow transplants compared with chemotherapy alone, particularly for patients with longer first remission (Besinger, 1996).Therefore, allogeneic-HSCT from an unrelated or related donor is indicated in children with relapse AML in CR2, as it may provide long-term survival, particularly those in first relapse that are in remission.

Autologous HSCT has been used as consolidation in children with AML in CR1 after induction therapy and represents a valid alternative for high-risk children lacking a matched sibling donor. Nevertheless, results of pediatric studies comparing autologous HSCT with chemotherapy are conflicting. The use of peripheral blood stem cells in children with AML given autologous HSCT is infrequent. Further prospective clinical trials are needed to address the pivotal clinical question of whether autologous HSCT is better than chemotherapy or allograft as consolidation treatment for childhood AML in first CR (Miano et al., 2007).

2.1.2 Acute lymphoblastic leukemia (ALL)

ALL is not a uniform disease, but consists of different subtypes with different clinical prognostic and cytogenetic features. The prognosis of childhood ALL has improved dramatically over the past quarter of a century. Currently, over 2500 children in the United States are diagnosed each year with ALL and almost 95% attain a clinical remission after three or four drug induction chemotherapy (Clavell, 1986; Pui, 1998; Reiter, et al., 1994; Rivera, 1993). Over 83% of children with newly diagnosed ALL treated with multi-agent chemotherapy with or without clinical radiotherapy are alive and disease free at 5 years (Gaynon, 2000; Silverman, 2001; Vilmer, 2000).

Despite recent advances in the diagnosis and treatment of childhood ALL, there are several subpopulations of patients that have molecular biological markers or chromosomal abnormalities and biological factors that include poor prednisone response and resistance to initial chemotherapy including persistence minimal residual disease, that makes them very high risk of failing current multi-agent chemotherapy regimens. These very high risk patients require alternative treatment strategies to prevent progression and/or relapse of their disease (Kersey, 1997; Pui,1995). Table 2 defines the very high risk ALL patients.

The indication for HSCT from a match sibling or an unrelated donor for children with ALL in CR1 is limited to the subpopulation of patients that have clinical and biological features that identifies them as very high risk of relapse, as most studies quote an event-free survival (EFS) of less than 50% and a relapse rate of up to 50% (Reiter et al., 1994; Rivera, 1993). Children's oncology group conducted a clinical research study from 1993 to 1996 to investigate the toxicity and efficacy of HSCT in newly diagnosed children with very high risk features of ALL at diagnosis and/or during initial induction chemotherapy and their findings support the current indication of HSCT for very high risk ALL in CR1, especially patients with primary induction failure and Philadelphia chromosome positive ALL (Satwani, 2007).

HSCT should also be considered as an option for relapse ALL. The decision to perform an allogeneic matched related or unrelated donor HSCT for patients with relapse ALL depends on many factors which can be considered strong predictors of outcome as suggested from a number of literature reports. Different sites of relapse and the duration of first remission may be the most important factors predicting outcome after a first relapse. Patients with late relapse (over 6 months from therapy withdrawal) may have relatively good outcome with conventional chemotherapy alone (Borgmann et al., 1995; Ritchey, 1999; Uderzo et al., 1990). In contrast, children who relapse (isolated/combined medullary) during therapy or within 30 months of diagnosis seem to benefit more from HSCT than chemotherapy with an event-free survival rates of 40-50% reported for patients in CR2 who underwent a HSCT (Kawakami et al.,1990).

It has been difficult to compare outcomes of patients treated with chemotherapy or HSCT, since patient populations are not necessarily equivalent. Patients with aggressive disease die earlier and may not be included in studies of marrow transplantation, resulting in selection bias (Tichelli et al., 1999). To address this question, matched-pair analyses have been performed for ALL CR2 patients treated with chemotherapy or HSCT (Dreger et al., 1997; Novotny et al., 1998). For patients with early first relapse, HSCT resulted in significantly better EFS rates at 5 years compared with chemotherapy alone (40% vs 17%; p<0.001) (Novotny et al., 1998). Marrow transplantation was associated with a reduced risk of relapse that was not negated by increased treatment related deaths. The difference between chemotherapy and HSCT for patients who experienced a late marrow relapse (45% DFS vs

65%) (Chessells et al., 1986; Hoogerbrugge et al., 1995) was evident but not statistically significant.

Another factor to consider when deciding whether HSCT is an option for relapse ALL is the phase of leukemia at the time of transplant because it is also highly predictive for the risk of leukemia relapse and death from non-relapse causes. In particular, patients transplanted in relapse with over 30% circulating blast, have very poor survival following HSCT (Kessinger, 1989). Patients transplanted in remission compared to those in relapse have a two to five fold reduction in risk of relapse (p=0.0001) (36).

In summary the current opinion is that the earlier the relapse the more difficult is to obtain and maintain a second complete remission, so HSCT should be consider as an elective therapeutic option in order to eradicate a resistant disease. Relapse patients who fail to achieve remission prior to transplant have very poor outcome, so HSCT should not be undertaken.

Any one or more of the following:
 	
- Cytogenetics
  t(9;22) (q34, q11) or BCR-ABL molecular rearrangement
  t(4;11) (q21, q23) or 11q23 molecular rearrangement
  Hypodiploidy ($\leq$44 chromosomes)
- Age $\geq$10 years and WBC $\geq$200 x10^9/L
- Induction failure (day 28 M2 or M3 BM)
- Infant ALL (2-12 months) with any one or more of the following:
  CD10 negative (CALLA) ALL phenotype
  WBC $\geq$100 x10^9/L at diagnosis
  Day 14 M2 or M3 BM

Table 2. Ultra High-Risk Criteria of Childhood ALL in CR1.

2.1.3 Chronic myelogenous leukemia (CML)

CML is rare in childhood and accounts for less than 10% of all childhood leukemia. The treatment of CML has undergone dramatic changes in recent years. Before introduction of HSCT, the standard treatment approach for chronic phase CML was single-agent chemotherapy such as busulfan, hydroxyurea and interferon-alpha, however, treatment rarely produced a true complete remission. After 1980's, allogenic-HSCT was introduced as the only curative therapy for patients with CML. Five large multi-institutional retrospective studies have shown a high rate of long-term disease free survival (55-75% after myeloablative allogeneic HSCT), but survival was accompanied by significant treatment-related mortality, especially when unrelated donor allografts were used (Creutzig, 1996; Cwynarski et al., 2003; Millot et al., 2003; Weisdorf et al., 2002). From the 1980's to 2000, allogeneic HSCT was the treatment of choice for younger patients in first chronic phase if an HLA-matched donor was available. Before 1999, CML was the most frequent indication for allogeneic HSCT worldwide. With the approval of imatinib by the FDA in 2001, this tyrosine kinase inhibitor soon became the frontline therapy for newly diagnosed CML patients and transplant rates in CML dropped quickly worldwide (Muramatsu et al., 2010).

Dramatic responses to oral imatinib administration were observed in adult patients with CML (Druker et al., 2001; Hughes et al., 2003). However, clinical experience with imatinib in the pediatric population is limited. Several studies have shown that treatment with imatinib has resulted in prolonged molecular response with limited drug toxicity with comparable results with those in adult patients (Millot et al., 2006). Imatinib is now implemented in the primary treatment regimen for children, but the paucity of evidence on its ability to result in permanent cure and the potential complications that may arise from long-term treatment with imatinib have prevented imatinib from superseding HSCT as the primary means of curative treatment in children. The results of allogeneic HSCT in children with CML are similar to those observed in adults; HSCT-related complications such as transplant-related mortality and graft versus host disease remain significant challenges.

There is a general consensus for the need for HSCT in patients with imatinib resistance or those with advance-phase (accelerated and blast phase). (Table 3). However, issues such as when to undertake HSCT in chronic-phase CML pediatric patients or how best to treat patients who have relapsed after HSCT are still controversial. When considering HSCT vs imatinib in pediatric CML patients in early chronic phase, one must consider that the objective for treatment of childhood CML is not palliation, but cure. Hence, the possible adverse effects that stem from long-term tyrosine kinase weigh more heavily in the childhood CML population. HSCT still remains an important treatment option especially for younger patients with CML depending on physician and patient preferences. As a result of multiple clinical trials in adults that have documented great results with the use of imatinib in CML in chronic phase (87% of patients treated with imatinib showed complete cytogenetic response at 18 months with 3.3% disease progression) (O'Brian et al., 2003), this results have been applied to children, and imatinib is now also the front-line treatment for childhood CML.

World Health Organization (WHO) Criteria	International Bone Marrow Transplant Registry Criteria
Accelerated phase	Accelerated phase
1) Persistent or increasing WBC (>10×10^9/L) and/or persistent or increasing splenomegaly	1) Leucocyte count difficult to control with hydroxyurea or busulfan
2) Persistent thrombocytosis (>1,000×10^9/L) uncontrolled by therapy	2) Rapid leucocyte doubling time (<5 days)
3) Persistent thrombocytopenia (<100×10^9/L) unrelated to therapy	3) PB or marrow blasts ≥10%
4) Clonal cytogenetic evolution occuring after the initial diagnostic karyotype	4) PB or marrow blasts and promyelocytes ≥20%
5) Peripheral blood (PB) basophils ≥20%	5) PB basophils and eosinophils ≥20%
6) 10-19% myeloblasts in the PB or bone marrow (BM)	6) Anemia or thrombocytopenia unresponsive to hydroxyurea or busulfan
Blast phase	7) Persistent thrombocytopenia
1) Blasts equal or are greater than 20% or the PB WBC or the nucleated cells of the BM,	8) Clonal evolution
or	9) Progressive splenomegaly
2) Extramedullary blast proliferation	10) Development of myelofibrosis
3) Accumulation of blats occupy focal but significant areas of the BM	Blast phase
	1) ≥30% blasts in the PB, marrow, or both
	2) Extramedullary infiltrates of leukemic cells

Adapted from Swerdlow, 2008; Speck, 1984.

Table 3. Definition of Accelerated Phase and Blast Phase Chronic Myeloid Leukemia (by WHO2008 and IBMTR Criteria)

The evaluation of the response to tyrosine kinase treatment is made through hematologic, cytogenetic and molecular testing (table 4). The overall evaluation should lead to a classification of treatment response as optimal, suboptimal or failure (table 5). For patients in early chronic phase who achieve an optimal response, the drug should be continued until allogeneic HSCT is undertaken. In those patients who fail to respond, second-generation tyrosine kinase inhibitors and HSCT need to be considered. In suboptimal responders, imatinib may be continued, possibly at a higher dosage, or second-generation tyrosine kinase inhibitors may be introduced (Lee & Chung, 2011) Prospective cooperative studies are needed to address this complex issue in young patients with CML.

Complete hematologic response

1. Complete normalization of peripheral blood counts with leukocyte count $<10 \times 10^9/L$
2. Platelet count $<450 \times 10^9/L$
3. No immature cells, such as blasts, promyelocytes, metamyelocyte
4. No signs or symptoms of disease with disappearance of palpable splenomegaly

Partial hematologic response
- Same as those for complete hematologic response, except for

1. persistence of immature cells or
2. platelet count <50% of the pretreatment count but $>450 \times \times 10^9/L$
3. persistent splenomegaly but <50% of the pretreatment extent

Cytogenetic response (in patients with complete hematologic response)

1. Complete response; No Ph-positive metaphase cells
2. Major response; 0-35% Ph-positive metaphase cells (complete+partial)
3. Partial response; 1-34% Ph-positive metaphase cells
4. Minor response; 35-90% Ph-positive metaphase cells

Molecular response

1. Complete molecular response; bcr-abl mRNA undetectable by RT-PCR
2. Major molecular response; $\geq$ 3-log reduction of bcr-abl mRNA

Adapted from Faderls, et al, 1999.

Table 4. Criteria for Cytogenetic and Hematologic Remission in CML.

Time	Response			
	Optimal	Suboptimal	Failure	Warning
At diagnosis	NA	NA	NA	Advanced phase
3 months	CHR	Less than CHR	No hematologic response ; Stable disease or disease progression No CyR (Ph+> 95%)	
6 months	At least PCyR (Ph+≤ 35%)	Less than PCyR (Ph+> 35%)		
9 months	At least PCyR (Ph+≤ 35%)	Less than PCyR (Ph+> 35%)	No CyR (Ph+> 95%)	
12 months	CCyR	PCyR (Ph+, 1-35%)	Less than PCyR (Ph+> 35%)	Less than MMolR
18 months	MMolR	Less than MMolR	Less than CCyR	
Any time during treatment	Stable or improving MMolR[†]	Loss of MMolR, mutations in bcr-abl kinase domain	Disease progression, mutations in bcr-abl kinase domain	Disease progression, new clonal cytogen-etic abnormalities

Abbreviations: NA, not applicable; CHR, complete hematologic response, CyR; Cytogenetic response, PCyR; partial cytogenetic response, CCyR; complete cytogenetic response, MMolR; major molecular response, Ph+; philadelphia chromosome positive
[†]MMolR indicated a ratio of BCR-ABL1 to ABL1 or other housekeeping genes of ≤0.1% on the international scale.

Table 5. Recommendation for Definitions of Treatment Response to Imatinib Used in Early Chronic Phase. Modified from Suttorp M, et al, 2011 and Baccarani M et al, 2009.

2.2 Lymphomas

2.2.1 Non hodgkin's lymphoma (NHL)

Children suffering from NHL(Burkitt, lymphoblastic, diffuse large B cell and anaplastic large cell lymphoma) even with stages III/IV have excellent results when treated with first-line chemotherapy and radiation therapy. Long term EFS is between 60-90%(Cairo et al., 2007; Gerrad et al., 2008; Link, 1997; Patte et al., 2007). However, for refractory or recurrent Burkitt's, diffuse large cell and lymphoblastic lymphoma, the long term survival is only 10-20% (Atr, 2001; Cairo, 2003) In contrast, for refractory or recurrent anaplastic large lymphoma, up to 60% of patients may achieve long-term survival (53).

Several studies have shown that patients with chemosensitive recurrent diseases can achieve long-term disease free survival after HSCT. In a recent study by Thomas Gross published in 2010, he examined the role of HSCT for patients less than 18 years with the four different histologic subtypes receiving autologous or allogeneic HSCT (sibling & unrelated) from 1990-2005. To date this is the largest study done for refractory/relapse NHL. He concluded that EFS rates were lower for patients not in complete remission at HSCT, regardless of donor type. After adjusting for disease status, 5-year EFS were similar after allogeneic and autologous HSCT for diffuse large B cell (50% vs 52%), Burkitt's (31% vs 27% and anaplastic large cell lymphoma (46% vs 35%). However, EFS was higher for lymphoblastic lymphoma after allogeneic HSCT (40% vs 4% p<0.01). Predictors of EFS for progressive or recurrent disease after HSCT included disease status at HSCT and use of allogeneic donor for lymphoblastic lymphoma.

HSCT (auto & allo) can be effective in salvaging children and adolescents with refractory or recurrent NHL and results are superior if complete remission can be achieved prior to HSCT. Allogeneic donor is preferred for patients with lymphoblastic lymphoma.

2.2.2 Hodgkin's disease (HD)

Autologous HSCT is the standard therapy for patients with HD in first chemosensitive relapse or second complete remission (CR) as shown by two prospective randomized clinical trials (Linch et al., 1993; Schmitz et al., 2002)

Currently, there is no indication for autologous HSCT in first CR, even in patients with bad prognostic features at diagnosis (Federico et al., 2003; Proctor et al., 2002).

For primary refractory patients or for patients in chemorefractory relapse, autologous HSCT has only a small chance of inducing long-term remission (Lazarus et al., 1999; Sweetenham et al., 1999). As part of a clinical protocol for patients with resistant HD, autologous HSCT might be considered as an initial debulking therapy to be followed by an allogeneic HSCT as consolidation therapy (Carella et al., 2000).

Allogeneic HSCT has mainly been used as salvage therapy for multiply relapsed or refractory HD. A retrospective analysis indicates that reduced intensity conditioning allogeneic HSCT can improve the outcome of HD patients that relapse after an autologous HSCT (Thomson et al., 2008). Its impact in the long term outcome of these patients has still to be prospectively evaluated. HSCTs from HLA-identical sibling donors and well-matched unrelated donors give a similar outcome (Anderlini et al., 2008).

2.3 Myelodysplastic syndrome (MDS)

MDS is rare in children an allogeneic HSCT from a sibling donor or a well-matched unrelated donor is currently the only curative therapy that is available for children with de novo MDS, JMML or secondary MDS. MDS is a heterogeneous disorder, characterized by a clonal stem cell disease with ineffective hematopoiesis which is morphologically abnormal. MDS in children differs from MDS in adults, as children more frequently suffer from hypocellular MDS. De novo MDS can be further classified as refractory cytopenia (RC; previously known as refractory anemia or RA), RA with excess of blast (RAEB) and RAEB in transformation (RAEBt).

The European working party on myelodysplastic syndrome (EWOG-MDS) reported their retrospective results on 63 children with RC (Kardos et al., 2003). Over 40% of patients had hypocellular marrows. Almost 50% of children with monosomy 7 progressed to advanced MDS within 2 years from diagnosis. By contrast, patients with hypocellular RC with a normal karyotype, may experience a long stable course before progression to generalized marrow failure occurs. Therefore, in patients with monosomy 7, HSCT should be performed soon after the diagnosis has been established. This is also advised for patients with advanced MDS (RAEB or RAEBt), and for patients with hypercellular RC, or with other clonal aberrations. In some patients the differentiation between hypocellular RC with a normal karyotype and aplastic anemia may be difficult, and in such patients a "watch and wait" strategy may be considered with repeated bone marrow evaluation before a final decision on diagnosis and therapy is made.

After the introduction of the new WHO definition of acute myeloid leukemia, which lowered the threshold to diagnose AML from 30 to 20% blasts, there has been a debate whether RAEBt should be classified and treated as MDS or AML (VArdiman, 2002). One approach is to build in some observation time to assess progression, and to look for signs indicative of AML, such as organomegaly or non-random chromosomal aberrations such as t(8;21) or inversion(16).

Another relevant question in this respect is whether patients with advanced MDS benefit from pre-HSCT chemotherapy or not. Current results indicate this is not the case, as outcome did not differ according to blast percentage <5%, 5-19% or >20% in directly transplanted patients (Stary, 2005).

In summary, patients diagnosed with advanced MDS should be treated with allogeneic-HSCT, which may even include less suitable donors such as mismatched or haploidentical donors if this is the only available choice for a particular patient.

2.4 Solid tumors

Neuroblastoma (stage IV beyond the age of 1 year, or high risk factors in lower stage) is still the only indication where the benefit of high-dose therapy with autologous HSCT has been shown by randomized trials (Ladenstein et al., 2008; Matthay et al., 2009).

Although to date the published results do not show an unequivocal benefit for consolidation with high-dose therapy, children and adolescents with solid tumors might undergo autologous HSCT after high-dose chemotherapy within clinical research trial, preferably as part of first –line treatment strategies in the following situations:

- Neuroblastoma (high risk, >CR1)
- Ewing's sarcoma (high risk or >CR1).
- Brain tumors: children with medulloblastoma and high-grade gliomas responsive to chemotherapy in an attempt to avoid or postpone radiotherapy.
- Soft tissue sarcoma: stage IV or in responding relapse.
- Germ cell tumors: after a relapse or with progressive disease.
- Wilm's tumor: relapse.
- Osteogenic sarcoma: the value of HSCT is not yet clear.

In general, allogeneic HSCT cannot be recommended in children with solid tumors. Allogeneic HSCT may be undertaken in the context of a clinical protocol in specialized centers.

2.5 Bone marrow failure (BMF)

BMF syndromes include a broad group of diseases of varying etiologies in which hematopoiesis is abnormal or completely arrested in one or more cell lines. BMF can be acquired aplastic anemia (AA) or can be congenital, as part of such syndromes as Fanconi anemia (FA), Diamond Blackfan anemia (DBA), and Shwachman Diamond syndrome (SDS). The estimated incidence of BMF is 2 per million in Europe, with higher rates in Asia, perhaps resulting from environmental factors.

2.5.1 Acquired severe aplastic anemia (AA)

HSCT using an HLA-matched related donor is the treatment of choice for severe acquired aplastic anemia, resulting in long-term survival rates of over 90% If an HLA-compatible family donor is not available, most patients are treated with high-dose immunosuppression, using antithymocyte globulin (ATG) plus cyclosporine, with or without granulocyte colony-stimulating factor (G-CSF). Approximately 70-80% of patients respond to immunosuppression, although the actuarial 10-year survival rate is about 40%. Marrow transplantation from unrelated donors is reserved for those patients who do not respond to or who relapse after immunosuppressive therapy.

2.5.2 Inherited bone marrow failure syndromes (IBMFS)

IBMFS should be considered for all patients presenting with AA, regardless of the presence or absence of characteristic physical findings. IBMFS require specific approaches to management. Sensitive and specific diagnostic tests, including identification of mutations in specific genes, are available for many disorders.

2.5.2.1 Fanconi anemia (FA)

FA is the most common IBMFS and consists of a complex disorder of increased sensitivity to DNA damage characterized by congenital anomalies, progressive BMF, and high risk of MDS, malignant transformation to acute leukemia and solid tumors. Significantly, a large percentage of affected persons (25% to 40%) have no visible anomalies, and FA cannot be excluded without specific testing for mutagen sensitivity. BMF in FA typically presents between the ages of 5 and 10 years, with an actuarial risk of developing bone marrow failure of 50% to 90% by age 40 years (Kutler et al., 2003; Rosenberg, 2008). The median age of patients who develop AML is 14 years (Alter, 2003), and cumulative incidence of hematologic malignancy by age 40 years is 22% to 33% (Kutler et al., 2003; Rosenberg, 2008). Symptomatic transfusion, G-CSF, and androgens can be used to treat cytopenias; however, HSCT is the only current definitive therapy to restore normal hematopoiesis.

Commonly agreed-upon indications for HSCT in these patients include evidence of severe marrow failure as manifested by an ANC less then $1000 \times 10^9/L$ with or without G-CSF support, or hemoglobin of less than 8 g/dl or platelet count less than $50,000 \times 10^9/L$ or requirement of blood transfusion on regular basis. HSCT is also indicated for FA patients with evidence of progression to MDS or AML. Patients with FA who have an HLA-identical related donor, early HSCT is now the first-line treatment of choice for BMF, and preferably before transfusion dependence develops, to limit the risk of graft failure.

Preparative regimens for HSCT in FA patients are modified from standard approaches because of the chromosomal instability present in all FA cells, including nonhematopoietic tissues. In vitro studies have shown that FA cells are hypersensitive to DNA cross-linking agents, such as cytoxan (Berger, 1980). In addition, patients with FA are at increased risk of severe GVHD compared with patients with severe AA because of defective DNA repair mechanisms, leading to prolonged tissue damage after targeting by an alloreactive response (Guardiola et al., 2004).

Elaine Gluckman's group at St Louis, Paris investigated the use of reduced-dose cytoxan (20 to 40mg/kg) and reduced-dose thoracoabdominal irradiation or total body irradiation (TBI) (400-450 cGy) and reported a long-term survival of 58.5% after sibling donor transplantation, although with high incidences of aGVHD (55%) and cGVHD (70%). Later series modified the Gluckman regimen with the addition of ATG, resulting in less aGVHD and cGVHD and improved survival (Ayas et al., 2001). A recent series of 35 FA patients undergoing matched-related HSCT using this regimen along with peri transplantation ATG reported an excellent 10-year actuarial survival of 89%, with aGVHD in 23% of cases and cGVHD in 12% of cases (Farzin et al., 2007).

These studies have used low dose radiation because patients with FA have an increased risk of posttransplantation malignancy, but what about avoiding radiation altogether? A recent retrospective review of experience with matched related HSCT in FA patients in Saudi Arabia by Ayas et al (Ayas et al., 2008) found significantly greater OS in patients receiving non radiation, low dose cytoxan and ATG regimens compared with those undergoing preparative regimens with cytoxan and additional thoracoabdominal radiation (72.5% vs 96.9%; p=0.013). The availability of fludarabine, a highly immunosuppressive nucleoside analog that is well tolerated by patients with FA, has allowed the elimination of radiation with good results. Tan et al in 2006, recently reported an actual OS of 82%, transplant related mortality of 9% and minimal GVHD in a cohort of 11 patients who underwent transplantation with low dose cytoxan, fludarabine and ATG with T cell-depleted bone marrow or umbilical cord cells.

HSCT from an unrelated donor for patients with FA remains a key treatment strategy. Historically, outcomes of alternative donor transplantation in FA have been discouraging, with high incidences of graft failure, aGVHD and cGVHD and organ toxicity related to preparative regimens. Many regimens have been looked at over the years for unrelated transplants including increasing the dose of radiation, adding ATG without significant improvement in overall survival. The advent of fludarabine based preparative regimens has resulted in considerable progress, improving engraftment without significant toxicity attributable to the drug. However, although fludarabine regimens have had some success in treating FA, concerns regarding reduced intensity conditioning (RIC) regimens persist; residual FA cells that survive the preparative regimen may present as AML as much as 10 years later (Ayas et al., 2001).Despite these data, (Chaudhury et al., 2008), in a study of 18 high-risk patients with transfusion dependent AA, MDS and AML receiving either related mismatched or unrelated matched or mismatched HSCT using fludarabine, TBI and cytoxan for preparative regimens with T-cell depleted stem cell sources, found 100% engraftment, OS 72.2% and DFS of 66.6% with a median follow up of 4.2 years, suggesting that a RIC preparative regimen might be sufficient to control malignancy in FA. Cord blood is an alternative stem cells source for patients with FA who lack an HLA-matched unrelated bone marrow donor, as umbilical cord blood transplant has decreased incidence of GVHD.

Despite the improved survival, identifying the ideal time for HSCT in FA patients requiring alternative donor transplantations remains challenging, given the still-significant peri transplantation mortality and the possibility of long lasting androgen response or survival with AA for a significant period without progression to MDS/AML. Referral and transplantation before exposure to large amounts of blood products or prolonged periods of severe neutropenia are likely to lead to the best outcomes.

2.5.2.2 Shwachman-diamond syndrome (SDS)

SDS is a rare autosomal recessive disorder characterized by exocrine pancreatic insufficiency, skeletal abnormalities and BMF with a predisposition to MDS and leukemia, especially AML. Although most patients with SDS have some hematologic abnormalities, most of them do not require HSCT. In the largest reported series, 20% of cases developed pancytopenia and 6% progressed to MDS (Ginzberg et al., 1999).

HSCT is the only curative treatment for bone marrow dysfunction associated with SDS. However, the timing of HSCT remains a subject of controversy, and the apparent lack of genotype-phenotype correlation makes selection of patients for early preemptive HSCT difficult at present. In addition, SDS patients, like FA patients, have increased toxicity with intensive conditioning regimens. Overall, the available literature on HSCT in SDS patients is limited and consists mainly of case reports (Cesaro et al., 2001; Fleitz et al., 2002). Preliminary data indicates that HSCT with reduced intensity conditioning is feasible in patients with SDS and is associated with excellent donor cell engraftment and modest morbidity.

2.5.2.3 Dyskeratosis congenita (DS)

DC is a disorder of diverse inheritance with chromosomal instability related to a defect in telomere maintenance, characterized by a triad of reticulate skin pigmentation, mucosal leukoplakia and nail dystrophy, along with BMF. Between 80% and 90% of persons with DC will develop hematopoietic abnormalities by age 30 years, and BMF is the leading cause of early mortality in this population (Dokal, 2000). In addition, DC patients are at increased risk for MDS/AML and solid tumors, especially squamous cell carcinomas, as well as progressive pulmonary fibrosis (Dokal, 2000).

Allogeneic HSCT remains the only curative approach for marrow failure in patients with DC; however outcomes have been poor due to early and late complications. Initial attempts at HSCT in DC patients with myeloablative regimens had poor results, with significant morbidity and mortality, including increased incidences of chronic pulmonary and vascular complications, likely related to these patients underlying tendency to develop restrictive pulmonary disease. Non-myeloablative transplants using low-dose Cytoxan and fludarabine and ATG have produced successful engraftment and good short term outcomes, largely in case reports (de laFuente, 2007). Regardless of the potential reduction in toxicity associated with non-myeloablative regimens, preexisting conditions characteristic of DC (e.g. pulmonary disease) may ultimately limit the effectiveness of HSCT in DC patients.

2.5.2.4 Diamond-blackfan anemia (DBA)

DBA is a rare inherited form of pure red blood cell aplasia that presents early in infancy. Mutations in one of a number of ribosomal proteins have been identified in approximately 50% of DBA patients, implicating ribosomal biogenesis or function in the disorder. Clinically, DBA is associated with macrocytosis, reticulocytopenia, and normal marrow cellularity with erythroblastopenia. Characteristically, these patients have elevated fetal hemoglobin and erythrocyte adenosine deaminase activity, and up to 35% have an associated congenital anomaly, with craniofacial and thumb abnormalities the most common.

Corticosteroids remain the mainstay of initial therapy in DBA, with 80% response rate. Only 20% of patients achieve remission; 40% require continued therapy with steroids, which can have significant side effects, and another 40% remain transfusion and chelation dependent (Vlachos et al., 2008). Steroid-intolerant or transfusion-dependent patients may be considered for HSCT, which although curative for DBA, remains controversial, because most of these patients can achieve long-term survival with supportive therapy alone.

A series of 36 patients from the DBA registry who underwent HSCT (main indication transfusion dependence) yielded 5-year survival rates of 72.7% in matched sibling donor recipients and 19% in alternative donor recipients (p=0.01) (Lipton et al., 2006). Similar results were reported in an international bone marrow transplant registry series of 61 patients with DBA undergoing HSCT with conventional cytoxan containing preparative regimens; 3-year survival was 76% after sibling donor transplantation compared with 39% after alternative donor transplantation (Roy et al., 2005). In both studies, the alternative donor recipients were more likely to have received a TBI-containing regimen or to have a longer time from diagnosis to transplantation, suggesting that TBI should be avoided. In addition, patients with DBA have an increased risk of malignancy compared to the general population, another reason why TBI-containing regimens should be avoided in this population. There also are encouraging case reports of successful HSCT in DBA with RIC fludarabine containing preparative regimens; however, the data are scanty and reflect short follow-up times; further study is needed in this area (Berndt, 2004; Ostronoff, 2004).

2.5.2.5 Congenital Amegakaryocytic Thrombocytopenia (CAMT)

CAMT is a rare autosomal recessive disorder caused by mutations in the thrombopoietin receptor. It is usually diagnosed early in childhood, presenting with isolated nonimmune thrombocytopenia with decreased marrow megakaryocytes. Approximately 50% of CAMT patients develop marrow aplasia, and some develop MDS or leukemia.

Although transient responses to steroids, cyclosporine and growth factors in CAMT have been documented, HSCT remains the only curative treatment. Good short-term survival has been reported after matched related donor HSCT in small case series. Reports of unrelated donor HSCT are largely case reports and describe significant engraftment challenges.

2.6 Immunodeficiencies

Primary cellular immunodeficiencies are a group of inherited disorders characterized by severe impairment of the innate or adaptive immune systems, which generally leads to early death from infectious complications. These disorders can be further categorized by the cell lineage primarily affected (table 6). Supportive care can extend the life span of patients affected by these diseases, definitive cure is generally only achieved by allogeneic hematopoietic stem cell transplantation, though recent advances in gene therapy hold significant promise that this may soon be a viable alternative. Allogeneic HSCT is indicated for severe primary immunodeficiencies from both HLA-identical and alternative donors.

Absent T- and B-lymphocyte function	Defective T and B lymphocytes	Dysfunctional T lymphocytes with predisposition to HLH	Absent or dysfunctional granulocytes
SCID	Wiskott–Aldrich syndrome	Familial HLH (defects in *perforin*, *MUNC*, etc.)	Severe congenital neutropenia
	HIGM1	Chediak–Higashi syndrome	Leukocyte adhesion disorder
		Griscelli syndrome	Chronic granulomatous disease
		XLP	

Abbreviations: HIGM1 = hyper IgM syndrome (CD40 ligand deficiency); HLH = hemophagocytic lymphohistiocytosis; XLP = X-linked lymphoprolifera-tive disease.

Table 6. Primary Immunodeficiencies Potentially Treated with HSCT.

2.6.1 Severe combined immunodeficiency (SCID)

SCID is a rare disorder caused by a group of genetic disorders with a shared phenotype of deficient T and B lymphocyte infunction (with or without abnormal natural killer (NK) cell development) that leads to early death from recurrent infections in affected children (table 7). Except for those patients with SCID due to deficiency of adenosine deaminase (ADA), for which replacement enzyme exists, the only curative therapy for SCIS is allogeneic HSCT. However, early results with gene insertion into autologous hematopoietic stem cells for children with x-linked SCID and ADA deficiency (Cavazzana-Calco, 2007) suggest that eventually this will become a more common form of curative treatment for many primary immunodeficiency diseases.

Name	Defect	Phenotype	Special
X-linked	Common γ chain	T-B + NK –	
JAK3 deficiency	Janus kinase 3	T-B + NK –	
Rag 1 or 2	Recombinase-activating proteins 1 or 2	T-B – NK +	Frequently associated with Omenn's syndrome: autoreactive GVHD
Artemis deficiency	Artemis (also known as DCLREIC)	T-B – NK +	Athabascan-speaking Native Americans, radiosensitive
Ligase 4 deficiency	Ligase 4	T-B – NK +	Radiosensitive
IL-7Rα deficiency	IL-7 receptorα	T-B + NK +	
CD45 deficiency	CD45	T-B + NK +	
CD3δ deficiency	CD3δ subunit	T-B + NK +	
CD3ε deficiency	CD3ε subunit	T-B + NK +	
CD3ς deficiency	CD3ς subunit	T-B + NK +	
Cartilage hair hypoplasia	Endoribonuclease	T-B + NK +	Dwarfism, hypoplastic hair Finnish, Amish
p56lck deficiency	p56lck Protein tyrosine kinase	T-B + NK +	
ADA deficiency	Adenosine deaminase	T-B – NK –	
PNP deficiency	Purine nucleoside phosphorylase	T-B – NK –	Neurologic dysfunction, ataxia
Reticular dysgenesis	Unknown	T-B – NK –	Impaired myeloid and erythroid development, sensorineural deafness
ZAP70 deficiency	ς-chain-associated protein kinase	CD4+, CD8– B+, NK +	
Bare lymphocyte Syndrome type II	HLA class II	CD4–(mild), CD8 + B+, NK +	North African
SCID with bowel atresia	Unknown	CD4+, CD8 +, B + NK +	

Abbreviations: ADA = adenosine deaminase; DCLREIC = DNA cross-link repair enzyme 1C; HLA = human leukocyte antigen.

Table 7. Genetic Sub-Types of Severe Combined Immunodeficiency.

HSCT should be done as soon as the diagnosis is confirmed because these patients are at risk of developing a life-threatening infection, particularly pulmonary infections. For all stem cell sources, successful outcomes are more likely to be achieved when the patient is still very young, preferably less than 6 months of age.(Buckley et al., 1999), demonstrated that infants transplanted less than 3.5 months of age had a 95% overall survival compared to only 76% overall survival in older children. The preferred choice of stem cell donor for a patient with SCID is an HLA-identical sibling, in which the overall survival now exceeds 90%, if the transplant is performed promptly. In patients without a matched sibling, the choice is whether to use an immediately available T cell depleted haplocompatible family member or to perform a search for an HLA matched unrelated donor or cord blood unit. Table 8 lists the reports on transplantation with different stem cell sources.

2.6.2 Wiskott-Aldrich syndrome (WAS)

WAS is characterized by a trial of thrombocytopenia with small platelets, eczema and recurrent infections. The T cell immunodeficiency predisposes to the development of autoimmune phenomena and lymphoma. Affected males rarely survive past the second decade of life. The only curative strategy is allogeneic HSCT. The international bone marrow registry and national marrow donor program demonstrated in 170 patients that while the 5-year OS of patients transplanted from HLA-identical siblings was 87%, the results for unrelated HSCT were significantly related to the age at transplant (Filipovich et al., 2001). Unrelated donors less than 5 years of age had an 85% 5-year OS, while all 15 patients greater than 5 years of age died (Filipovich et al., 2001). Haploidentical related transplants have been less successful with an OS of 45-52%.

	Year	Reference	MRD	Haplo	Haplo	MUD	MUD	Cord
Conditioning			None	None	MA	MA	RI	MA
Dror et al.	1993	3	—	67% (12)	50% (12)	—	—	—
Buckley et al.	1999	5	100% (12)	78% (77)	—	—	—	66% (3)
Bertrand et al.	1999	4	—	46% (50)	54% (129)	—	—	—
Dalal et al.	2000	15	—	—	—	67% (9)	—	—
Knutsen and Wall	2000	16	—	—	—	—	—	88% (8)
Antoine et al.	2003	6	81% (104)	—	—	63% (28)	—	—
Rao et al.	2005	17	—	—	—	71% (7)	83% (6)	—
Bhattacharya et al.	2005	18	—	—	—	—	—	80% (10)*
Grunebaum et al.	2006	14	92% (13)	—	53% (40)	81% (41)	—	—

Stem cell source: MRD (matched related donor) vs haplo (haplocompatible family donor) vs MUD (matched unrelated donor) vs Cord (unrelated cord blood stem cells). Conditioning: none vs MA (myeloablative) vs RI (reduced intensity). Percentage indicates overall survival (absolute number of patients). *Some patients received no conditioning.

Table 8. Survival Following HSCT For SCID Based on Stem Cell Source and Conditioning Regimen.

2.6.3 Familial hemophagocytic lymphohistiocytosis (HLH)

Familial HLH is characterized by episodes of fever, hepatosplenomegaly and cytopenias. An autosomal recessive defect in one of the several genes including those encoding perforin or Munc 13, causes reduced NK and T cell cytotoxicity. This leads to a widespread accumulation of lymphocytes and mature macrophages with hypercytokinemia. Familial HLH is invariably fatal. The only curative strategy for treatment of familial HLH is allogeneic HSCT. A report from a multicenter prospective trial, HLH-94, demonstrated a 62% 3-year EFS in 65 children undergoing allogeneic HSCT with a variety of stem cell sources (Henter et al., 2002).

2.6.4 Chronic granulomatous disease (CGD)

CGD is characterized by recurrent pyogenic infections in patients with normal neutrophil numbers. A defect in one of the four genes encoding subunits of the nicotinamide adenine dinucleotide phosphate-oxidase complex leads to insufficient production of free protons from which to make hydrogen peroxide. With good supportive care, including therapy with interferon gamma, affected individuals can live up to the fourth decade of life, but suffer early mortality from recurrent pulmonary infections.

Allogeneic HSCT is the only curative strategy. A report from the European group for Blood and Marrow Transplantation demonstrated in 23 patients that myeloablative conditioning prior to matched sibling HSCT can be safely performed (85%OS), especially if the patient were free of infection at the time of HSCT (100% OS) (Seger et al., 2002). Given the current success rates, some favor transplantation in all patients with CGD who have an appropriate donor at the earliest opportunity.

Recent data, (Kuhn's et al., 2010) showed that patients with very low superoxide production had worse long-term survival than those with higher levels of NADPH oxidase activity suggesting that these patients should be considered appropriate candidates for early HSCT, particularly if a sibling matched donor is available. An increased alkaline phosphatase level, a history of liver abscesses, and a decrease in platelet count reflecting portal hypertension are adverse prognostic indicators (Feld et al., 2008). These patients might also be considered for early transplantation. Even with improved survival and longevity caused by better infection and inflammation management, complications and their consequences can accumulate over time. However, HSCT is probably better before infections and inflammatory damage accumulates. Transplantation has aloes reversed some of the inflammatory and autoimmune complications associated with CGD and might prevent their development (Seger et al., 2002). Allogeneic HSCT has improved dramatically over the last decade because of improved conditioning regimens and GVHD prophylaxis, high-resolution sequence-based matching and improved pre transplantation, peri transplantation and post transplantation management and as a result it has become a successful and sensible option for many patients with CGD.

2.7 Inherited metabolic diseases (IMD)

IMD is a diverse group of diseases arising from genetic defects in lysosomal enzymes or peroxisomal function. The lysosome is an intracellular sorting, recycling and digestion of organic molecules. Loss of functional activity of lysosomal enzymes results in accumulation of substrates, such as glycoprotein or mucopolysaccharides (MPS). The clinical manifestations vary depending on the specific enzymatic deficiency, level of residual activity, and site of substrate accumulation.

Allogeneic HSCT can prolong life and improve its quality in patients with IMD. HSCT offers a permanent source of enzyme replacement therapy and also might mediate nonhematopoietic cell regeneration or repair. The likely processes responsible for the effectiveness of HSCT for IMD includes cytoreduction to ablate myeloid and immune elements, engraftment of donor-derived hematopoietic and immune system, donor leukocytes production of enzyme, distribution of enzyme through blood circulation, migration of cells to brain, cross blood-brain barrier, many develop microglia, replacement of enzyme in the brain by cross-correction and nonhematopoietic cell engraftment (Prasad and Kurtzberg, 2008).HSCT has been performed in almost 20 of the 40 known lysosomal storage disorders and peroxisomal storage disorders. However, the majority of transplant experience to date is in patients with MPS I (Hurler Syndrome), other MPS syndromes (MPSII, MPSIII, A & B, MPSVI), adrenal leukodystrophy (ALD), metachromic leukodystrophy (MLD), and globoid leukodystrophy (Krabbe disease), accounting for more than 80% of the cases. Table 9 identifies the IMD for which allogeneic HSCT is currently indicated or under investigation. The response to HSCT varies from disease to disease, within patients with same disease, and within different organ systems in the same patient.

2.7.1 Hurler syndrome (MPS IH)

MPS IH, the most sever phenotype of alpha-l-iduronidase deficiency, is an autosomal recessive disorder characterized by progressive accumulation of stored glycosaminoglycans (GAGs). Hurler and other phenotypes of MPS I are a broad continuous clinical spectrum. Accumulation of GAGs results in progressive, multisystem dysfunction that includes psychomotor retardation, severe skeletal malformations, life-threatening cardiopulmonary complications, and early death.

Disorder	Enzyme/Protein	HSCT Indication	Comments
Mucopolysaccharidoses			
Hurler (MPS IH)	α-ʟ-Iduronidase	Standard therapy	
Hurler/Scheie (MPS IH/S)	α- ʟ-Iduronidase	Optional	ERT first-line therapy
Scheie (MPS IS)	α- ʟ-Iduronidase	Optional	ERT first-line therapy
Hunter: severe (MPS IIA)	Iduronate-2-sulfatase	Investigational	Only early or asymptomatic
Hunter: attenuated (MPS IIB)	Iduronate-2-sulfatase	Investigational	Only early or asymptomatic
Sanfilippo (MPS IIIA)	Heparan-N-sulfatase	Investigational	Only early or asymptomatic
Sanfilippo (MPS IIIB)	N-Acetylglucosaminidase	Investigational	Only early or asymptomatic
Sanfilippo (MPS IIIC)	AcetylCoA:N-acetyltransferase	Investigational	Only early or asymptomatic
Sanfilippo (MPS IIID)	N-Acetylglucosamine 6-sulfatase	Investigational	Only early or asymptomatic
Maroteaux-Lamy (MPS VI)	Arylsulfatase B	Optional	ERT first-line therapy
Sly (MPS VII)	β-Glucuronidase	Optional	
Leukodystrophies			
X-ALD, cerebral	ALD protein	Standard therapy	Not for advanced disease
MLD: early onset	ARSA	Unknown	Only early or asymptomatic
MLD: late onset	ARSA	Standard therapy	
GLD: early onset	GALC	Standard therapy	Neonate, screening diagnosis, or second case in known family; not for advanced disease
GLD: late onset	GALC	Optional	
Glycoprotein metabolic and miscellaneous disorders			
Fucosidosis	Fucosidase	Optional	
α-Mannosidosis	α-Mannosidase	Optional	
Aspartylglucosaminuria	Aspartylglucosaminidase	Optional	
Farber	Ceraminidase	Optional	
Tay-Sachs: early onset	Hexosaminidase A	Unknown	Neonate, screening diagnosis, or second case in known family
Tay-Sachs: juvenile	Hexosaminidase A	Unknown	
Sandhoff: early onset	Hexosaminidase A & B	Unknown	Neonate, screening diagnosis, or second case in known family
Sandhoff: juvenile	Hexosaminidase A & B	Unknown	
Gaucher 1 (nonneuronopathic)	Glucocerebrosidase	Optional	ERT first-line therapy
Gaucher 2 (acute neuronopathic)	Glucocerebrosidase	Unknown	
Gaucher 3 (subacute neuronopathic)	Glucocerebrosidase	Unknown	Limited benefit of ERT
Gaucher 3 (Norrbottnian)	Glucocerebrosidase	Optional	
Pompe	Glucosidase	Investigational	ERT available
Niemann-Pick: type A	Acid sphingomyelinase	Unknown	
Niemann-Pick: type B	Acid sphingomyelinase	Unknown	ERT in clinical trial
Niemann-Pick: type C	Cholesterol trafficking	Optional for C-2	
Mucolipidosis: type II (I-cell)	N-Acetylglucosamine-1-phosphotransferase	Investigational	Only early or asymptomatic
Wolman syndrome	Acid lipase	Optional	May be viewed as standard
MSD	Sulfatases	Investigational	

Table does not include diseases where HSCT is not indicated. Standard therapy: HSCT applied routinely. Considerable published research evidence from registries and institutions shows efficacy. Delayed diagnosis or advanced disease may preclude transplant for individual patients. Optional: HSCT is effective but other therapy is increasingly considered first choice. Or, insufficient published evidence for HSCT to be considered standard. Investigational: possible a priori reason for HSCT. Further published evidence needed to support the use of HSCT in clinical practice. Unknown: no published evidence that HSCT is beneficial.

Table 9. IMD for which HSCT may be indicated

Data from the CIBMTR and EBMT indicate that more than 500 allogeneic HSCTs have been performed worldwide for children with MPS IH since 1980, making it the most commonly transplanted IMD. HSCT is effective, resulting in increased life expectancy and improvement of clinical parameters if performed early in the disease course before the onset of irreversible damage. Donor engraftment after HSCT has resulted in improvement of the following clinical symptoms: rapid reduction of obstructive airway symptoms, and hepatomegaly; improvement in cardiovascular function as well as hearing, vision and linear growth; finally hydrocephalus is either prevented or stabilized. In addition, cerebral damage already present before HSCT seems to be irreversible, but HSCT is able to prevent progressive psychomotor deterioration and improve cognitive function (Peters, 1998; Vellodi et al., 1997).

A matched normal sibling is the preferred HSCT donor. In the past decade an unrelated cord blood (CB) has been used with increasing frequency in patients without a sibling donor. CB offers several potential advantages compared with bone marrow or peripheral blood for HSCT, including better availability, greater tolerance for HLA mismatches, lower incidence and severity of GVHD and reduced likelihood of transmitting viral infections (Staba et al., 2004; Prasad et al., 2008). The use of CB for children with MPS IH has been associated with high rates of chimerism, engraftment and overall survival (Staba et al., 2004; Prasad et al., 2008). Similar results are noted for CB in other selected IMD (Escolar et al., 2005). As a result of this data, the EBMT developed transplantation guidelines for patients with MPS IH in 2005. These guidelines are widely used today and include a standardized busulfan/cytoxan (BU/CY) conditioning regimen, an enzymatically normal matched sibling bone marrow donor if available, and if not, cord blood as the preferred graft source. A recent EUROCORD- Duke university MPS IH collaborative study showed that early transplant (i.e., within 4.6 months from diagnosis) with CB and BU/Cy conditioning was associated with improved engraftment and overall survival. Furthermore, 94% of engrafted survivors achieved full donor chimerism. (Boelens et al., 2007).

Despite the overall success from HSCT, some disease manifestations persists or can even progress after HSCT, and this includes the musculoskeletal disorders secondary to the IMD that does not resolve and often requires orthopedic surgical intervention. In addition, neurocognitive dysfunction and corneal clouding that developed before HSCT may be irreversible. The outcome of HSCT for children with MPS IH is promising, yet variable from child to child. The variability is presumably caused by factors such as genotype, age and clinical status before HSCT, donor enzyme activity level, donor chimerism (mixed or full) stem cell source (CB, BM,PB) and resultant enzyme activity level in the recipient (Aldenhoven, 2008). An international long-term follow up study involving Europe and North America is underway to evaluate the influence of these various factors. Overall progress has been made. HSCT for children with MPS IH has become a safer procedure, with recent survival rates exceeding 90%.

2.7.2 Other mucopolysaccharidosis syndromes

Compared with MPS IH, experience with HSCT for treatment of other MPS disorders is limited. Small numbers and lack of detailed functional outcome data hamper the development of specific therapy guidelines. Conceptually, the basis for the effectiveness of HSCT in these children is the same as those with MPS IH. However, the kinetics of cellular migration, differentiation, distribution, and effective enzyme delivery may differ. Also, there is wide clinical variability within and across specific MPS diseases. As with HSCT for other IMD, important factors in the outcome may be timing of transplant, graft source, and the underlying severity of the phenotype in a given child. To date, most of the published experience is in recipients of BMT (Guffon et al., 2009). Recently, survival has been reported in small cohorts undergoing CBT, but their functional outcomes are not yet published.

The role of HSCT in MPS II remains controversial because of lack of convincing evidence of neurocognitive benefit. The status of HSCT for Sanfilippo Syndrome (MPS III) is similar to that of MPS II with inadequate data and inability to make specific recommendations about timing of transplant, graft source, and potential neurological benefit. Eleven long-term survivors of BMT have been reported, but all showed declined in neurocognitive function

(Gungor,1995; Vellodi et al., 1992). On the other hand, the results of HSCT for Maroteaux-Lamy Syndrome (MPS VI) have been promising. MPS VI has multiple clinical phenotypes, but generally patients live into the second to fourth decade. HSCT in 4 patients with MPS VI lead to improvement in cardiopulmonary function, facial features, and quality of life (Herskhovitz et al., 1999). HSCT can be considered a therapeutic option for patients with MPS VI that are intolerant or fail ERT.

2.7.3 Adrenal leukodystrophy (ALD)

X-ALD is a peroxisomal disorder involving defective beta-oxidation of very long chain fatty acids (VLCFA). The affected gene in X-ALD is ABCD1 and the peroxisomal membrane protein for which it codes is ALDP. More than 500 mutations in the gene are described, but there is no relationship between the nature of the mutation and the clinical presentation of illness. X-ALD has a variable clinical presentation. Patients can be asymptomatic or present with adrenal insufficiency and/or non inflammatory axonopathy (AMN) and/or cerebral disease. The clinical course is so variable with some individuals never developing symptoms so therefore, HSCT can not be recommended based on the presence or absence of the genetic mutation. HSCT is indicated only in those patients with clear evidence of early cerebral inflammatory disease as determined by a gadolinium enhanced MRI. (Peters, 2003). Cerebral disease may manifest itself during childhood or adolescence. Approximately 40% of genetically affected boys develop childhood cerebral X-ALD. Many of the remainder develops AMN. Cerebral disease is usually progressive, although clinical stabilization without HSCT can occur. HSCT is not currently indicated for asymptomatic individuals as prophylaxis. In view of the natural history of the disease such a practice would mean that some boys would undergo HSCT (with its short-term mortality and long-term morbidity risks) who might otherwise have been healthy. Nor is indicated for those individuals with advanced cerebral disease because HSCT does not reverse and may even worsen, established disease.

In this disease, judicious timing of the transplant is paramount. Asymptomatic boys should be regularly screened for signs of inflammatory brain disease, a potential donor identified, and HSCT rapidly performed if and when such symptoms appear. The presence of brain MRI abnormalities and the presence or absence of enhancement with gadolinium has been shown to be of prognostic value. A 34-point MRI scoring system specific for X-ALD that was designed by Loes and colleagues (Loes et al., 1994; Loes et al., 2003) is now used worldwide for patient evaluation and treatment decisions. An MRI severity score as low as 1 with gadolinium enhancement in a young boy is highly predictive of subsequent progressive demyelination and is an indication for transplant. However, the identification of an HSCT donor for asymptomatic boys should not await MRI anomalies, but should done immediately after diagnosis to prevent delays if a follow up MRI indicates disease progression.

Review of the literature supports that most boys that have been transplanted from the best available donor have received full intensity chemotherapy-only preparative regimen (Peters, 2004); most unrelated donors have been adult bone marrow donors, but some CB donors have been used (Beam, 2007); donor-derived engraftment rates seem higher than seen in patients transplanted for MPS IH syndrome (86% of 93 evaluable patients at a median follow-up of 11 months; 93% of related donor transplants; 80% of unrelated donor transplant) (Peters,1998,2004); outcome is affected by disease status, donor source and HLA matching (Peters, 2004). The most common causes of death are progressive cerebral X-ALD disease and GVHD. TRM is 10% in related donors and 18% in unrelated donors. Five-year survival rates for recipients of related donor and unrelated donor transplants have been reported at 64% and 53%, respectively (Peters, 2004); and finally, survival is clearly affected by disease status at time of transplant as assessed by the number of neurologic deficits and MRI severity score. In those with 0 or 1 neurologic deficit and MRI score of less than 9, the 5-year survival was 92% compare to 45% in all other patients (Peters, 2004).

2.7.4 Globoid leukodystrophy (GLD)

GLD or Krabbe disease is an autosomal recessive lysosomal storage disorder caused by deficiency of galactocerebrosidase (GALC), an enzyme responsible for degrading beta-galactocerebroside, a major component of myelin sheath. GALC deficiency causes defective and decreased myelination and inflammation in the CNS and peripheral nervous systems from catabolic derivatives of beta-galactocerebroside such as psychosine. These changes lead to progressive deterioration in neurologic and cognitive function, resulting in spasticity, mental deterioration, blindness, deafness, seizures and early death. In the most severe "early onset or infantile" form, children develop symptoms before 6 months of age and usually die by age 2. In the "late onset" form, symptoms appear in early to late childhood, but only a few children survive into teenage years.

HSCT is the only available therapy with potential to improve neurocognitive function, increase survival and alter the natural history of the disease. Krivit and colleagues (Krivit et al., 1998) described the use of allogeneic HSCT to treat 5 patients with GLD (4 received HLA-sibling HSCT & 1 unrelated cord). Two children with late onset GLD had substantial neurologic disability and they had resolution of their symptoms after transplant. Cognition, language and memory continued to develop normally in 3 children with late-onset disease. Most children had improvement in MRI, CSF protein levels, and all had normalization of enzyme activity. These findings support the use of allogeneic HSCT for children with GLD. If a matched related donor is not available, unrelated cord blood has also been shown to be beneficial (Escolar et al., 2005).

2.7.5 Metachromatic leukodystrophy (MLD)

MLD is an autosomal recessive lysosomal disorder arising from deficiency of arylsulfatase A (ARSA) enzyme activity and characterized by increased urinary sulfatides. The clinical phenotype is a broad continuous spectrum ranging from early-infantile MLD to adult-onset forms. Clinical symptoms vary depending on timing of presentation (infantile, juvenile or adult form), but all include abnormal cognitive skills, behavioral abnormalities with adults having mental regression and psychiatric symptoms, progressive spastic disease and increased CSF protein.

The first BMT for MLD was performed more than 20 years ago. According to the EBMT and CIBMTR registries, more than 100 transplants have since been performed for this disorder. Despite this number, the lack of graft-outcome and long-term follow up studies makes it difficult to draw firm conclusions regarding the efficacy of HSCT in MLD. In addition, data suggest that outcomes are less promising than those for MPS IH. It is not clear if MLD patients, or which phenotypes, might benefit from HSCT. For presymptomatic juvenile and adult onset patients there is positive evidence. Improved transplantation techniques and the prompt availability of CB grafts may positively influence long-term outcomes. An international registry would facilitate comparative evaluation of therapeutic options, leading to improved guidelines.

3. Expanding Indications for transplant

HSCT has been explored in a number of malignant and nonmalignant diseases. Currently, research is rapidly expanding in areas not historically considered for HSCT. Also, as morbidity and mortality decrease, HSCT is being reconsidered for many diseases in which HSCT was previously considered and rejected. Several potential indications are reported in this section.

3.1 Beta-thalassemia

Thalassemias result from mutations of the globin genes that cause reduced or absent hemoglobin production, reducing oxygen delivery. To treat the anemia and restore oxygen delivery to tissues, chronic lifelong transfusions are required in those who have thalassemia major. However, this promotes progressive iron overload and organ damage. The only definitive cure for thalassemia is to correct the genetic defect by HSCT. Transplantation is recommended early, if an allogeneic healthy related sibling donor or a related CB is available. Several studies have suggested that umbilical cord blood transplant (UCBT) recipients benefit from a lower risk of GVHD (Gluckman, 1997; Wagner, 1995) and a recent analysis comparing 113 children who received a UCBT from a compatible sibling with 2052 HLA-identical sibling marrow transplant recipients showed that children receiving UCB experienced a significantly reduced risk of developing aGVHD and cGVHD (Rocha, 2000).

Prior to transplant, the patient should be assigned to 1 of 3 Pesaro risk class to assess risk factors for BMT. This classification is based upon clinical features of thalassemia that include: (1) adherence to a program of regular iron chelation therapy, (2) the presence or absence of hepatomegaly and (3) the presence or absence of portal fibrosis observed by liver biopsy. The conditioning regimen is uniform for classes 1 and 2 patients, but is modified for those who have class 3 features due to an increased risk of transplant-related mortality (Lucarelli, 1990). As a result of this risk classification and the development of new conditioning regimens, the outcome of thalassemia patients have improved with thalassemia-free survival and EFS over 70% reported worldwide. When stratifying patients, initially those with Pesaro Class 1 characteristics < 17 years had a superior thalassemia-free survival; however, recent updates show that outcomes are very similar across all three risk categories after employing risk-based conditioning regimens (Bhatia, 2008). Unrelated donor transplants are also used in selected patients (Bhatia, 2008). Following transplant, iron overload may still be a problem; consequently, chelation or phlebotomy may still be necessary.

3.2 Sickle cell disease (SCD)

SCD contrasts with thalassemia major by its variable course of clinical severity. Its typical clinical manifestation include anemia, severe painful crisis, acute chest syndrome, splenic sequestration, stroke (clinically overt and silent), chronic pulmonary and renal dysfunction, growth retardation, neuropsychological deficits and premature death. Historically, the mainstays of treatment are both preventive and supportive. The three major therapeutic options available for children affected with SCD are: chronic blood transfusion, hydroxyurea and HSCT. Of these options, only HSCT affords patients the possibility of cure. The use of transplantation for the treatment of patients with SCD has been considered for many years. However, because of the morbidity and mortality of HSCT, it was considered too risky. Recently, due to advances in supportive care and immunosuppressive therapy, transplant is again being considered for SCD. The preliminary experience of HSCT for beta-thalassemia major has in part provided the rationale for extending this treatment to sickle cell anemia. Walter et al (Walter et al., 1996) used selection criteria similar to that applied to patients with beta thalassemia major and chose patients with debilitating clinical events, including stroke, recurrent acute chest syndrome and recurrent painful vaso-occlusive crises, but selected children rather than adults and before the development of permanent end organ damage. These recommendations are associated with significant morbidity and early mortality among patients with SCD and are the criteria upon which most early studies using HSCT are based.

Three major clinical series account for most of the experience of HSCT for SCD (Bernaudin et al, 2007; Walters et al, 2000; Vermylen et al, 1998). In all three series, the majority of patients received HLA-identical sibling donor allograft and all patients received the same conditioning regimen (busulfan 14-16mg/kg with cytoxan 200) and GVHD prophylaxis (ATG, cyclosporine and methotrexate). The results of these three studies were very similar. OS was 92-94% and EFS was 82-86% with a median follow-up range of 0.9-17.9 years. TRM from all three series was also similar and was approximately 7% with infections as the chief cause. Similarly, the incidence of aGVHD > grade II was approximately 15-20%. The rate of cGVHD was 20% in Vermylen et al study compared to 12 and 13.5% in the Walters et al and Bernaudin et al reports, respectively. While HSCT is curative in patients with SCD, only 14-18% of patients have a matched family donor. The use of unrelated donors in HSCT for SCD is under development. There are several limitations which restrict the uniform utilization of allogeneic adult donors that include donor availability, and the high risk of severe aGVHD. The use of unrelated cord blood transplantation is also being considered and recent studies have shown promising results, although g raft rejection and aGVHD still remain issues. In addition, efforts to expand the application of HSCT for SCD have been restricted not only by lacking suitable donors, but also by the risk of significant toxicity from the myeloablative conditioning regimen. With the advent of lower intensity conditioning regimens which rely on less myeloablation and more immunosuppression, many of the long-term effects, such as growth and endocrine dysfunction observed after myeloablative conditioning regimens, may be ameliorated.

3.3 Autoimmune disease

Autoimmune diseases are often controlled with treatments that act on the immune system. However, these therapies are usually not curative. Recently many autoimmune diseases have been treated with HSCT. The goal of autologous HSCT is to reset the immune system. Studies on thymic lymphocytes after auto HSCT have shown that, after a burst sustained by pre transplant memory cells, the organ is repopulated by likely harvest-derived naïve T cells, and also the T-lymphocyte repertoire may significantly differ before and after autografting, thus suggesting the possibility of achieving an immune resetting through autologous HSCT (Isaacs, 2004; Sun, 2004). Allogeneic probably results in the highest potential for cure. However, there is higher morbidity and mortality caused by GVHD. Marmont summarize several allogeneic transplant cases in which the patient achieved full post transplant donor chimerism but their autoimmune disease still relapsed. A European database, the International Autoimmune Disease Stem Cell Project Database, was established in 1996. The database contains 600 patients, most treated with autologous HSCT; 15% of the patients registered are children. Some of the autoimmune diseases in children that were treated with HSCT are juvenile idiopathic arthritis, immune cytopenias, systemic sclerosis, systemic lupus and Crohn's disease (Rabusin, 2008).

3.4 Other non-malignant disease

3.4.1 Autosomal recessive osteopetrosis (ARO)

ARO is a rare genetic bone disease in which a deficit in bone resorption by osteoclasts leads to increased bone density and secondary defects. The disease is often lethal early in life unless treated with HSCT. However, recently the dissection of the molecular bases of the disease has shown that ARO is genetically heterogeneous and has revealed the presence of subsets of patients which do not benefit from HSCT, highlighting the importance of molecular diagnosing ARO to identify and establish the proper therapies for better prognosis (Villa, 2008). EBMT conducted a retrospective analysis of 122 children who had received an allogeneic HSCT for ARO between 1980 and 2001. The actuarial probabilities of 5 years disease free survival were 73% for recipients of a genotype HLA-identical HSCT (n=40), 43% for recipients of a phenotype HLA-identical or one HLA antigen mismatch graft from a related donor (n=21), 40% for recipients of a graft from a matched unrelated donor (n=20) and 24% for patients who received a graft from an HLA-haplotype-mismatch related donor (n=41). Causes of death after HSCT were graft failure and early-TRM complications. Conservation of vision was better in children transplanted before the age of 3 months (Driessen, 2003). HSCT is the only curative treatment for ARO and should be offered as early as possible.

3.4.2 Congenital erythropoietic porphyria (CEP)

CEP is a rare autosomal recessive disorder of porphyrin metabolism in which the genetic defect is the deficiency of uroporphyrinogen III cosynthase (UIIIC). Deficiency of this enzyme results in an accumulation of high amounts of uroporphyrin I in all tissues leading to hemolytic anemia, splenomegaly, erythrodontia, bone fragility, exquisite photosensitivity and mutilating skin lesions. The vital prognosis is very bad and until now, no treatment seems to be efficient. Bone marrow transplantation seems to be able to correct the enzymatic deficit that causes the disease because it is located in the bone marrow. A few cases of patients have been reported to be cured of the disease with stem cell transplantation (Shaw, 2001). HSCT should be strongly considered because this is currently the only known curative therapy.

3.4.3 Immune dysregulation, polyendocrinopathy, enteropathy, X-linked (IPEX) syndrome

IPEX syndrome is a rare, fatal autoimmune disorder caused by mutations in the forkhead box protein 3 (FOXP3) genes leading to the disruption of signaling pathways involved in regulatory T-Lymphocyte function. Patients with IPEX syndrome often present in early infancy and without therapeutic intervention, affected male patients usually die within the first or second year of life. These patients require supportive therapy including parental nutrition, insulin, antibiotics and blood transfusions. Immunosuppressive therapy has been used with variable improvement in symptoms. Correction of the dysregulated immune system can be achieved by allogeneic HSCT using a suitable donor. Although, HSCT is the only viable option for long-term survival, patients are usually very ill to tolerate traditional myeloablative conditioning regimens. Recent studies reported the successful outcome of HSCT using a low-intensity, nonmyeloablative conditioning regimen in 2 patients with IPEX syndrome and significant pre transplant risk factors (Burroughs, 2010; Rao, 2007).

3.4.4 Epidermolysis bullosa (EM)

EB is a group of blistering skin disorders resulting from mutations in genes encoding protein components of the cutaneous basement membrane zone. HSCT has been shown to ameliorate the deficiency of the skin-specific structural protein in children with EB (Fujita, 2010; Tolar, 2011).

4. Conclusion

The indications for HSCT are continually changing and expanding rapidly beyond the traditional use as a treatment for malignant and nonmalignant diseases. The inclusion of cord blood as a source of stem cells and the availability of reduce intensity regimens has allowed us to expand the indications for HSCT to patients who otherwise would not meet accepted criteria for conventional HSCT. The field of HSCT is continually growing and a great deal of additional research is needed to continue to improve our outcomes. This is an exciting time in HSCT with many new avenues becoming available for patients.

5. References

[1]   The role of cytotoxic therapy with hematopoietic stem cell transplantation in the therapy of acute myeloid leukemia in children. *Biol Blood Marrow Transplant.* Apr 2007;13(4):500-501.

[2]   Aldenhoven M, Boelens JJ, de Koning TJ. The clinical outcome of Hurler syndrome after stem cell transplantation. *Biol Blood Marrow Transplant.* May 2008; 14(5):485-498.

[3]   Anderlini P, Saliba R, Acholonu S, et al. Fludarabine-melphalan as a preparative regimen for reduced-intensity conditioning allogeneic stem cell transplantation in relapsed and refractory Hodgkin's lymphoma: the updated M.D. Anderson Cancer Center experience. *Haematologica.* Feb 2008; 93(2):257-264.

[4]   Apperley J. CML in pregnancy and childhood. *Best Pract Res Clin Haematol.* Sep 2009; 22(3):455-474.

[5] Arndt C, Tefft M, Gehan E, et al. A feasibility, toxicity, and early response study of etoposide, ifosfamide, and vincristine for the treatment of children with rhabdomyosarcoma: a report from the Intergroup Rhabdomyosarcoma Study (IRS) IV pilot study. *J Pediatr Hematol Oncol.* Mar-Apr 1997; 19(2):124-129.

[6] Atra A, Gerrard M, Hobson R, Imeson JD, Hann IM, Pinkerton CR. Outcome of relapsed or refractory childhood B-cell acute lymphoblastic leukaemia and B-cell non-Hodgkin's lymphoma treated with the UKCCSG 9003/9002 protocols. *Br J Haematol.* Mar 2001; 112(4):965-968.

[7] Ayas M, Al-Jefri A, Al-Seraihi A, Elkum N, Al-Mahr M, El-Solh H. Matched-related allogeneic stem cell transplantation in Saudi patients with Fanconi anemia: 10 year's experience. *Bone Marrow Transplant.* Aug 2008; 42 Suppl 1:S45-S48.

[8] Ayas M, Solh H, Mustafa MM, et al. Bone marrow transplantation from matched siblings in patients with fanconi anemia utilizing low-dose cyclophosphamide, thoracoabdominal radiation and antithymocyte globulin. *Bone Marrow Transplant.* Jan 2001; 27(2):139-143.

[9] Baccarani M, Cortes J, Pane F, Niederwieser D, Saglio G, Apperley J, et al. Chronic myeloid leukemia: an update of concepts and management recommendations of European Leukemia Net. *J Clin Oncol 2009; 27:6041-51.*

[10] Bader P, Kreyenberg H, Hoelle W, et al. Increasing mixed chimerism defines a high-risk group of childhood acute myelogenous leukemia patients after allogeneic stem cell transplantation where pre-emptive immunotherapy may be effective. *Bone Marrow Transplant.* Apr 2004; 33(8):815-821.

[11] Beam D, Poe MD, Provenzale JM, et al. Outcomes of unrelated umbilical cord blood transplantation for X-linked adrenoleukodystrophy. *Biol Blood Marrow Transplant.* Jun 2007; 13(6):665-674.

[12] Bensinger WI, Buckner CD, Demirer T, Storb R, Appelbaum FA. Transplantation of allogeneic peripheral blood stem cells. *Bone Marrow Transplant.* Mar 1996; 17 Suppl 2:S56-57.

[13] Bensinger WI, Weaver CH, Appelbaum FR, et al. Transplantation of allogeneic peripheral blood stem cells mobilized by recombinant human granulocyte colony-stimulating factor. *Blood.* Mar 15 1995; 85(6):1655-1658.

[14] Berger R, Bernheim A, Gluckman E, Gisselbrecht C. In vitro effect of cyclophosphamide metabolites on chromosomes of Fanconi anaemia patients. *Br J Haematol.* Aug 1980;45(4):565-568.

[15] Bernaudin F, Socie G, Kuentz M, et al. Long-term results of related myeloablative stem-cell transplantation to cure sickle cell disease. *Blood.* Oct 1 2007; 110(7):2749-2756.

[16] Berndt A, Helwig A, Ehninger G, Bornhauser M. Successful transplantation of CD34+ selected peripheral blood stem cells from an unrelated donor in an adult patient with Diamond-Blackfan anemia and secondary hemochromatosis. *Bone Marrow Transplant.* Jan 2005; 35(1):99-100.

[17] Bhatia M, Walters MC. Hematopoietic cell transplantation for thalassemia and sickle cell disease: past, present and future. *Bone Marrow Transplant.* Jan 2008;41(2):109-117.

[18] Boelens JJ, Rocha V, Aldenhoven M, et al. Risk factor analysis of outcomes after unrelated cord blood transplantation in patients with hurler syndrome. *Biol Blood Marrow Transplant.* May 2009; 15(5):618-625.

[19] Borgmann A, Hartmann R, Schmid H, et al. Isolated extramedullary relapse in children with acute lymphoblastic leukemia: a comparison between treatment results of chemotherapy and bone marrow transplantation. BFM Relapse Study Group. *Bone Marrow Transplant.* Apr 1995; 15(4):515-521.

[20] Buckley RH, Schiff SE, Schiff RI, et al. Hematopoietic stem-cell transplantation for the treatment of severe combined immunodeficiency. *N Engl J Med.* Feb 18 1999;340(7):508-516.

[21] Burroughs LM, Torgerson TR, Storb R, et al. Stable hematopoietic cell engraftment after low-intensity nonmyeloablative conditioning in patients with immune dysregulation, polyendocrinopathy, enteropathy, X-linked syndrome. *J Allergy Clin Immunol.* Nov 2010; 126(5):1000-1005.

[22] Cairo MS, Gerrard M, Sposto R, et al. Results of a randomized international study of high-risk central nervous system B non-Hodgkin lymphoma and B acute lymphoblastic leukemia in children and adolescents. *Blood.* Apr 1 2007;109(7):2736-2743.

[23] Cairo MS, Sposto R, Hoover-Regan M, et al. Childhood and adolescent large-cell lymphoma (LCL): a review of the Children's Cancer Group experience. *Am J Hematol.* Jan 2003; 72(1):53-63.

[24] Cairo MS, Sposto R, Perkins SL, et al. Burkitt's and Burkitt-like lymphoma in children and adolescents: a review of the Children's Cancer Group experience. *Br J Haematol.* Feb 2003;120(4):660-670.

[25] Carella AM, Cavaliere M, Lerma E, et al. Autografting followed by nonmyeloablative immunosuppressive chemotherapy and allogeneic peripheral-blood hematopoietic stem-cell transplantation as treatment of resistant Hodgkin's disease and non-Hodgkin's lymphoma. *J Clin Oncol.* Dec 1 2000; 18(23):3918-3924.

[26] Cavazzana-Calvo M, Fischer A. Gene therapy for severe combined immunodeficiency: are we there yet? *J Clin Invest.* Jun 2007; 117(6):1456-1465.

[27] Cesaro S, Guariso G, Calore E, et al. Successful unrelated bone marrow transplantation for Shwachman-Diamond syndrome. *Bone Marrow Transplant.* Jan 2001; 27(1):97-99.

[28] Chaudhury S, Auerbach AD, Kernan NA, et al. Fludarabine-based cytoreductive regimen and T-cell-depleted grafts from alternative donors for the treatment of high-risk patients with Fanconi anaemia. *Br J Haematol.* Mar 2008;140(6):644-655.

[29] Chessells JM, Rogers DW, Leiper AD, et al. Bone-marrow transplantation has a limited role in prolonging second marrow remission in childhood lymphoblastic leukaemia. *Lancet.* May 31 1986; 1(8492):1239-1241.

[30] Clavell LA, Gelber RD, Cohen HJ, et al. Four-agent induction and intensive asparaginase therapy for treatment of childhood acute lymphoblastic leukemia. *N Engl J Med.* Sep 11 1986; 315(11):657-663.

[31] Creutzig U, Ritter J, Zimmermann M, Klingebiel T. [Prognosis of children with chronic myeloid leukemia: a retrospective analysis of 75 patients]. *Klin Padiatr.* Jul-Aug 1996;208(4):236-241.

[32] Creutzig U, Zimmermann M, Ritter J, et al. Treatment strategies and long-term results in paediatric patients treated in four consecutive AML-BFM trials. *Leukemia*. Dec 2005; 19(12):2030-2042.

[33] Cwynarski K, Roberts IA, Iacobelli S, et al. Stem cell transplantation for chronic myeloid leukemia in children. *Blood*. Aug 15 2003; 102(4):1224-1231.

[34] de la Fuente J, Dokal I. Dyskeratosis congenita: advances in the understanding of the telomerase defect and the role of stem cell transplantation. *Pediatr Transplant*. Sep 2007; 11(6):584-594.

[35] Dokal I. Dyskeratosis congenita in all its forms. *Br J Haematol*. Sep 2000; 110(4):768-779.

[36] Dreger P, Glass B, Uharek L, Zeis M, Schmitz N. Allogenic transplantation of mobilized peripheral blood progenitor cells: towards tailored cell therapy. *Int J Hematol*. Jul 1997;66(1):1-11.

[37] Druker BJ, Talpaz M, Resta DJ, et al. Efficacy and safety of a specific inhibitor of the BCR-ABL tyrosine kinase in chronic myeloid leukemia. *N Engl J Med*. Apr 5 2001;344(14):1031-1037.

[38] Escolar ML, Poe MD, Provenzale JM, et al. Transplantation of umbilical-cord blood in babies with infantile Krabbe's disease. *N Engl J Med*. May 19 2005; 352(20):2069-2081.

[39] Farzin A, Davies SM, Smith FO, et al. Matched sibling donor haematopoietic stem cell transplantation in Fanconi anaemia: an update of the Cincinnati Children's experience. *Br J Haematol*. Feb 2007; 136(4):633-640.

[40] Federico M, Bellei M, Brice P, et al. High-dose therapy and autologous stem-cell transplantation versus conventional therapy for patients with advanced Hodgkin's lymphoma responding to front-line therapy. *J Clin Oncol*. Jun 15 2003; 21(12):2320-2325.

[41] Feld JJ, Hussain N, Wright EC, et al. Hepatic involvement and portal hypertension predict mortality in chronic granulomatous disease. *Gastroenterology*. Jun 2008; 134(7):1917-1926.

[42] Filipovich AH, Stone JV, Tomany SC, et al. Impact of donor type on outcome of bone marrow transplantation for Wiskott-Aldrich syndrome: collaborative study of the International Bone Marrow Transplant Registry and the National Marrow Donor Program. *Blood*. Mar 15 2001;97(6):1598-1603.

[43] Fleitz J, Rumelhart S, Goldman F, et al. Successful allogeneic hematopoietic stem cell transplantation (HSCT) for Shwachman-Diamond syndrome. *Bone Marrow Transplant*. Jan 2002; 29(1):75-79.

[44] Fujita Y, Abe R, Inokuma D, et al. Bone marrow transplantation restores epidermal basement membrane protein expression and rescues epidermolysis bullosa model mice. *Proc Natl Acad Sci U S A*. Aug 10 2010; 107(32):14345-14350.

[45] Gaynon PS, Trigg ME, Heerema NA, et al. Children's Cancer Group trials in childhood acute lymphoblastic leukemia: 1983-1995. *Leukemia*. Dec 2000; 14(12):2223-2233.

[46] Gerrard M, Cairo MS, Weston C, et al. Excellent survival following two courses of COPAD chemotherapy in children and adolescents with resected localized B-cell non-Hodgkin's lymphoma: results of the FAB/LMB 96 international study. *Br J Haematol*. Jun 2008; 141(6):840-847.

[47] Gibson BE, Wheatley K, Hann IM, et al. Treatment strategy and long-term results in paediatric patients treated in consecutive UK AML trials. *Leukemia.* Dec 2005; 19(12):2130-2138.

[48] Gibson BE, Wheatley K, Hann IM, et al. Treatment strategy and long-term results in paediatric patients treated in consecutive UK AML trials. *Leukemia.* Dec 2005;19(12):2130-2138.

[49] Ginzberg H, Shin J, Ellis L, et al. Shwachman syndrome: phenotypic manifestations of sibling sets and isolated cases in a large patient cohort are similar. *J Pediatr.* Jul 1999; 135(1):81-88.

[50] Gluckman E, Auerbach AD, Horowitz MM, et al. Bone marrow transplantation for Fanconi anemia. *Blood.* Oct 1 1995; 86(7):2856-2862.

[51] Gluckman EG, Roch VV, Chastang C. Use of Cord Blood Cells for Banking and Transplant. *Oncologist.* 1997; 2(5):340-343.

[52] Gross TG, Hale GA, He W, et al. Hematopoietic stem cell transplantation for refractory or recurrent non-Hodgkin lymphoma in children and adolescents. *Biol Blood Marrow Transplant.* Feb 2010; 16(2):223-230.

[53] Guardiola P, Socie G, Li X, et al. Acute graft-versus-host disease in patients with Fanconi anemia or acquired aplastic anemia undergoing bone marrow transplantation from HLA-identical sibling donors: risk factors and influence on outcome. *Blood.* Jan 1 2004; 103(1):73-77.

[54] Guffon N, Bertrand Y, Forest I, Fouilhoux A, Froissart R. Bone marrow transplantation in children with Hunter syndrome: outcome after 7 to 17 years. *J Pediatr.* May 2009; 154(5):733-737.

[55] Gungor N, Tuncbilek E. Sanfilippo disease type B. A case report and review of the literature on recent advances in bone marrow transplantation. *Turk J Pediatr.* Apr-Jun 1995;37(2):157-163.

[56] Henter JI, Samuelsson-Horne A, Arico M, et al. Treatment of hemophagocytic lymphohistiocytosis with HLH-94 immunochemotherapy and bone marrow transplantation. *Blood.* Oct 1 2002; 100(7):2367-2373.

[57] Herskhovitz E, Young E, Rainer J, et al. Bone marrow transplantation for Maroteaux-Lamy syndrome (MPS VI): long-term follow-up. *J Inherit Metab Dis.* Feb 1999;22(1):50-62.

[58] Hoogerbrugge PM, Gerritsen EJ, vd Does-van den Berg A, et al. Case-control analysis of allogeneic bone marrow transplantation versus maintenance chemotherapy for relapsed ALL in children. *Bone Marrow Transplant.* Feb 1995; 15(2):255-259.

[59] Hughes TP, Kaeda J, Branford S, et al. Frequency of major molecular responses to imatinib or interferon alfa plus cytarabine in newly diagnosed chronic myeloid leukemia. *N Engl J Med.* Oct 9 2003; 349(15):1423-1432.

[60] Isaacs JD, Thiel A. Stem cell transplantation for autoimmune disorders. Immune reconstitution. *Best Pract Res Clin Haematol.* Jun 2004; 17(2):345-358.

[61] Kardos G, Baumann I, Passmore SJ, et al. Refractory anemia in childhood: a retrospective analysis of 67 patients with particular reference to monosomy 7. *Blood.* Sep 15 2003;102(6):1997-2003.

[62] Kawakami M, Tsutsumi H, Kumakawa T, et al. Levels of serum granulocyte colony-stimulating factor in patients with infections. *Blood.* Nov 15 1990; 76(10):1962-1964.

[63] Kersey JH. Fifty years of studies of the biology and therapy of childhood leukemia. *Blood.* Dec 1 1997;90(11):4243-4251.

[64] Kessinger A, Smith DM, Strandjord SE, et al. Allogeneic transplantation of blood-derived, T cell-depleted hemopoietic stem cells after myeloablative treatment in a patient with acute lymphoblastic leukemia. *Bone Marrow Transplant.* Nov 1989; 4(6):643-646.

[65] Krivit W, Shapiro EG, Peters C, et al. Hematopoietic stem-cell transplantation in globoid-cell leukodystrophy. *N Engl J Med.* Apr 16 1998;338(16):1119-1126.

[66] Kuhns DB, Alvord WG, Heller T, et al. Residual NADPH oxidase and survival in chronic granulomatous disease. *N Engl J Med.* Dec 30 2010;363(27):2600-2610.

[67] Kutler DI, Singh B, Satagopan J, et al. A 20-year perspective on the International Fanconi Anemia Registry (IFAR). *Blood.* Feb 15 2003; 101(4):1249-1256.

[68] Ladenstein R, Potschger U, Hartman O, et al. 28 years of high-dose therapy and SCT for neuroblastoma in Europe: lessons from more than 4000 procedures. *Bone Marrow Transplant.* Jun 2008; 41 Suppl 2:S118-127.

[69] Lange BJ et al. Distinctive demography, biology, and outcome of acute myeloid leukemia and myelodysplastic syndrome in children with Down syndrome: Children's Cancer Group Studies 2861 and 2891. *Blood.* 1998 Jan 15; 91 (2): 608-15.

[70] Lazarus HM, Rowlings PA, Zhang MJ, et al. Autotransplants for Hodgkin's disease in patients never achieving remission: a report from the Autologous Blood and Marrow Transplant Registry. *J Clin Oncol.* Feb 1999; 17(2):534-545.

[71] Lee JW, Chung NG. The treatment of pediatric chronic myelogenous leukemia in the imatinib era. *Korean J Pediatr.* Mar 2011; 54(3):111-116.

[72] Linch DC, Winfield D, Goldstone AH, et al. Dose intensification with autologous bone-marrow transplantation in relapsed and resistant Hodgkin's disease: results of a BNLI randomised trial. *Lancet.* Apr 24 1993; 341(8852):1051-1054.

[73] Link MP, Shuster JJ, Donaldson SS, Berard CW, Murphy SB. Treatment of children and young adults with early-stage non-Hodgkin's lymphoma. *N Engl J Med.* Oct 30 1997; 337(18):1259-1266.

[74] Lipton JM, Atsidaftos E, Zyskind I, Vlachos A. Improving clinical care and elucidating the pathophysiology of Diamond Blackfan anemia: an update from the Diamond Blackfan Anemia Registry. *Pediatr Blood Cancer.* May 1 2006;46(5):558-564.

[75] Ljungman P, Bregni M, Brune M, et al. Allogeneic and autologous transplantation for haematological diseases, solid tumours and immune disorders: current practice in Europe 2009. *Bone Marrow Transplant.* Feb 2010; 45(2):219-234.

[76] Ljungman P, Urbano-Ispizua A, Cavazzana-Calvo M, et al. Allogeneic and autologous transplantation for haematological diseases, solid tumours and immune disorders: definitions and current practice in Europe. *Bone Marrow Transplant.* Mar 2006; 37(5):439-449.

[77] Locatelli F, Zecca M, Pession A, et al. The outcome of children with Fanconi anemia given hematopoietic stem cell transplantation and the influence of fludarabine in the conditioning regimen: a report from the Italian pediatric group. *Haematologica.* Oct 2007;92(10):1381-1388.

[78] Loes DJ, Fatemi A, Melhem ER, et al. Analysis of MRI patterns aids prediction of progression in X-linked adrenoleukodystrophy. *Neurology.* Aug 12 2003; 61(3):369-374.

[79] Loes DJ, Hite S, Moser H, et al. Adrenoleukodystrophy: a scoring method for brain MR observations. *AJNR Am J Neuroradiol.* Oct 1994; 15(9):1761-1766.

[80] Mack DR, Forstner GG, Wilschanski M, Freedman MH, Durie PR. Shwachman syndrome: exocrine pancreatic dysfunction and variable phenotypic expression. *Gastroenterology.* Dec 1996; 111(6):1593-1602.

[81] Marks DI, Khattry N, Cummins M, et al. Haploidentical stem cell transplantation for children with acute leukaemia. *Br J Haematol.* Jul 2006; 134(2):196-201.

[82] Marmont AM. Allogeneic haematopoietic stem cell transplantation for severe autoimmune diseases: great expectations but controversial evidence. *Bone Marrow Transplant.* Jul 2006; 38(1):1-4.

[83] Matthay KK, Reynolds CP, Seeger RC, et al. Long-term results for children with high-risk neuroblastoma treated on a randomized trial of myeloablative therapy followed by 13-cis-retinoic acid: a children's oncology group study. *J Clin Oncol.* Mar 1 2009; 27(7):1007-1013.

[84] Miano M, Labopin M, Hartmann O, et al. Haematopoietic stem cell transplantation trends in children over the last three decades: a survey by the paediatric diseases working party of the European Group for Blood and Marrow Transplantation. *Bone Marrow Transplant.* Jan 2007; 39(2):89-99.

[85] Millot F, Esperou H, Bordigoni P, et al. Allogeneic bone marrow transplantation for chronic myeloid leukemia in childhood: a report from the Societe Francaise de Greffe de Moelle et de Therapie Cellulaire (SFGM-TC). *Bone Marrow Transplant.* Nov 2003; 32(10):993-999.

[86] Millot F, Guilhot J, Nelken B, et al. Imatinib mesylate is effective in children with chronic myelogenous leukemia in late chronic and advanced phase and in relapse after stem cell transplantation. *Leukemia.* Feb 2006; 20(2):187-192.

[87] Muramatsu H, Kojima S, Yoshimi A, et al. Outcome of 125 children with chronic myelogenous leukemia who received transplants from unrelated donors: the Japan Marrow Donor Program. *Biol Blood Marrow Transplant.* Feb 2010; 16(2):231-238.

[88] Neudorf S, Sanders J, Kobrinsky N, et al. Allogeneic bone marrow transplantation for children with acute myelocytic leukemia in first remission demonstrates a role for graft versus leukemia in the maintenance of disease-free survival. *Blood.* May 15 2004;103(10):3655-3661.

[89] Novotny J, Kadar J, Hertenstein B, et al. Sustained decrease of peripheral lymphocytes after allogeneic blood stem cell aphereses. *Br J Haematol.* Mar 1998;100(4):695-697.

[90] O'Brien SG, Guilhot F, Larson RA, et al. Imatinib compared with interferon and low-dose cytarabine for newly diagnosed chronic-phase chronic myeloid leukemia. *N Engl J Med.* Mar 13 2003;348(11):994-1004.

[91] Oliansky DM, Rizzo JD, Aplan PD, et al. The role of cytotoxic therapy with hematopoietic stem cell transplantation in the therapy of acute myeloid leukemia in children: an evidence-based review. *Biol Blood Marrow Transplant.* Jan 2007; 13(1):1-25.

[92] Ostronoff M, Florencio R, Campos G, et al. Successful nonmyeloablative bone marrow transplantation in a corticosteroid-resistant infant with Diamond-Blackfan anemia. *Bone Marrow Transplant.* Aug 2004; 34(4):371-372.

[93] Patte C, Auperin A, Gerrard M, et al. Results of the randomized international FAB/LMB96 trial for intermediate risk B-cell non-Hodgkin lymphoma in children and adolescents: it is possible to reduce treatment for the early responding patients. *Blood.* Apr 1 2007; 109(7):2773-2780.

[94] Peters C, Charnas LR, Tan Y, et al. Cerebral X-linked adrenoleukodystrophy: the international hematopoietic cell transplantation experience from 1982 to 1999. *Blood.* Aug 1 2004;104(3):881-888.

[95] Peters C, Shapiro EG, Anderson J, et al. Hurler syndrome: II. Outcome of HLA-genotypically identical sibling and HLA-haploidentical related donor bone marrow transplantation in fifty-four children. The Storage Disease Collaborative Study Group. *Blood.* Apr 1 1998; 91(7):2601-2608.

[96] Peters C, Steward CG. Hematopoietic cell transplantation for inherited metabolic diseases: an overview of outcomes and practice guidelines. *Bone Marrow Transplant.* Feb 2003; 31(4):229-239.

[97] Prasad VK, Kurtzberg J. Emerging trends in transplantation of inherited metabolic diseases. *Bone Marrow Transplant.* Jan 2008; 41(2):99-108.

[98] Prasad VK, Mendizabal A, Parikh SH, et al. Unrelated donor umbilical cord blood transplantation for inherited metabolic disorders in 159 pediatric patients from a single center: influence of cellular composition of the graft on transplantation outcomes. *Blood.* Oct 1 2008; 112(7):2979-2989.

[99] Proctor SJ, Mackie M, Dawson A, et al. A population-based study of intensive multi-agent chemotherapy with or without autotransplant for the highest risk Hodgkin's disease patients identified by the Scotland and Newcastle Lymphoma Group (SNLG) prognostic index. A Scotland and Newcastle Lymphoma Group study (SNLG HD III). *Eur J Cancer.* Apr 2002; 38(6):795-806.

[100] Pui CH. Childhood leukemias. *N Engl J Med.* Jun 15 1995; 332(24):1618-1630.

[101] Pui CH, Evans WE. Acute lymphoblastic leukemia. *N Engl J Med.* Aug 27 1998; 339(9):605-615.

[102] Rabusin M, Andolina M, Maximova N. Haematopoietic SCT in autoimmune diseases in children: rationale and new perspectives. *Bone Marrow Transplant.* Jun 2008; 41 Suppl 2:S96-99.

[103] Rao A, Kamani N, Filipovich A, et al. Successful bone marrow transplantation for IPEX syndrome after reduced-intensity conditioning. *Blood.* Jan 1 2007; 109(1):383-385.

[104] Reiter A, Schrappe M, Ludwig WD, et al. Chemotherapy in 998 unselected childhood acute lymphoblastic leukemia patients. Results and conclusions of the multicenter trial ALL-BFM 86. *Blood.* Nov 1 1994; 84(9):3122-3133.

[105] Ritchey AK, Pollock BH, Lauer SJ, Andejeski Y, Barredo J, Buchanan GR. Improved survival of children with isolated CNS relapse of acute lymphoblastic leukemia: a pediatric oncology group study. *J Clin Oncol.* Dec 1999; 17(12):3745-3752.

[106] Rivera GK, Pinkel D, Simone JV, Hancock ML, Crist WM. Treatment of acute lymphoblastic leukemia. 30 years' experience at St. Jude Children's Research Hospital. *N Engl J Med.* Oct 28 1993; 329(18):1289-1295.

[107] Rocha V, Wagner JE, Jr., Sobocinski KA, et al. Graft-versus-host disease in children who have received a cord-blood or bone marrow transplant from an HLA-identical sibling. Eurocord and International Bone Marrow Transplant Registry Working Committee on Alternative Donor and Stem Cell Sources. *N Engl J Med.* Jun 22 2000; 342(25):1846-1854.

[108] Rosenberg PS, Alter BP, Ebell W. Cancer risks in Fanconi anemia: findings from the German Fanconi Anemia Registry. *Haematologica.* Apr 2008,93(4):511-517.

[109] Roy V, Perez WS, Eapen M, et al. Bone marrow transplantation for diamond-blackfan anemia. *Biol Blood Marrow Transplant.* Aug 2005; 11(8):600-608.

[110] Satwani P, Sather H, Ozkaynak F, et al. Allogeneic bone marrow transplantation in first remission for children with ultra-high-risk features of acute lymphoblastic leukemia: A children's oncology group study report. *Biol Blood Marrow Transplant.* Feb 2007; 13(2):218-227.

[111] Schmit-Pokorny K. Expanding indications for stem cell transplantation. *Semin Oncol Nurs.* May 2009; 25(2):105-114.

[112] Schmitz N, Pfistner B, Sextro M, et al. Aggressive conventional chemotherapy compared with high-dose chemotherapy with autologous haemopoietic stem-cell transplantation for relapsed chemosensitive Hodgkin's disease: a randomised trial. *Lancet.* Jun 15 2002;359(9323):2065-2071.

[113] Seger RA, Gungor T, Belohradsky BH, et al. Treatment of chronic granulomatous disease with myeloablative conditioning and an unmodified hemopoietic allograft: a survey of the European experience, 1985-2000. *Blood.* Dec 15 2002;100(13):4344-4350.

[114] Silverman LB, Gelber RD, Dalton VK, et al. Improved outcome for children with acute lymphoblastic leukemia: results of Dana-Farber Consortium Protocol 91-01. *Blood.* Mar 1 2001;97(5):1211-1218.

[115] Staba SL, Escolar ML, Poe M, et al. Cord-blood transplants from unrelated donors in patients with Hurler's syndrome. *N Engl J Med.* May 6 2004; 350(19):1960-1969.

[116] Stary J, Locatelli F, Niemeyer CM. Stem cell transplantation for aplastic anemia and myelodysplastic syndrome. *Bone Marrow Transplant.* Mar 2005; 35 Suppl 1:S13-16.

[117] Sun W, Popat U, Hutton G, et al. Characteristics of T-cell receptor repertoire and myelin-reactive T cells reconstituted from autologous haematopoietic stem-cell grafts in multiple sclerosis. *Brain.* May 2004; 127(Pt 5):996-1008.

[118] Suttorp M, Yaniv I, Schultz KR. Controversies in the treatment of CML in children and adolescents: TKIs versus BMT? *Biol Blood Marrow Transplant.* Jan 2011; 17(1 Suppl):S115-122.

[119] Sweetenham JW, Carella AM, Taghipour G, et al. High-dose therapy and autologous stem-cell transplantation for adult patients with Hodgkin's disease who do not enter remission after induction chemotherapy: results in 175 patients reported to the European Group for Blood and Marrow Transplantation. Lymphoma Working Party. *J Clin Oncol.* Oct 1999; 17(10):3101-3109.

[120] Tan PL, Wagner JE, Auerbach AD, Defor TE, Slungaard A, Macmillan ML. Successful engraftment without radiation after fludarabine-based regimen in Fanconi anemia patients undergoing genotypically identical donor hematopoietic cell transplantation. *Pediatr Blood Cancer.* May 1 2006; 46(5):630-636.

[121] Thomson KJ, Peggs KS, Smith P, et al. Superiority of reduced-intensity allogeneic transplantation over conventional treatment for relapse of Hodgkin's lymphoma following autologous stem cell transplantation. *Bone Marrow Transplant.* May 2008; 41(9):765-770.

[122] Tichelli A, Passweg J, Hoffmann T, et al. Repeated peripheral stem cell mobilization in healthy donors: time-dependent changes in mobilization efficiency. *Br J Haematol.* Jul 1999;106(1):152-158.

[123] Tolar J, Blazar BR, Wagner JE. Concise review: Transplantation of human hematopoietic cells for extracellular matrix protein deficiency in epidermolysis bullosa. *Stem Cells.* Jun 2011;29(6):900-906.

[124] Uderzo C, Grazia Zurlo M, Adamoli L, et al. Treatment of isolated testicular relapse in childhood acute lymphoblastic leukemia: an Italian multicenter study. Associazione Italiana Ematologia ed Oncologia Pediatrica. *J Clin Oncol.* Apr 1990; 8(4):672-677.

[125] Vardiman JW, Harris NL, Brunning RD. The World Health Organization (WHO) classification of the myeloid neoplasms. *Blood.* Oct 1 2002; 100(7):2292-2302.

[126] Vellodi A, Young E, New M, Pot-Mees C, Hugh-Jones K. Bone marrow transplantation for Sanfilippo disease type B. *J Inherit Metab Dis.* 1992;15(6):911-918.

[127] Vellodi A, Young EP, Cooper A, et al. Bone marrow transplantation for mucopolysaccharidosis type I: experience of two British centres. *Arch Dis Child.* Feb 1997; 76(2):92-99.

[128] Vermylen C, Cornu G, Ferster A, et al. Haematopoietic stem cell transplantation for sickle cell anaemia: the first 50 patients transplanted in Belgium. *Bone Marrow Transplant.* Jul 1998; 22(1):1-6.

[129] Vilmer E, Suciu S, Ferster A, et al. Long-term results of three randomized trials (58831, 58832, 58881) in childhood acute lymphoblastic leukemia: a CLCG-EORTC report. Children Leukemia Cooperative Group. *Leukemia.* Dec 2000; 14(12):2257-2266.

[130] Vlachos A, Ball S, Dahl N, et al. Diagnosing and treating Diamond Blackfan anaemia: results of an international clinical consensus conference. *Br J Haematol.* Sep 2008;142(6):859-876.

[131] Wagner JE, Eapen M, MacMillan ML, et al. Unrelated donor bone marrow transplantation for the treatment of Fanconi anemia. *Blood.* Mar 1 2007; 109(5):2256-2262.

[132] Wagner JE, Kernan NA, Steinbuch M, Broxmeyer HE, Gluckman E. Allogeneic sibling umbilical-cord-blood transplantation in children with malignant and non-malignant disease. *Lancet.* Jul 22 1995;346(8969):214-219.

[133] Walters MC, Patience M, Leisenring W, et al. Barriers to bone marrow transplantation for sickle cell anemia. *Biol Blood Marrow Transplant.* May 1996; 2(2):100-104.

[134] Walters MC, Storb R, Patience M, et al. Impact of bone marrow transplantation for symptomatic sickle cell disease: an interim report. Multicenter investigation of bone marrow transplantation for sickle cell disease. *Blood.* Mar 15 2000; 95(6):1918-1924.

[135] Weisdorf DJ, Anasetti C, Antin JH, et al. Allogeneic bone marrow transplantation for chronic myelogenous leukemia: comparative analysis of unrelated versus matched sibling donor transplantation. *Blood.* Mar 15 2002; 99(6):1971-1977.

7

Detection of CMV Infection in Allogeneic SCT Recipients: The Multiple Assays

Pilar Blanco-Lobo, Omar J. BenMarzouk-Hidalgo and Pilar Pérez-Romero
Unit of Infectious Disease, Microbiology and Preventive Medicine,
Instituto de Biomedicina de Sevilla (IBiS)/CSIC/Universidad de Sevilla,
University Hospital Virgen del Rocio, Sevilla,
Spain

1. Introduction

Cytomegalovirus (CMV) end-organ disease is a serious complication after stem cell transplantation (SCT) (Boeckh M, 2003). Within the first one hundred days after SCT, 50% of recipients develop CMV infection determined by positive antigenemia and 65 to 86.5% when viral replication is determined by real-time PCR (RT-PCR) (Ljungman et al., 2006; Solano et al., 2001). Described risk factors for CMV infection concern donor type, graft source, positive CMV serostatus of donor and recipient, CD34+ graft selection, preconditioning regimen, GvHD prophylaxis regimen, incidence of acute and chronic GvHD and prophylaxis and treatment for GvHD (Ljungman et al., 2002; Ozdemir et al., 2007). Pre-emptive therapy is currently based on viral replication determined by either antigenemia or RT-PCR (Drew, 2007). Although antigenemia has been extensively used (Drew, 2007), RT-PCR has been shown to be more sensitive (Hakki et al., 2003; Solano et al., 2001).

The use of techniques based on nucleic acid amplification for the detection of CMV in clinical samples are in expansion and in many hospitals have replaced the use of other assays such as viral cultures or pp65 antigenemia. Several studies have assessed the performance between the different CMV viral load assays available. However, no many studies have compared the differences between the DNA extraction methods used (Fahle & Fischer, 2000; Caliendo et al., 2007; Kalpoe et al., 2004; Leruez-Ville et al., 2003; Avetisyan et al., 2006; Boeckh et al., 2009; Gerna et al., 2008; Gimeno et al., 2008). Although during the DNA extraction the majority of the methods use internal controls as a measurement of the DNA loss during the extraction procedure, in the downstream amplification not many of the assays use DNA standards that will facilitate the comparison among the different kits and standardization of the results between hospitals. In fact the availability of an optimal and efficient DNA extraction procedure that can use a broad type of samples with minimum modifications in the procedure may be practical and affordable for use in the clinical practice (Fahle & Fischer, 2000).

One of the differences between results using the methods available is type of clinical specimen used to perform the CMV DNA extraction. Samples collected vary from plasma, whole blood or leukocytes, with the optimal sample for monitoring CMV viral being controversial. Since CMV infect cells, the viral load results obtained from leukocytes isolated from peripheral blood or whole blood samples tend to be higher than the results obtained from plasma. However, it has been reported a high correlation between CMV viral load results from plasma samples and whole blood samples (Caliendo et al., 2007; Kalpoe et al., 2004; Leruez-Ville et al., 2003). Moreover, some authors believe that the presence of CMV particles in plasma is related with the level of viral replication (Kalpoe et al., 2004), representing the infectious viral particles able to spread to other host cells. Thus whole blood and plasma samples are equally suitable for testing CMV infection in SCT recipients.

Molecular techniques for CMV quantification such as RT-PCR have been shown to be useful for the rapid diagnosis of CMV infection and for monitoring clinical responses to antiviral therapy. This technique offers some advantages over others PCR methods, including increased precision, accuracy, reproducibility and a shorter turnaround time. To date, the clinical utility of using the RT-PCR test to guide preemptive therapy in transplant recipients has been mainly studied in SCT recipients (Avetisyan et al., 2006; Boeckh M, 2009; Gerna et al., 2008; Gimeno et al., 2008; Harrington et al., 2007; Kalpoe et al., 2004; Lilleri et al., 2004; Limaye et al., 2001; Machida et al., 2000; Ruell et al., 2007; Verkruyse et al., 2006). However, it has not been established a cutoff threshold for initiating antiviral therapy against CMV probably due to the significant differences between the different techniques used to determine the CMV viral load. In the absence of standardization the current clinical guidelines recommend to each individual laboratory to establish their own viral thresholds for CMV management (Kotton et al., 2010; Razonable & Emery, 2004).

2. DNA extraction methods

CMV extraction assays can be performed manually and automated. While manual extraction assays use non-corrosive reagents, are generally inexpensive and are easy to use, they require more labour intensive manipulation increasing the risk for contamination of the samples. In addition, this type of extraction procedures requires highly trained laboratory personnel to ensure reproducible results. Another limitation of the manual assays is the use of ethanol to precipitate the DNA, which may inhibit subsequent RT-PCR assays if not properly removed (Valentine-Thon, 2002). The manual assays are mostly used in research laboratories where the number of samples used at once is not high and the personnel are highly qualified for the procedures.

Automated extraction methods are not widely extended although there are commonly used in clinical services where the number of clinical samples to process every day is high. The main feature of the automated extraction systems is the increase in reproducibility of the extraction among different samples, in addition to a reduction of the risk of contamination and the high number of samples that could be performed at the same time. However, the main handicap of this technology is the elevated cost of the instruments, as well as the high-costs of instruments` reagents and maintenance and the necessary laboratory space required (Espy et al., 2006).

While recently reports have shown improvement in the sensibility obtained by the automated extraction instruments in comparison with the manual extraction kits (Gartner et al., 2004; Mengelle et al., 2011), and several studies performed on different herpesviruses have shown increased sensibility when automated extraction was performed compared to manual extraction kits (Nicholson et al.; 1997; Griffiths et al.; 1984), our laboratory recently demonstrated that the DNA extraction method from Affigene was more efficient than the automated system from Abbott providing a more accurate estimation of CMV DNA load (Gracia-Ahufinger et al., 2010). Our data proving that the manual DNA extraction method from Affigene resulted in a more efficient DNA extraction in comparison with that of an automated procedure from Abbott were somewhat surprising and are in contrast to previously published studies showing just the opposite (Kalpoe et al., 2004; Limaye et al., 2001). In this context, our data underscore the fact that the DNA extraction efficiency of distinct automated systems may not be comparable and should be thoroughly evaluated. This finding translates into critical therapeutic consequences, as patients would be treated depending on a threshold viral load, which will be different depending on the method used. In this context, these data reinforce the idea that local guidelines for the initiation of pre-emptive therapy based on commercial assays must be established as long as universally accepted standards for quantitative analysis of CMV DNAemia are not available.

3. Detection of CMV infection

CMV viral load determination is used to diagnose active CMV infection, to adopt treatment strategies to prevent CMV infection after transplantation and to monitor CMV after therapy. For this reason it is necessary to establish robust and reproducible assays to make possible to detect CMV levels within a wide range from low to very high number of copies (Abbate et al., 2008).

3.1 CMV detection using antigemia assays

The pp65 antigenemia developed in the late 1980s was the first non-cell culture based quantitative assay used in clinic to detect CMV infection (Atkinson & Emery), making obsolete the previous techniques such as shell vial assays (Gleaves et al., 1984; Nicholson et al., 1997), or the detection of early antigen fluorescent foci (DEAFF) test (Griffiths et al., 1984). The pp65 antigenemia assay is based on the detection of the pp65 phosphoprotein of CMV in peripheral blood leukocytes (Van der Bij et al., 1988), and it has been widely used for years to quantify and guiding the administration of therapy and monitoring active CMV infection of STC recipients (Bonon et al., 2005; Tormo et al., 2010). However, the antigenemia assay has many disadvantages such as, it requires quite a lot blood volume as well as intensive labour and need to process samples within 6h from the time of collection to achieve optimal sensitivity (Kim et al., 2007; Mhiri et al., 2007), it restricts the numbers of samples that can be analyzed simultaneously and it requires a high number of leukocytes (at least more than 200 leukocytes) for acceptable performance of the assay (Preiser et al., 2001), being unfeasible during periods of severe neutropenia. In addition, due to the fact that antigenemia results can be elevated after following ganciclovir treatment despite of a decrease of DNAemia levels, results using antigenemia for monitoring efficacy of the pre-emptive therapy of CMV infection in SCT recipients may be mislead (Sia et al., 2000). Other molecular techniques have reduced the turnaround time for monitoring CMV infection.

3.2 Qualitative PCR assays

In the past few years new sensitive PCR based techniques have been developed for earlier detection of CMV infection. The new assays developed were initially qualitative and they were able to detect CMV viremia in plasma of SCT recipients, and were compared with antigenemia assay (Boeckh et al., 1997; Boivin et al., 2000; Ksouri et al., 2007; Mori et al., 2000; Preiser et al., 2001). Results from Boivin et al. found a higher sensitivity in antigenemia test, while Boeckh et al. suggested a similar sensibility in both techniques. Most of these studies used in-house PCR assays (Boeckh et al., 1997; Boivin et al., 2000; Preiser et al., 2001), which made difficult to compare results and to conclude the clinical value of the methods (Solano et al., 2001).

The AMPLICOR CMV DNA PCR assay (Roche Diagnostics, Branchburg, N.J.) was the first qualitative technique commercialized. However, despite of being a more sensitive technique, antigenemia was found to be a more suitable technique both for guiding the initiation of preemptive therapy and for monitoring the efficacy of ganciclovir treatment (Solano et al., 2001).

3.3 Quantitative PCR assays

The quantitative PCR assays have demonstrated to be more suitable and clinically relevant than qualitative PCR for the detection of CMV DNA (Sia et al., 2000), providing useful information for the management of patients at high risk for developing CMV infection. Quantitative results may facilitate the establishment of a threshold for CMV viral load and the discrimination between patients who had symptomatic CMV infection and those who do not. Thus, allowing to establish the degree of viral replication and to distinguish between low and high level of CMV infection that may lead to disease after SCT (Preiser et al., 2001). Although there are many different commercially available quantitative PCR assays for CMV detection, the COBAS AMPLICOR CMV MONITOR test is one of the more commonly used in the clinical practice. This quantitative PCR developed by Roche included an internal quantification standard. The performance of the assay was found to be more sensitive compared with other qualitative tests (Boivin et al., 2000; Caliendo et al., 2001), with a lower limit of detection of 400 copies/ml of plasma and a dynamic range up to 50,000CMV DNA copies/ml. This assay has been widely used for early detection of CMV infection in a variety of clinical specimens and clinical studies (Ghisetti et al., 2004; Lehto et al., 2005; Martin-Davila et al., 2005; Piiparinen et al., 2005; Sia et al., 2000; Westall et al., 2004). However, it shows some disadvantages, due to the fact that it requires manual extraction it has a low number of sample processing (24 per run) and a long performance (approximately 8 h). In addition, the limit of detection has been established in 2.78 log10 cop/ml, value that is high especially for the early detection of CMV replication (Kerschner et al., 2011).

The use of quantitative PCR to detect CMV infection has been highly controversial regarding the specimen used (plasma, whole blood or leukocytes) for the quantification of the CMV viral load (Boeckh et al., 1997; Boivin et al., 2000; Caliendo et al., 2000; Flexman et al., 2001; Kaiser et al., 2002; Machida et al., 2000; Razonable et al., 2002; Tanaka et al., 2000; Weinberg, Schissel, & Giller, 2002). Some studies have suggested that quantitative PCR measurements for monitoring CMV viral load in whole-blood have a higher sensitivity compared to using cells or plasma during CMV disease in immunocompromised patients (Razonable et al., 2002) (von Muller et al., 2007). The authors consider that whole blood includes all the compartments in which the virus can replicate (Deback et al., 2007). In addition, Cortez et al found that quantitative PCR performed in whole blood provided a higher number of positive results (58.2% vs. 39.5%) compared to plasma (Cortez et al., 2003). However, Leruez-Ville et al. compared the performance of a RT-PCR specifically to amplify high conserved region of CMV UL93 gene in plasma and whole blood, demonstrating that both plasma and whole blood were equally suitable for monitoring active CMV infection (Leruez-Ville et al., 2003).

3.4 RT-PCR assays

In the mid 1990s become available the first two commercialized RT-PCR platforms. In the last years, different companies have tried to improve the technique including faster cycling, higher throughput and flexibility, new optical systems and more accessible software (Table 1). For example, it has been developed several versions of the LightCycler instruments such as Roche LightCycler™ PCR or SmartCycler (Cepheid) for performing sensitive, specific and rapid assays for the detection of CMV, time- and cost-effectiveness and with low contamination risk (Schaade et al., 2000). RT-PCR based on TaqMan probes and related technologies have proven higher dynamic range, precision, accuracy, reproducibility, a shorter turnaround time and a low risk of contamination, offering many advantages over quantitative-competitive PCR assays. With the use of these techniques, the quantification of CMV in clinically relevant samples could be reproducibly achieved in 2h allowing to understand CMV replication kinetics in humans (Atkinson & Emery, 2011). In addition, other advantages have been described about the use of RT-PCR to evaluate the CMV load in HSCT including the ability to test blood during episodes of neutropenia and subsequent disease that had been missed by antigenemia (Kaiser et al., 2002).

On the contrary, RT-PCR also has some disadvantages compared with conventional PCR such as the start-up expense of the assay and the incompatibility of some platforms with certain reagents (Mackay, Arden, & Nitsche, 2002).

Although most of RT-PCR assays for monitoring CMV infection in SCT recipients have been laboratory developed (Boeckh et al., 2004; Griscelli et al., 2001; Herrmann et al., 2004; Hong et al., 2004; Kalpoe et al., 2004; Leruez-Ville et al., 2003; Lilleri et al., 2004; Limaye et al., 2001; Nitsche et al., 2000; Pumannova et al., 2006; Ruell et al., 2007; Schaade et al., 2000; Tanaka et al., 2000; Tanaka et al., 2002; Yakushiji et al., 2002; Yun et al., 2003), several commercial tests are available and have been used in different clinical diagnostic laboratories. However, there are not many studies based on the application of these commercial assays in SCT recipients (Bravo et al.; Gimeno et al., 2008; Gouarin et al., 2007; Gracia-Ahufinger et al., 2010; Hanson et al., 2007). As it will be described below, these studies evaluated the suitability of the commercial assays for the surveillance of active CMV infection in these patients and compared the performance of the different tests.

LABORATORY DEVELOPED REAL TIME PCR	
ADVANTAGES	**REF**
Less expensive and with the possibility of being personally established by developers.	[10, 11, 17, 18, 20, 56, 61, 63-71]

COMMERCIAL REAL TIME PCR				
NAME	**MANUFACTURER**	**VIRAL TARGET**	**ADVANTAGES**	**REF**
COBAS Amplicor CMV Monitor	Roche	UL54	Sensitive, low limit of detection and broad dynamic range.	[40-45, 51]
LightCycler® CMV Quantitative Kit	Roche	UL54	Reasonably accurate, sensitive, specific and linear. Suitable for the detection of CMV DNA early after transplantation.	[74,75]
Artus CMV PCR test	QIAGEN	UL122	Reliable CMV diagnostic early after transplantation. High sensitivity and performance.	74
CMV R-gene™	Argene	UL83	Accurate quantification in SCT patients, good correlation with other RT-PCR assays and pp65 antigenemia. Validated with several types of specimen and DNA purification systems (automatic and manual).	73
Abbott CMV real-time PCR Kit	Abbott Diagnosis	UL122	High sensitivity and very low limit of detection (25 cps/mL). Good correlation with antigenemia and suitable to monitoring active CMV infection in SCT patients.	[15, 72]
Affigene CMV Trender	Cepheid	Not specified	Robust, reproducible and sensitive. Better analytical performance than the Abbot test and accurate estimation of the viral load.	[29,28]

Table 1. Technical advantages of the laboratory developed and commercially available RT-PCR methods.

3.4.1 Commercial RT-PCR assays

There are several commercially available RT-PCR assays developed for the detection of CMV infection in clinical samples. Most of these assays use specific targets, such as UL83, UL123 genes or the HXFL4 region (Alain et al.; Caliendo et al., 2007; Gault et al., 2001; Gouarin et al., 2007; Mengelle et al., 2003). The most common targets used for the detection of CMV by RT-PCR are the immediate early (IE) gene (Nitsche et al., 1999), the polymerase (UL54) gene (Schaade et al., 2000) , the glycoprotein B gene (UL55) (Espy et al., 2006) and the pp65 gene (UL83) (Stocher et al., 2003). Among the commercially available standardized methods to detect CMV infection, the LightCycler® CMV Quantitative Kit (Roche), the RealArt CMV LightCycler PCR reagent test (QIAGEN, Germantown, MD), CMV R-gene™ (Argene, France), Affigene CMV Trender (Cepheid, Sweden) and the Abbott CMV real-time PCR Kit (Abbott Diagnosis, USA) have been evaluated in SCT.

The LightCycler® CMV Quantitative assay (Roche) is a standardized RT-PCR test based on analyte-specific reagents (ASR) designed to detect a fragment of 240 pb within the polymerase gene (UL54) (Alain et al.). This test has been compared with the RealArt CMV LightCycler PCR reagent test (QIAGEN) that detects a fragment of 105 pb within the IE gene (Hanson et al., 2007). They made the comparison using OptiQuant CMV DNA panels (AcroMetrix Corp.) that contained four concentrations of CMV strain AD169 and with plasma specimens collected from SCT recipients. Although both tests were suitable to detect CMV DNA early after transplantation, the results using the Qiagen test showed higher sensitivity as well as a better performance at the lower standard concentration (Hanson et al., 2007).

Other remarkable CMV RT-PCR assay is the CMV R-gene™ (Argene, France) that targets the pp65 gene (UL83). This test has been evaluated in SCT recipients from four centers showing an accurate quantification, as well as a good correlation with other laboratory-developed RT-PCR assays and pp65 antigenemia, thus the authors suggest that the R-gene test is a good alternative method to diagnose and monitor CMV infection (Gouarin et al., 2007). The Affigene CMV Trender kit was developed by Cepheid and it has been shown to be robust, reproducible and sensitive enough for routine measurement of patient samples (Abbate et al., 2008). The analytical performance of this assay was also evaluated in our laboratory compared with the Abbott CMV RT-PCR Kit, using samples obtained from SCT recipients. The Affigene CMV Trender assay yielded higher viral load than the Abbot test, suggesting a better analytical performance. The comparison was also performed using the OptiQuant CMV DNA quantification panel showing that the Affigene test provides a more accurate estimation of the CMV DNA load (Gracia-Ahufinger et al., 2010). The test manufactured by Abbott, was previously evaluated in plasma samples from SCT recipients (Gimeno et al., 2008).

However the assay was compared with the antigenemia test to monitoring active CMV infection in SCT patients. Results showed a good correlation of the results but higher sensitivity for the RT-PCR assay (Gimeno et al., 2008). More recently the Abbott CMV RT-PCR assay was also evaluated in SCT recipients compared with other two commercial tests (Roche and Nanogen) (Bravo et al., 2011). The results found variations in the performance of the tests which limited to establish a common cutoff between different assays. This issue will be discussed below.

4. CMV viral load threshold for treatment initiation

The development of antiviral strategies has resulted in a large decrease in the incidence of CMV disease. Two main therapeutic strategies have been developed for the control of CMV infection and prevention of CMV disease, prophylaxis and pre-emptive therapy. Both strategies have been shown to be equally effective to protect against CMV infection. In the prophylaxis strategy antiviral treatment is administered to all patients after transplantation for a period of time between 100 and 200 days. (Boeckh M, 2003; Hebart & Einsele, 2004; Meijer et al., 2003; Zaia, 2002). In the pre-emptive strategy treatment is administered only when the CMV viral load reaches an established threshold (Gimeno et al., 2008; Machida et al., 2000). The preemptive administration of treatment consequently requires the use of highly sensitive assay for monitoring CMV viral load.

The International Consensus Guidelines on the Management of CMV after transplantation considered necessary the establishment of a universal cut-off value for initiating therapy (Razonable & Emery, 2004). Several studies have tried to establish the clinical utility of using the RT-PCR test to guide preemptive therapy in SCT recipients (Avetisyan et al., 2006; Boeckh M, 2009; Gerna et al., 2008; Gimeno et al., 2008; Harrington et al., 2007; Kalpoe et al., 2004; Lilleri et al., 2004; Limaye et al., 2001; Machida et al., 2000; Ruell et al., 2007; Verkruyse et al., 2006). However as stated earlier, there are significant differences between the different techniques used to determine the CMV viral load, thus the standardization of specific cutoff values is limited by the variations in the performance of the test, the assay design, and the diversity in the patient population studied thus results can not be extrapolated. So, it would be necessary an international reference standard between viral loads obtained with different tests. Currently, each laboratory must establish its own cutoff value and monitor clinical outcomes to verify the trigger points used.

Some authors have suggested that pre-emptive therapy should be initiated after two consecutive increased viral load values (Boeckh M, 2009; Gimeno et al., 2008). However, the inter- and intra-assay variability in some cases with variations over 30% that may represent a risk for using this treatment initiation strategy (Boeckh & Boivin, 1998; Boeckh & Nichols, 2004), with variations of the viral load less than 0.5 log may not be significant. Other authors propose considering CMV replication kinetics for the initiation of treatment. In these cases, it needs to be considered that while CMV duplicate within 1-2 days on average, the time for replication is shorter in the presence of immunosuppressant drugs, which may result in faster increase of the viral loads. In addition in these cases may be necessary taking into account the initial viral load since it is predictive of risk for developing CMV disease (Emery & Griffiths, 2000).

Some studies have established optimal cut-offs for treatment initiation, classifying patients according to the risk for developing CMV disease. A recent publication by Boeckh and Ljungman recommends initiating treatment with viral loads over 100 copies/ml in SCT recipients at high risk for CMV infection that received the transplant within the last 100 days, and 500 copies/ml for patients at low risk. For long-term SCT recipients initiation of treatment is recommended with viral loads over 1,000 copies/ml (Boeckh M, 2009).

Most of the studies to establish thresholds for the control of CMV infection have been performed using plasma for testing CMV viral load with a wide range of cut-off viral loads varying from 550 copies/ml to 10,000 copies/ml (Avetisyan et al., 2006; Gimeno et al., 2008;

Hong et al., 2004; Yakushiji et al., 2002). Other studies have established thresholds for the control of CMV infection of 1,000 copies/ml (Boeckh M, 2009; Harrington et al., 2007), and 10,000 (Gerna et al., 2008; Lilleri et al., 2004; Verkruyse et al., 2006) using whole blood. These cut-off values were defined to be protective independently of their CMV sero-status. Few studies have established a protective cut-off for CMV infection in leukocytes; one of these established a cut off of 1,000 CMV genomes copies per 200,000 leukocytes (Avetisyan et al., 2006).

Another important issue after transplantation is the optimal frequency of CMV monitoring which has not been defined for SCT. Most authors recommend a weekly periodicity increased twice a week once CMV replication is detected and during treatment administration, while treatment administration should be interrupted after two consecutive negative determinations (Boeckh M, 2009).

In summary, it has not been established a cutoff threshold for initiating antiviral therapy against CMV maybe due to differences in CMV serological status, immunosuppressive drug regimens and period of treatment. Further studies are necessary in large series of SCT recipients assessing safety of viral load thresholds.

5. Standardization of CMV viral load quantification

Since CMV viral loads (in copies per milliliter of body fluid) correlate with the development of CMV disease (Emery & Griffiths, 2000; Humar et al., 1999), the use of molecular diagnostics based on the measurement of the viral load has contributed to patients' management after transplantation for more than a decade. During preemptive administration of treatment, antiviral therapy is initiated when CMV replication reaches an established threshold in the peripheral blood (Lilleri et al., 2009), prior to develop clinical symptoms. Therefore, the use methods such as RT-PCR can be useful to determine when to initiate the preemptive therapy and its duration (Emery & Griffiths, 2000; Humar et al., 1999; Humar et al., 2002; Sia & Patel, 2000) as well as to monitor the response to the administered therapy. However, as previously stated the most important handicap of the available RT-PCR techniques is the high variability of CMV viral load results among different laboratories. Pang et al designed a comparative study among thirty laboratories to evaluate the reproducibility of in-house and commercial assays to detect CMV infection. They prepared a panel of samples with different CMV DNA concentrations that were evaluated in different laboratories, with several commercial available assays. While the intra-laboratory coefficient of variation was considered acceptable (around 17%), they inter-laboratory variability resulted higher than 140%. These authors considered that differences in viral load lower at <0.5 log10 are not considered clinically relevant. This difference limits the comparisons inter-laboratories and prevents the establishment of a determinate cut-off broadly applicable for making clinical decisions and monitoring the initiation of pre-emptive therapy (Caliendo et al., 2009). These discrepancies result into clinical therapeutic consequences, as a number of patients may receive treatment in one hospital while not in other hospital using a different assay (Gracia-Ahufinger et al., 2010).

The differences among assays are based on the method for nucleic acid extraction, the specimen type, the target genomic region, primers and probes used for amplification and detection (Caliendo et al., 2009; Ikewaki et al., 2005). Although, the variability in the results obtained with commercial assays (kits or ASRs) are proven to be lower than when using in-house developed methods (Pang et al., 2009).

The most critical factor for standardization is the lack of using an universally accepted standard for CMV quantification will make possible the comparison among results thus establishing a common management of patients in different centers (Atkinson & Emery, 2011). The reference material used as a calibrator have to be traceable and commutable to achieve accurate clinical results ensuring consistency with clinical samples (Caliendo et al., 2009). While many laboratories produce their own calibrator as an attempt of standardizing some CMV reference material is under development and in fact there are standards commercially available for quantification. For instance, the National Institute of Standards and Technology (NIST) started the development of a reference standard for CMV based on pure CMV DNA from a Towne strain from which after some modification, the final construct will be used to produce viral DNA (Wang et al., 2004). Moreover, the OptiQuant® CMV DNA Quantification Panel from AcroMetrix has been carefully formulated to mimic naturally occurring human specimens containing CMV viral DNA. It consists of cultured CMV that has been diluted in defibrinated, delipidized normal human plasma at different concentrations. The panel can be used with any test procedure designed for measuring CMV DNA in human serum or plasma and it has been widely used as a standard in several studies (Bravo et al.; Forman et al., 2011; Hanson et al., 2007; Raggam et al., 2010) to compare techniques with the same laboratory and inter-laboratory.

In the absence of standardization the current clinical guidelines recommend to each individual laboratory to establish their own viral thresholds for CMV management, (Kotton et al., 2010; Razonable & Emery, 2004), threshold that cover a wide range of viral loads varying from 200-500 copies/mL in some laboratories (Ikewaki et al., 2005; Mori et al., 2002) to 2000-5000 copies/mL in others (Humar et al., 1999).

6. Conclusions

In conclusion, the quantitative PCR assays have demonstrated to be more suitable and clinically relevant for the monitoring of the CMV viral load, and the management of patients that develop CMV infection. Although there are several commercially available RT-PCR assays developed for the detection of CMV infection in clinical samples, there are variations in the performance of these tests which limit to establish a common cutoff between different assays. Each laboratory must establish its own cutoff value and monitor clinical outcomes to verify the trigger points used. Using universally accepted standards for CMV quantification will make possible the comparison among results establishing a common management of patients in different centers. However, in the absence of standardization the current clinical guidelines recommend to each individual laboratory to establish their own viral thresholds for CMV management. Further studies are still necessary to establish standardized cut-off values in large series of transplant recipients.

7. Acknowledgement

The authors thank other members of the laboratory. P.P-R. was funded by Instituto de Salud Carlos III, Programa Miguel Servet CP05/00226.

8. References

Abbate, I.; Finnstrom, N.; Zaniratti, S.; Solmone, M. C.; Selvaggini, S.; Bennici, E.; Neri, S.; Brega, C.; Paterno, M.; & Capobianchi, M. R. (2008). Evaluation of an automated extraction system in combination with Affigene CMV Trender for CMV DNA quantitative determination: comparison with nested PCR and pp65 antigen test. *J Virol Methods* Vol.151, No.1, pp. 61-5, ISSN 0166-0934

Alain, S.; Lachaise, V.; Hantz, S.; & Denis, F. Comparison between the LightCycler CMV Quant Kit (Roche Diagnostics) with a standardized in-house Taqman assay for cytomegalovirus blood viral load quantification. *Pathol Biol (Paris)* Vol.58, No.2, pp. 156-61, ISSN 1768-3114

Atkinson, C.; & Emery, V. C. (2011). Cytomegalovirus quantification: Where to next in optimising patient management? *J Clin Virol* Vol.51, No.4, pp. 223-8, ISSN 1873-5967

Avetisyan, G.; Larsson, K.; Aschan, J.; Nilsson, C.; Hassan, M.; & Ljungman, P. (2006). Impact on the cytomegalovirus (CMV) viral load by CMV-specific T-cell immunity in recipients of allogeneic stem cell transplantation. *Bone Marrow Transplant* Vol.38, No.10, pp. 687-92, ISSN 0268-3369

Boeckh, M.; & Boivin, G. (1998). Quantitation of cytomegalovirus: methodologic aspects and clinical applications. *Clin Microbiol Rev* Vol.11, No.3, pp. 533-54, ISSN 0893-8512

Boeckh, M.; Gallez-Hawkins, G. M.; Myerson, D.; Zaia, J. A.; & Bowden, R. A. (1997). Plasma polymerase chain reaction for cytomegalovirus DNA after allogeneic marrow transplantation: comparison with polymerase chain reaction using peripheral blood leukocytes, pp65 antigenemia, and viral culture. *Transplantation* Vol.64, No.1, pp. 108-13, ISSN 0041-1337

Boeckh, M.; Huang, M.; Ferrenberg, J.; Stevens-Ayers, T.; Stensl&, L.; Nichols, W. G.; & Corey, L. (2004). Optimization of quantitative detection of cytomegalovirus DNA in plasma by real-time PCR. *J Clin Microbiol* Vol.42, No.3, pp. 1142-8, ISSN 0095-1137

Bocckh M. (2009). How we treat cytomegalovirus in hematopoietic cell transplant recipients. *Blood* Vo.113, No.23, pp. 5711-9, ISSN 1528-0020

Boeckh, M.; & Nichols, W. G. (2004). The impact of cytomegalovirus serostatus of donor & recipient before hematopoietic stem cell transplantation in the era of antiviral prophylaxis and preemptive therapy. *Blood* Vol.103, No.6, pp. 2003-8, ISSN 0006-4971

Boeckh, M.; Papanicolaou, G.; Rubin, R.; Wingard, J.R.; Zaia, J. (2003). CMV in hematopoietic stem cell transplant recipients: Current status, known challenges, and future strategies. *Biol. Blood Marrow Transplant* Vol.5, pp. 543-558, ISSN 1083-8791

Boivin, G.; Belanger, R.; Delage, R.; Beliveau, C.; Demers, C.; Goyette, N.; & Roy, J. (2000). Quantitative analysis of cytomegalovirus (CMV) viremia using the pp65 antigenemia assay and the COBAS AMPLICOR CMV MONITOR PCR test after blood & marrow allogeneic transplantation. *J Clin Microbiol* Vol.38, No.12, pp. 4356-60, ISSN 0095-1137

Bonon, S. H.; Menoni, S. M.; Rossi, C. L.; De Souza, C. A.; Vigorito, A. C.; Costa, D. B.; & Costa, S. C. (2005). Surveillance of cytomegalovirus infection in haematopoietic stem cell transplantation patients. *J Infect* Vol.50, No.2, pp. 130-7, ISSN 0163-4453

Bravo, D.; Clari, M. A.; Costa, E.; Munoz-Cobo, B.; Solano, C.; Jose Remigia, M.; & Navarro, D. (2011). Comparative Evaluation of Three Automated Systems for DNA Extraction in Conjunction with Three Commercially Available Real-Time PCR

Assays for Quantitation of Plasma Cytomegalovirus DNAemia in Allogeneic Stem Cell Transplant Recipients. *J Clin Microbiol* Vol.49, No.8, pp. 2899-904, ISSN 1098-660X

Caliendo, A. M.; Ingersoll, J.; Fox-Canale, A. M.; Pargman, S.; Bythwood, T.; Hayden, M. K.; Bremer, J. W.; & Lurain, N. S. (2007). Evaluation of real-time PCR laboratory-developed tests using analyte-specific reagents for cytomegalovirus quantification. *J Clin Microbiol* Vol.45, No.6, pp. 1723-7, ISSN 0095-1137

Caliendo, A. M.; Schuurman, R.; Yen-Lieberman, B.; Spector, S. A.; &ersen, J.; Manjiry, R.; Crumpacker, C.; Lurain, N. S.; & Erice, A. (2001). Comparison of quantitative & qualitative PCR assays for cytomegalovirus DNA in plasma. *J Clin Microbiol* Vol.39, No.4, pp. 1334-8, ISSN 0095-1137

Caliendo, A. M.; Shahbazian, M. D.; Schaper, C.; Ingersoll, J.; Abdul-Ali, D.; Boonyaratanakornkit, J.; Pang, X. L.; Fox, J.; Preiksaitis, J.; & Schonbrunner, E. R. (2009). A commutable cytomegalovirus calibrator is required to improve the agreement of viral load values between laboratories. *Clin Chem* Vol.55, No.9, pp. 1701-10, ISSN 1530-8561

Caliendo, A. M.; St George, K.; Kao, S. Y.; Allega, J.; Tan, B. H.; LaFontaine, R.; Bui, L.; & Rinaldo, C. R. (2000). Comparison of quantitative cytomegalovirus (CMV) PCR in plasma & CMV antigenemia assay: clinical utility of the prototype AMPLICOR CMV MONITOR test in transplant recipients. *J Clin Microbiol* Vol.38, No.6, pp. 2122-7, ISSN 0095-1137

Cortez, K. J.; Fischer, S. H.; Fahle, G. A.; Calhoun, L. B.; Childs, R. W.; Barrett, A. J.; & Bennett, J. E. (2003). Clinical trial of quantitative real-time polymerase chain reaction for detection of cytomegalovirus in peripheral blood of allogeneic hematopoietic stem-cell transplant recipients. *J Infect Dis* Vol.188, No.7, pp. 967-72, ISSN 0022-1899

Deback, C.; Fillet, A. M.; Dhedin, N.; Barrou, B.; Varnous, S.; Najioullah, F.; Bricaire, F.; & Agut, H. (2007). Monitoring of human cytomegalovirus infection in immunosuppressed patients using real-time PCR on whole blood. *J Clin Virol* Vol.40, No.3, pp. 173-9, ISSN 1386-6532

Drew, W. L. (2007). Laboratory diagnosis of cytomegalovirus infection and disease in immunocompromised patients. *Curr Opin Infect Dis* Vol.20, No.4, pp. 408-11, ISSN 0951-7375

Emery, V. C.; & Griffiths, P. D. (2000). Prediction of cytomegalovirus load and resistance patterns after antiviral chemotherapy. *Proc Natl Acad Sci U S A* Vol.97, No.14, pp. 8039-44, ISSN 0027-8424

Espy, M. J.; Uhl, J. R.; Sloan, L. M.; Buckwalter, S. P.; Jones, M. F.; Vetter, E. A.; Yao, J. D.; Wengenack, N. L.; Rosenblatt, J. E.; Cockerill, F. R. 3rd; & Smith, T. F. (2006). Real-time PCR in clinical microbiology: applications for routine laboratory testing. *Clin Microbiol Rev* Vol.19, No.1, pp. 165-256, ISSN 0893-8512

Fahle, G. A.; & Fischer, S. H. (2000). Comparison of six commercial DNA extraction kits for recovery of cytomegalovirus DNA from spiked human specimens. *J Clin Microbiol* Vol.38, No.10, pp. 3860-3, ISSN 0095-1137

Flexman, J.; Kay, I.; Fonte, R.; Herrmann, R.; Gabbay, E.; & Palladino, S. (2001). Differences between the quantitative antigenemia assay and the cobas amplicor monitor quantitative PCR assay for detecting CMV viraemia in bone marrow and solid organ transplant patients. *J Med Virol* Vol.64, No.3, pp. 275-82, ISSN 0146-6615

Forman, M.; Wilson, A.; & Valsamakis, A. (2011). Cytomegalovirus DNA quantification using an automated platform for nucleic Acid extraction & real-time PCR assay setup. *J Clin Microbiol* Vol.49, No.7, pp. 2703-5, ISSN 1098-660X

Gartner, B. C.; Fischinger, J. M.; Litwicki, A.; Roemer, K.; & Mueller-Lantzsch, N. (2004). Evaluation of a new automated, st&ardized generic nucleic acid extraction method (total nucleic acid isolation kit) used in combination with cytomegalovirus DNA quantification by COBAS AMPLICOR CMV MONITOR. *J Clin Microbiol* Vol.42, No.8, pp. 3881-2, ISSN 0095-1137

Gault, E.; Michel, Y.; Dehee, A.; Belabani, C.; Nicolas, J. C.; & Garbarg-Chenon, A. (2001). Quantification of human cytomegalovirus DNA by real-time PCR. *J Clin Microbiol* Vol.39, No.2, pp. 772-5, ISSN 0095-1137

Gerna, G.; Lilleri, D.; Caldera, D.; Furione, M.; Zenone Bragotti, L.; & Aless&rino, E. P. (2008). Validation of a DNAemia cutoff for preemptive therapy of cytomegalovirus infection in adult hematopoietic stem cell transplant recipients. *Bone Marrow Transplant* Vol.41, No.10, pp. 873-9, ISSN 0268-3369

Ghisetti, V.; Barbui, A.; Franchello, A.; Varetto, S.; Pittaluga, F.; Bobbio, M.; Salizzoni, M.; & Marchiaro, G. (2004). Quantitation of cytomegalovirus DNA by the polymerase chain reaction as a predictor of disease in solid organ transplantation. *J Med Virol* Vol.73, No.2, pp. 223-9, ISSN 0146-6615

Gimeno, C.; Solano, C.; Latorre, J. C.; Hern&ez-Boluda, J. C.; Clari, M. A.; Remigia, M. J.; Furio, S.; Calabuig, M.; Tormo, N.; & Navarro, D. (2008). Quantification of DNA in plasma by an automated real-time PCR assay (cytomegalovirus PCR kit) for surveillance of active cytomegalovirus infection and guidance of preemptive therapy for allogeneic hematopoietic stem cell transplant recipients. *J Clin Microbiol* Vol.46, No.10, pp. 3311-8, ISSN 1098-660X

Gleaves, C. A.; Smith, T. F.; Shuster, E. A.; & Pearson, G. R. (1984). Rapid detection of cytomegalovirus in MRC-5 cells inoculated with urine specimens by using low-speed centrifugation and monoclonal antibody to an early antigen. *J Clin Microbiol* Vol.19, No.6, pp. 917-9, ISSN 0095-1137

Gouarin, S.; Vabret, A.; Scieux, C.; Agbalika, F.; Cherot, J.; Mengelle, C.; Deback, C.; Petitjean, J.; Dina, J.; & Freymuth, F. (2007). Multicentric evaluation of a new commercial cytomegalovirus real-time PCR quantitation assay. *J Virol Methods* Vol.146, No.1-2, pp. 147-54, ISSN 0166-0934

Gracia-Ahufinger, I.; Tormo, N.; Espigado, I.; Solano, C.; Urbano-Ispizua, A.; Clari, M. A.; de la Cruz-Vicente, F.; Navarro, D.; & Perez-Romero, P. (2010). Differences in cytomegalovirus plasma viral loads measured in allogeneic hematopoietic stem cell transplant recipients using two commercial real-time PCR assays. *J Clin Virol* Vol.48, No.2, pp. 142-6, ISSN 1873-5967

Griffiths, P. D.; Panjwani, D. D.; Stirk, P. R.; Ball, M. G.; Ganczakowski, M.; Blacklock, H. A.; & Prentice, H. G. (1984). Rapid diagnosis of cytomegalovirus infection in immunocompromised patients by detection of early antigen fluorescent foci. *Lancet* Vol.2, No.8414, pp. 1242-5, ISSN 0140-6736

Griscelli, F.; Barrois, M.; Chauvin, S.; Lastere, S.; Bellet, D.; & Bourhis, J. H. (2001). Quantification of human cytomegalovirus DNA in bone marrow transplant recipients by real-time PCR. *J Clin Microbiol* Vol.39, No.12, pp. 4362-9, ISSN 0095-1137

Hakki, M.; Riddell, S. R.; Storek, J.; Carter, R. A.; Stevens-Ayers, T.; Sudour, P.; White, K.; Corey, L.; & Boeckh, M. (2003). Immune reconstitution to cytomegalovirus after allogeneic hematopoietic stem cell transplantation: impact of host factors, drug therapy, and subclinical reactivation. *Blood* Vol.102, No.8, pp. 3060-7, ISSN 0006-4971

Hanson, K. E.; Reller, L. B.; Kurtzberg, J.; Horwitz, M.; Long, G.; & Alex&er, B. D. (2007). Comparison of the Digene Hybrid Capture System Cytomegalovirus (CMV) DNA (version 2.0), Roche CMV UL54 analyte-specific reagent, and QIAGEN RealArt CMV LightCycler PCR reagent tests using AcroMetrix OptiQuant CMV DNA quantification panels and specimens from allogeneic-stem-cell transplant recipients. *J Clin Microbiol* Vol.45, No.6, pp. 1972-3, ISSN 0095-1137

Harrington, S. M.; Buller, R. S.; Storch, G. A.; Li, L.; Fischer, S. H.; Murray, P. R.; & Gea-Banacloche, J. C. (2007). The effect of quantification standards used in real-time CMV PCR assays on guidelines for initiation of therapy in allogeneic stem cell transplant patients. *Bone Marrow Transplant* Vol.39, No.4, pp. 237-8, ISSN 0268-3369

Hebart, H.; & Einsele, H. (2004). Clinical aspects of CMV infection after stem cell transplantation. *Hum Immunol* 65(5), pp. 432-6.

Herrmann, B.; Larsson, V. C.; Rubin, C. J.; Sund, F.; Eriksson, B. M.; Arvidson, J.; Yun, Z.; Bondeson, K.; & Blomberg, J. (2004). Comparison of a duplex quantitative real-time PCR assay and the COBAS Amplicor CMV Monitor test for detection of cytomegalovirus. *J Clin Microbiol* Vol.42, No.5, pp. 1909-14, ISSN 0095-1137

Hong, K. M.; Najjar, H.; Hawley, M.; & Press, R. D. (2004). Quantitative real-time PCR with automated sample preparation for diagnosis & monitoring of cytomegalovirus infection in bone marrow transplant patients. *Clin Chem* Vol.50, No.5, pp. 846-56, ISSN 0009-9147

Humar, A.; Gregson, D.; Caliendo, A. M.; McGeer, A.; Malkan, G.; Krajden, M.; Corey, P.; Greig, P.; Walmsley, S.; Levy, G.; & Mazzulli, T. (1999). Clinical utility of quantitative cytomegalovirus viral load determination for predicting cytomegalovirus disease in liver transplant recipients. *Transplantation* Vol.68, No.9, pp. 1305-11, ISSN 0041-1337

Humar, A.; Kumar, D.; Boivin, G.; & Caliendo, A. M. (2002). Cytomegalovirus (CMV) virus load kinetics to predict recurrent disease in solid-organ transplant patients with CMV disease. *J Infect Dis* Vol.186, No.6, pp. 829-33, ISSN 0022-1899

Ikewaki, J.; Ohtsuka, E.; Satou, T.; Kawano, R.; Ogata, M.; Kikuchi, H.; & Nasu, M. (2005). Real-time PCR assays based on distinct genomic regions for cytomegalovirus reactivation following hematopoietic stem cell transplantation. *Bone Marrow Transplant* Vol.35, No.4, pp. 403-10, ISSN 0268-3369

Kaiser, L.; Perrin, L.; Chapuis, B.; Hadaya, K.; Kolarova, L.; Deffernez, C.; Huguet, S.; Helg, C.; & Wunderli, W. (2002). Improved monitoring of cytomegalovirus infection after allogeneic hematopoietic stem cell transplantation by an ultrasensitive plasma DNA PCR assay. *J Clin Microbiol* Vol.40, No.11, pp. 4251-5, ISSN 0095-1137

Kalpoe, J. S.; Kroes, A. C.; de Jong, M. D.; Schinkel, J.; de Brouwer, C. S.; Beersma, M. F.; & Claas, E. C. (2004). Validation of clinical application of cytomegalovirus plasma DNA load measurement and definition of treatment criteria by analysis of correlation to antigen detection. *J Clin Microbiol* Vol.42, No.4, pp. 1498-504, ISSN 0095-1137

Kerschner, H.; Bauer, C.; Schlag, P.; Lee, S.; Goedel, S.; & Popow-Kraupp, T. (2011). Clinical evaluation of a fully automated CMV PCR assay. *J Clin Virol* Vol.50, No.4, pp. 281-6, ISSN 1873-5967

Kim, D. J.; Kim, S. J.; Park, J.; Choi, G. S.; Lee, S.; Kwon, C. D.; Ki, C.; & Joh, J. (2007). Real-time PCR assay compared with antigenemia assay for detecting cytomegalovirus infection in kidney transplant recipients. *Transplant Proc* Vol.39, No.5, pp. 1458-60, ISSN 0041-1345

Kotton, C. N.; Kumar, D.; Caliendo, A. M.; Asberg, A.; Chou, S.; Snydman, D. R.; Allen, U.; & Humar, A. (2010). International consensus guidelines on the management of cytomegalovirus in solid organ transplantation. *Transplantation* Vol.89, No.7, pp. 779-95, ISSN 1534-6080

Ksouri, H.; Eljed, H.; Greco, A.; Lakhal, A.; Torjman, L.; Abdelkefi, A.; Ben Othmen, T.; Ladeb, S.; Slim, A.; Zouari, B.; Abdeladhim, A.; & Ben Hassen, A. (2007). Analysis of cytomegalovirus (CMV) viremia using the pp65 antigenemia assay, the amplicor CMV test, and a semi-quantitative polymerase chain reaction test after allogeneic marrow transplantation. *Transpl Infect Dis* Vol.9, No.1, pp. 16-21, ISSN 1398-2273

Lehto, J. T.; Lemstrom, K.; Halme, M.; Lappalainen, M.; Lommi, J.; Sipponen, J.; Harjula, A.; Tukiainen, P.; & Koskinen, P. K. (2005). A prospective study comparing cytomegalovirus antigenemia, DNAemia and RNAemia tests in guiding pre-emptive therapy in thoracic organ transplant recipients. *Transpl Int* Vol.18, No.12, pp. 1318-27, ISSN 0934-0874

Leruez-Ville, M.; Ouachee, M.; Delarue, R.; Sauget, A. S.; Blanche, S.; Buzyn, A.; & Rouzioux, C. (2003). Monitoring cytomegalovirus infection in adult and pediatric bone marrow transplant recipients by a real-time PCR assay performed with blood plasma. *J Clin Microbiol* Vol.41, No.5, pp. 2040-6, ISSN 0095-1137

Lilleri, D.; Baldanti, F.; Gatti, M.; Rovida, F.; Dossena, L.; De Grazia, S.; Torsellini, M.; & Gerna, G. (2004). Clinically-based determination of safe DNAemia cutoff levels for preemptive therapy or human cytomegalovirus infections in solid organ and hematopoietic stem cell transplant recipients. *J Med Virol* Vol.73, No.3, pp. 412-8, ISSN 0146-6615

Lilleri, D.; Lazzarotto, T.; Ghisetti, V.; Ravanini, P.; Capobianchi, M. R.; Baldanti, F.; & Gerna, G. (2009). Multicenter quality control study for human cytomegalovirus DNAemia quantification. *New Microbiol* Vol.32, No.3, 245-53, ISSN 1121-7138

Limaye, A. P.; Huang, M. L.; Leisenring, W.; Stensl&, L.; Corey, L.; & Boeckh, M. (2001). Cytomegalovirus (CMV) DNA load in plasma for the diagnosis of CMV disease before engraftment in hematopoietic stem-cell transplant recipients. *J Infect Dis* Vol.183, No.3, pp. 377-82, ISSN 0022-1899

Ljungman, P.; Griffiths, P.; & Paya, C. (2002). Definitions of cytomegalovirus infection and disease in transplant recipients. *Clin Infect Dis* Vol.34, No.8, pp. 1094-7, ISSN 1537-6591

Ljungman, P.; Perez-Bercoff, L.; Jonsson, J.; Avetisyan, G.; Sparrelid, E.; Aschan, J.; Barkholt, L.; Larsson, K.; Winiarski, J.; Yun, Z.; & Ringden, O. (2006). Risk factors for the development of cytomegalovirus disease after allogeneic stem cell transplantation. *Haematologica* Vol.91, No.1, pp. 78-83, ISSN 1592-8721

Mackay, I. M.; Arden, K. E.; & Nitsche, A. (2002). Real-time PCR in virology. *Nucleic Acids Res* Vol.30, No.6, pp. 1292-305, ISSN 1362-4962

Machida, U.; Kami, M.; Fukui, T.; Kazuyama, Y.; Kinoshita, M.; Tanaka, Y.; K&a, Y.; Ogawa, S.; Honda, H.; Chiba, S.; Mitani, K.; Muto, Y.; Osumi, K.; Kimura, S.; & Hirai, H. (2000). Real-time automated PCR for early diagnosis and monitoring of cytomegalovirus infection after bone marrow transplantation. *J Clin Microbiol* Vol.38, No.7, pp. 2536-42, ISSN 0095-1137

Martin-Davila, P.; Fortun, J.; Gutierrez, C.; Marti-Belda, P.; C&elas, A.; Honrubia, A.; Barcena, R.; Martinez, A.; Puente, A.; de Vicente, E.; & Moreno, S. (2005). Analysis of quantitative PCR assay for CMV infection in liver transplant recipients: an intent to find the cut-off value. *J Clin Virol* Vol.33, pp. 138-144, ISSN 1386-6532

Meijer, E.; Bol&, G. J.; & Verdonck, L. F. (2003). Prevention of cytomegalovirus disease in recipients of allogeneic stem cell transplants. *Clin Microbiol Rev* Vol.16, No.4, pp. 647-57, ISSN 0893-8512

Mengelle, C.; Mansuy, J. M.; Da Silva, I.; Davrinche, C.; & Izopet, J. (2011). Comparison of 2 highly automated nucleic acid extraction systems for quantitation of human cytomegalovirus in whole blood. *Diagn Microbiol Infect Dis* Vol.69, No.2, pp. 161-6, ISSN 1879-0070

Mengelle, C.; Pasquier, C.; Rostaing, L.; S&res-Saune, K.; Puel, J.; Berges, L.; Righi, L.; Bouquies, C.; & Izopet, J. (2003). Quantitation of human cytomegalovirus in recipients of solid organ transplants by real-time quantitative PCR and pp65 antigenemia. *J Med Virol* Vol.69, No.2, pp. 225-31, ISSN 0146-6615

Mhiri, L.; Kaabi, B.; Houimel, M.; Arrouji, Z.; & Slim, A. (2007). Comparison of pp65 antigenemia, quantitative PCR and DNA hybrid capture for detection of cytomegalovirus in transplant recipients & AIDS patients. *J Virol Methods* Vol.143, No.1, pp. 23-8, ISSN 0166-0934

Mori, T.; Okamoto, S.; Watanabe, R.; Yajima, T.; Iwao, Y.; Yamazaki, R.; Nakazato, T.; Sato, N.; Iguchi, T.; Nagayama, H.; Takayama, N.; Hibi, T.; & Ikeda, Y. (2002). Dose-adjusted preemptive therapy for cytomegalovirus disease based on real-time polymerase chain reaction after allogeneic hematopoietic stem cell transplantation. *Bone Marrow Transplant* Vol.29, No.9, pp. 777-82, ISSN 0268-3369

Mori, T.; Sato, N.; Watanabe, R.; Okamoto, S.; & Ikeda, Y. (2000). Erythema exsudativum multiforme induced by granulocyte colony-stimulating factor in an allogeneic peripheral blood stem cell donor. *Bone Marrow Transplant* Vol.26, No.2, pp. 239-40, ISSN 0268-3369

Nicholson, V. A.; Whimbey, E.; Champlin, R.; Abi-Said, D.; Przepiorka, D.; Tarr&, J.; Chan, K.; Bodey, G. P.; & Goodrich, J. M. (1997). Comparison of cytomegalovirus antigenemia & shell vial culture in allogeneic marrow transplantation recipients receiving ganciclovir prophylaxis. *Bone Marrow Transplant* Vol.19, No.1, pp. 37-41, ISSN 0268-3369

Nitsche, A.; Steuer, N.; Schmidt, C. A.; L&t, O.; Ellerbrok, H.; Pauli, G.; & Siegert, W. (2000). Detection of human cytomegalovirus DNA by real-time quantitative PCR. *J Clin Microbiol* Vol.38, No.7, pp. 2734-7, ISSN 0095-1137

Nitsche, A.; Steuer, N.; Schmidt, C. A.; O.; & Siegert, W. (1999). Different real-time PCR formats compared for the quantitative detection of human cytomegalovirus DNA. *Clin Chem* Vol.45, No.11, pp. 1932-7, ISSN 0009-9147

Ozdemir, E.; Saliba, R. M.; Champlin, R. E.; Couriel, D. R.; Giralt, S. A.; de Lima, M.; Khouri, I. F.; Hosing, C.; Kornblau, S. M.; Anderlini, P.; Shpall, E. J.; Qazilbash, M. H.; Molldrem, J. J.; Chemaly, R. F.; & Komanduri, K. V. (2007). Risk factors associated with late cytomegalovirus reactivation after allogeneic stem cell transplantation for hematological malignancies. *Bone Marrow Transplant* Vol.40, No.2, pp. 125-36, ISSN 0268-3369

Pang, X. L.; Fox, J. D.; Fenton, J. M.; Miller, G. G.; Caliendo, A. M.; & Preiksaitis, J. K. (2009). Interlaboratory comparison of cytomegalovirus viral load assays. *Am J Transplant* Vol.9, No.2, pp. 258-68, ISSN 1600-6143

Piiparinen, H.; Helantera, I.; Lappalainen, M.; Suni, J.; Koskinen, P.; Gronhagen-Riska, C.; & Lautenschlager, I. (2005). Quantitative PCR in the diagnosis of CMV infection and in the monitoring of viral load during the antiviral treatment in renal transplant patients. *J Med Virol* Vol.76, No.3, pp. 367-72, ISSN 0146-6615

Preiser, W.; Brauninger, S.; Schwerdtfeger, R.; Ayliffe, U.; Garson, J. A.; Brink, N. S.; Franck, S.; Doerr, H. W.; & Rabenau, H. F. (2001). Evaluation of diagnostic methods for the detection of cytomegalovirus in recipients of allogeneic stem cell transplants. *J Clin Virol* Vol.20, No.1-2, pp. 59-70, ISSN 1386-6532

Pumannova, M.; Roubalova, K.; Vitek, A.; & Sajdova, J. (2006). Comparison of quantitative competitive polymerase chain reaction-enzyme-linked immunosorbent assay with LightCycler-based polymerase chain reaction for measuring cytomegalovirus DNA in patients after hematopoietic stem cell transplantation. *Diagn Microbiol Infect Dis* Vol.54, No.2, pp. 115-20, ISSN 0732-8893

Raggam, R. B.; Bozic, M.; Salzer, H. J.; Hammerschmidt, S.; Homberg, C.; Ruzicka, K.; & Kessler, H. H. (2010). Rapid quantitation of cytomegalovirus DNA in whole blood by a new molecular assay based on automated sample preparation & real-time PCR. *Med Microbiol Immunol* Vol.199, No.4, pp. 311-6, ISSN 1432-1831

Razonable, R. R.; Brown, R. A.; Wilson, J.; Groettum, C.; Kremers, W.; Espy, M.; Smith, T. F.; & Paya, C. V. (2002). The clinical use of various blood compartments for cytomegalovirus (CMV) DNA quantitation in transplant recipients with CMV disease. *Transplantation* Vol.73, No.6, pp. 968-73, ISSN 0041-1337

Razonable, R. R.; & Emery, V. C. (2004). Management of CMV infection and disease in transplant patients. 27-29 February 2004. *Herpes* Vol.11, No.3, pp. 77-86, ISSN 0969-7667

Ruell, J.; Barnes, C.; Mutton, K.; Foulkes, B.; Chang, J.; Cavet, J.; Guiver, M.; Menasce, L.; Dougal, M.; & Chopra, R. (2007). Active CMV disease does not always correlate with viral load detection. *Bone Marrow Transplant* Vol.40, No.1, pp. 55-61, ISSN 0268-3369

Schaade, L.; Kockelkorn, P.; Ritter, K.; & Kleines, M. (2000). Detection of cytomegalovirus DNA in human specimens by LightCycler PCR. *J Clin Microbiol* Vol.38, No.11, pp. 4006-9, ISSN 0095-1137

Sia, I. G.; & Patel, R. (2000). New strategies for prevention & therapy of cytomegalovirus infection and disease in solid-organ transplant recipients. *Clin Microbiol Rev* Vol.13, No.1, 83-121, ISSN 0893-8512

Sia, I. G.; Wilson, J. A.; Espy, M. J.; Paya, C. V.; & Smith, T. F. (2000). Evaluation of the COBAS AMPLICOR CMV MONITOR test for detection of viral DNA in specimens taken from patients after liver transplantation. *J Clin Microbiol* Vol.38, No.2, pp. 600-6, ISSN 0095-1137

Solano, C.; Munoz, I.; Gutierrez, A.; Farga, A.; Prosper, F.; Garcia-Conde, J.; Navarro, D.; & Gimeno, C. (2001). Qualitative plasma PCR assay (AMPLICOR CMV test) versus pp65 antigenemia assay for monitoring cytomegalovirus viremia & guiding preemptive ganciclovir therapy in allogeneic stem cell transplantation. *J Clin Microbiol* Vol.39, No.11, pp. 3938-41, ISSN 0095-1137

Stocher, M.; Leb, V.; Bozic, M.; Kessler, H. H.; Halwachs-Baumann, G.; O.; Stekel, H.; & Berg, J. (2003). Parallel detection of five human herpes virus DNAs by a set of real-time polymerase chain reactions in a single run. *J Clin Virol* Vol.26, No.1, pp. 85-93, ISSN 1386-6532

Tanaka, N.; Kimura, H.; Iida, K.; Saito, Y.; Tsuge, I.; Yoshimi, A.; Matsuyama, T.; & Morishima, T. (2000). Quantitative analysis of cytomegalovirus load using a real-time PCR assay. *J Med Virol* Vol.60, No.4, pp. 455-62, ISSN 0146-6615

Tanaka, Y.; K&a, Y.; Kami, M.; Mori, S.; Hamaki, T.; Kusumi, E.; Miyakoshi, S.; Nannya, Y.; Chiba, S.; Arai, Y.; Mitani, K.; Hirai, H.; & Mutou, Y. (2002). Monitoring cytomegalovirus infection by antigenemia assay & two distinct plasma real-time PCR methods after hematopoietic stem cell transplantation. *Bone Marrow Transplant* Vol.30, No.5, pp. 315-9, ISSN 0268-3369

Tormo, N.; Solano, C.; Benet, I.; Clari, M. A.; Nieto, J.; de la Camara, R.; Lopez, J.; Lopez-Aldeguer, N.; Hern&ez-Boluda, J. C.; Remigia, M. J.; Garcia-Noblejas, A.; Gimeno, C.; & Navarro, D. (2010). Lack of prompt expansion of cytomegalovirus pp65 and IE-1-specific IFNgamma CD8+ and CD4+ T cells is associated with rising levels of pp65 antigenemia and DNAemia during pre-emptive therapy in allogeneic hematopoietic stem cell transplant recipients. *Bone Marrow Transplant* Vol.45, No.3, pp. 543-9, ISSN 1476-5365

Valentine-Thon, E. (2002). Quality control in nucleic acid testing--where do we stand? *J Clin Virol* Vol.25, No.Suppl 3, pp. S13-21, ISSN 1386-6532

Van der Bij, W.; Schirm, J.; Torensma, R.; Van Son, W. J.; Tegzess, A. M.; & The, T. H. (1988). Comparison between Viremia and Antigenemia for Detection of Cytomegalovirus in Blood. *J Clin Microbiol* Vol.26, No.12, pp. 5, ISSN 0095-1137

Verkruyse, L. A.; Storch, G. A.; Devine, S. M.; Dipersio, J. F.; & Vij, R. (2006). Once daily ganciclovir as initial pre-emptive therapy delayed until threshold CMV load > or =10000 copies/ml: a safe and effective strategy for allogeneic stem cell transplant patients. *Bone Marrow Transplant* Vol.37, No.1, pp. 51-6, ISSN 0268-3369

von Muller, L.; Hinz, J.; Bommer, M.; Hampl, W.; Kluwick, S.; Wiedmann, M.; Bunjes, D.; & Mertens, T. (2007). CMV monitoring using blood cells and plasma: a comparison of apples with oranges? *Bone Marrow Transplant* Vol.39, No.6, pp. 353-7, ISSN 0268-3369

Wang, W.; Patterson, C. E.; Yang, S.; & Zhu, H. (2004). Coupling generation of cytomegalovirus deletion mutants and amplification of viral BAC clones. *J Virol Methods* Vol.121, No.2, pp. 137-43, ISSN 0166-0934

Weinberg, A.; Schissel, D.; & Giller, R. (2002). Molecular methods for cytomegalovirus surveillance in bone marrow transplant recipients. *J Clin Microbiol* Vol.40, No.11, 4203-6, ISSN 0095-1137

Westall, G. P.; Michaelides, A.; Williams, T. J.; Snell, G. I.; & Kotsimbos, T. C. (2004). Human cytomegalovirus load in plasma and bronchoalveolar lavage fluid: a longitudinal study of lung transplant recipients. *J Infect Dis* Vol.190, No.6, pp. 1076-83, ISSN 0022-1899

Yakushiji, K.; Gondo, H.; Kamezaki, K.; Shigematsu, K.; Hayashi, S.; Kuroiwa, M.; Taniguchi, S.; Ohno, Y.; Takase, K.; Numata, A.; Aoki, K.; Kato, K.; Nagafuji, K.; Shimoda, K.; Okamura, T.; Kinukawa, N.; Kasuga, N.; Sata, M.; & Harada, M. (2002). Monitoring of cytomegalovirus reactivation after allogeneic stem cell transplantation: comparison of an antigenemia assay and quantitative real-time polymerase chain reaction. *Bone Marrow Transplant* Vol.29, No.7, pp. 599-606, ISSN 0268-3369

Yun, Z.; Lewensohn-Fuchs, I.; Ljungman, P.; Ringholm, L.; Jonsson, J.; & Albert, J. (2003). A real-time TaqMan PCR for routine quantitation of cytomegalovirus DNA in crude leukocyte lysates from stem cell transplant patients. *J Virol Methods* Vol.110, No.1, pp. 73-9, ISSN 0166-0934

Zaia, J. A. (2002). Prevention of cytomegalovirus disease in hematopoietic stem cell transplantation. *Clin Infect Dis* Vol.35, No.8, pp. 999-1004, ISSN 1537-6591

8

Hematopoietic Stem Cell Potency for Cellular Therapeutic Transplantation

Karen M. Hall, Holli Harper and Ivan N. Rich
HemoGenix, Inc
U.S.A.

1. Introduction

Potency is the quantitative measurement of biological activity of a product (European Medicines Agency (EMA), 2008). Potency provides assurance that production and manufacture demonstrate consistency and provides information on stability and performance of the product. It also allows correlation with the clinical response and can help avoid product failure or toxicity due to the improper dose of the product being administered. For biopharmaceutical products such as drugs, growth factors and cytokines, vaccines etc., measurement of potency to predict dose has been a routine procedure for many years. Cells, on the other hand, are complex living entities that are continuously in flux. The potency of cells can change depending on numerous physiological and external environmental factors. Yet, with the increased number of cellular therapeutic applications and clinical regimen involving numerous cell types, the need to reliably and reproducibly measure biological and functional activity to meet the requirements of potency and ensure patient safety is of increasing importance (EMA, 2008; U.S. Food and Drug Administration, (FDA), 2011).

Determining the potency of a stem cell therapeutic can be a daunting task, especially if knowledge of the system biology, physiology and regulation is limited. In contrast, the hematopoietic system has proven to be not only an excellent model for stem cell biology, but also a model system for proliferation and differentiation in different applications. One of these applications is stem cell transplantation, a procedure that had its origins during the 1950s, became a quantitative assay in mice in 1961 (Till & McCulloch), and a routine clinical procedure in the 1970s (Santos et al. 1972; Thomas et al. 1977; Santos, 1983) Since that time, the number of human bone marrow transplantations reached a peak in the late 1990s (National Marrow Donor Program (NMDP); Pasquini & Wang, 2010) and has been declining to be replaced by alternative stem cell sources derived from mobilized peripheral blood (Haas et al. 1990; Koerbling et al. 1990; Sohn et.al. 2002) and umbilical cord blood (Broxmeyer et al. 1989; Gluckman et al. 1989).

Regardless of the tissue source, a successful transplant of stem cells is dependent upon the ability of the transplanted stem cells to lodge or "seed" in the bone marrow and begin the process of proliferation to produce lineage-specific progenitor cells. These differentiate into functionally mature circulating neutrophils, platelets and erythroid cells, the number of which provides information on the time at which engraftment took place. Proper lympho-hematopoietic reconstitution occurs much later. The ability of the stem cells to engraft is dependent upon two primary factors. The first is the status and condition of the patient. The second is the proliferation ability and potential of the stem cells prior to being transplanted.

Proliferation ability is equivalent to the proliferation status of the stem cells at the time of testing. This parameter defines stem cell "quality". Proliferation potential, on the other hand, is the capacity or potential of the stem cells to proliferate. For a continuously proliferating system such as lympho-hematopoiesis, stem cell potential decreases from the most primitive to the most mature stem cells. Thus, the more primitive a stem cell, the greater its proliferation potential and therefore its potency. It follows that the primary goal of stem cell transplantation is to provide the patient with stem cells that exhibit varying degrees of proliferation potential or potency. In this way, the patient can be endowed with stem cells that provide both short- (Charbord, 1994; Civin et al. 1996; Leung et al. 1999; Zubair et al. 2006) and long-term (Civin et al. 1996; Leung et al. 1999; Zubair et al. 2006; Duggan et al. 2000) engraftment and reconstitution.

A product that is "balanced" to provide the correct amount of short- and long-term stem cell engraftment and reconstitution would be the ideal situation. Present technology is not, however, capable of measuring or delivering a "balanced" stem cell product. In many cases, the donor stem cell product is skewed towards a greater proportion of mature rather than primitive stem cells or visa versa. However, it is possible to quantitatively measure both stem cell quality and potency of representative stem cell populations to provide a reasonably good approximation of the overall quality and potency of the stem cell product. These parameters would then predict the potential of the stem cells to engraft and reconstitute the system.

In 2009, the U.S. Food and Drug Administration (FDA, 2009) designated umbilical cord blood as a drug because, when transplanted into a patient, it results in systemic effects. The consequence of this designation has meant that virtually every aspect from cord blood collection to transplantation must be validated and documented according to regulatory requirements. Included in this process are the tests and assays to monitor the procedures and characterize the product prior to use. Besides histocompatability testing, the most important parameter that should be measured just prior to the stem cell product being used is potency. The FDA guidance on potency for cellular therapeutic products specifically describes the regulations that define a potency assay as compliant (FDA, 2011). A potency assay must provide quantitative data demonstrating the biological activity of all "active ingredients" specific to the product. In the case of a stem cell product, the "active ingredients" are the stem cell themselves. The results must meet pre-defined acceptance and/or rejection criteria so that the test results provide information as to whether the product can be released for use. In addition, the assay(s) must include reference materials, standards and controls, since without these, the necessary validation parameters (accuracy, sensitivity, specificity, precision and robustness) cannot be measured and documented.

The present communication describes an *in vitro* assay that measures stem cell potency and quality and helps define release criteria for hematopoietic products derived from mobilized peripheral blood, umbilical cord blood or bone marrow. The assay was designed to comply with regulatory requirements. In the 3-step process, all of the data required is accumulated in the initial stem cell culture and measurement step. The data obtained provides a degree of stem cell quality and potency assurance that has hitherto not been possible using the traditional methods of total nucleated cell count (TNC), viability and viable CD34+ counts, which provide no indication of stem cell functionality or growth. To illustrate the steps of the assay, a small number of mobilized peripheral blood samples are used to demonstrate the procedure for determining potency, quality and release criteria. A larger cohort of umbilical cord blood samples is then used to show the applicability of the assay.

The assay relies on two basic characteristics of stem cells, namely proliferation ability (quality) and potential (potency). It had been previously demonstrated that when hematopoietic stem cells were stimulated to proliferate in the presence of growth factors and cytokines, the intracellular ATP (iATP) concentration increased proportionately to the cell concentration plated (Rich & Hall, 2005; Rich, 2007). The steepness or slope of the cell dose response was dependent upon the primitiveness and proliferation potential of the cells being examined. Stem cells have a greater proliferation potential than lineage-specific progenitor cells (Botnick e al. 1979). It would therefore be expected that the slope of the cell dose response would be steeper for stem cells than progenitor cells. In other words, the steeper the slope of the cell dose response, the greater the proliferation potential and the greater the potency. This biological phenomenon was incorporated into an assay that first estimates the potency ratio for two stem cell populations of a sample compared to a reference standard of the same material. The information obtained from the initial culture step was then used in the second step to substantiate the correlation between stem cell potency and quality. Finally, stem cell potency and quality were combined to determine release criteria of a sample. This information is provided when the iATP is released after culture by lysis of the cells. The iATP acts as a limiting substrate for the most sensitive, non-radioactive signal detection system available. This is a luciferin/luciferase reaction that produces bioluminescence, which is measured as light in a plate luminometer (Rich, 2003). The procedure and results described in this communication lay the foundation for future studies of stem cell potency and clinical outcome that might improve the risk of graft failure (Picardi & Arcese, 2010; Querol et al. 2010) as well as safety and efficacy for the patient.

2. Materials and methods

2.1 Cells

Several cryopreserved, mobilized peripheral blood (mPB) samples from different donors were obtained from AllCells, Inc (Berkley, CA) in accordance with the company's Internal Review Board (IRB) approval. Vials of cryopreserved umbilical cord blood (UCB) samples were provided and released for research purposes by the University of Colorado Cord Blood Bank (ClinImmune, Inc) in Aurora, CO with approval by the respective Internal Review Board. Additional mPB and UCB cells were obtained from each source to use as internal reference standards.

2.2 Reference standards (RS)

The establishment of RSs is an absolute requirement for performing a potency assay. For hematopoietic cell-based therapeutics the number of cells obtained from a single donor UCB unit, mPB procedure or bone marrow aspirate are limited. This poses severe restrictions on establishing cellular reference standards. From a practical viewpoint, there are two alternatives. The first would be to establish multiple aliquots from several different donors that could be used as reference standards. Although each batch of RS would be expected to exhibit different biological activity and therefore different potency and quality characteristics, one batch would be designated as the primary RS. A second (donor specific) batch of cells would be tested against the primary RS and designated the secondary RS. Similarly, a third batch of cells would be tested against the secondary RS and designated the tertiary RS. The most recent batch of cells established as the RS would be used for every day testing until a new RS is established and tested. In this way it would always be possible to prepare a new RS and compare it against and established RS. The second alternative would be to assay a statistically significant number of samples of the same material to establish a range and mean/median potency that could be used as a "combined" RS for individual samples. This type of RS would take considerable time to establish. It would also require multiple laboratories to use the same standardized and validated assay so that results could be compared. The advantage would be that a "global" reference standard might be established for different cellular products that would allow comparison and calculation of potency ratios and quality of samples processed by individual laboratories. Release criteria for use in transplantation could also be established. The regulatory requirement for reference standards needed to measure cell potency is probably one of the most important aspects that has to be addressed by the different cellular therapeutic communities and standards organizations.

For the present study, the first alternative to establish reference standards was used. Cells designated as reference standards were prepared by separating the mononuclear cells (MNC) by density gradient centrifugation (see below), adjusting the cell concentration so that 1 million MNC were prepared in 7.5% DMSO with 10% fetal bovine serum (FBS) and medium in 1ml. The cells were frozen in ampoules using an automated rate freezer and stored in liquid nitrogen (LN2).

2.3 Preparation of cells for culture

Cryopreserved cells were thawed in a 37°C water bath and the contents transferred to a tube containing 20mL of warmed Iscove's Modified Dulbecco's Medium (IMDM) supplemented with 10% FBS. After thawing and washing the cells once, followed by resuspension in 1mL IMDM and 2% DNase, a cell count was performed on 20µL using a cell counter (Z2, Beckman Coulter, Brea, CA). Another aliquot of 20µL was stained with 7-aminoactinomycin D (7-AAD, Beckman Coulter, Brea, CA) and the viability measured by flow cytometry using an EPICS XL/MCL flow cytometer (Beckman Coulter, Brea, CA). Samples exhibiting viability below 85% were not used since cells either demonstrated poor proliferation or did not proliferate. The MNCs from each sample were fractionated on density gradient medium (Nycoprep 1.077, Axis-Shield, Accurate Chemicals and Scientific, Westbury, NY) by centrifugation for 10 min at 1,000 x g at room temperature (RT). The cells were washed in IMDM, centrifuged at 300 x g for 10 min at RT and resuspended in IMDM. This additional step removed the contaminating and dead cells and increased the viability to above 90%. Since several internal studies indicated that 7-AAD could produce false positive results with respect to cell growth potential (data not shown), all samples were assessed for the production of iATP at 2,500, 5,000 and 7,500 cells/well to substantiate metabolic cell viability and functionality as described below.

2.4 *In vitro* cell culture of 2 stem cell populations to determine potency, quality and release criteria

The instrument-based, ATP bioluminescence assay used to determine potency, quality and release (HALO-96 PQR, HemoGenix, Inc, Colorado Springs, CO) has been previously described in detail (Hall & Rich, 2009). It is summarized here for completeness. In contrast to a previous study using cord blood cells and a methylcellulose assay format (Reems et al. 2008), the assay described below is a methylcellulose-free, 96-well culture system that incorporates Suspension Expansion Culture (SEC) technology (Rich, 2007; Hall & Rich, 2009; Olaharski et al. 2009) for detecting both primitive (high proliferative potential stem and progenitor cells, HPP-SP) and more mature multipotential hematopoietic stem cells (colony-forming cell granulocyte, erythroid, macrophage megakaryocyte, CFC-GEMM). The assay was performed as follows. For each sample, the cell concentration was adjusted to 7.5×10^5 cells/mL and a serial dilution performed in IMDM to produce 5×10^5 and 2.5×10^5 cells/mL. From each cell dilution, 0.1mL was added to two separate tubes containing 0.9mL of master mix, one for each stem cell population being determined. After mixing, 0.1mL of the culture master mix was dispensed into 8 replicate wells of a 96-well plate to achieve the final concentrations of 2,500, 5,000 and 7,500 cells/well. The cocktail to stimulate CFC-GEMM consisted of erythropoietin, granulocyte-macrophage and granulocyte colony-stimulating factor, stem cell factor, thrombopoietin, Flt3-ligand and interleukins 3 and 6. The cocktail to stimulate the HPP-SP stem cell population contained the same growth factors/cytokines as that for CFC-GEMM, but with the addition of interleukins 2 and 7. The plates were incubated for 5 days at 37°C in a fully humidified incubator containing 5% CO_2 and 5% O_2 (Rich & Kubanek, 1982).

2.5 Assay calibration, standardization and sample processing

Prior to measuring bioluminescence of the samples after culture incubation, an ATP standard curve was performed (Rich & Hall, 2005; Reems et al. 2008; Hall & Rich, 2009). Serial dilutions from a 10μM stock concentration were prepared so that the final dilutions were 5, 1, 0.5, 0.1, 0.05, 0.01 and 0.005μM. In addition, an IMDM background and high and low ATP controls were included. Each dilution was dispensed into 4 wells (0.1mL/well) of a 96-well plate. To each well, 0.1 mL of an ATP enumeration reagent containing a lysis buffer, luciferin and luciferase was added. The contents were mixed and the plate left to incubate for 2 min in a plate luminometer (SpectraMax L, Molecular Devices, Sunnyvale, CA) after which the bioluminescence was measured as light (photons). The resulting ATP standard curve was then used to automatically interpolate the output of the luminometer in relative luminescence units (RLU) into standardized ATP concentrations (μM) using the instrument software (SoftMax Pro v5.4, Molecular Devices, Sunnyvale, CA). Inclusion of high and low controls in addition to the ATP standard curve allowed the assay to be calibrated and standardized. After performing the ATP standard curve, the sample plate(s) were removed from the incubator and allowed to attain room temperature. Thereafter, 0.1mL of the ATP enumeration reagent was dispensed into each well and the contents mixed. After 10 min incubation in the instrument or in the dark, the bioluminescence was measured and the ATP concentrations automatically interpolated from the ATP standard curve.

2.6 Assay validation and statistics

The ATP bioluminescence assay has been previously validated in accordance with bioanalytical method validation (FDA, 2001). For this specific application, the assay exhibited an accuracy (proportion of correct outcomes) of greater than 90%. Sensitivity (proportion of correctly identified positive samples) and specificity (proportion of correctly identified negative samples) were determined using receiver operator characteristic (ROC) statistics (DeLong et al. 1985) in which the area under the curve (AUC) was determined for background (no stimulatory cocktail) versus CFC-GEMM and background versus HPP-SP. For the former, the AUC was 0.752 (95% confidence intervals; 0.71-0.8; $p < 0.0001$), while for the latter the AUC was 0.73 (95% confidence intervals; 0.68-0.78, $p<0.001$). Since the AUC must be between 0.5 and 1, the results demonstrated that the assay could differentiate between sensitivity and specificity. Assay precision (reliability and reproducibility) was performed on background, CFC-GEMM and HPP-SP over a cell dose range from 2,500 to 10,000 cells/well and demonstrated coefficients of variation (CV) of 15% or less. This was in compliance with regulatory requirements (FDA, 2011). Robustness, in this case transferability of the assay from one laboratory to another, had been previously reported (Reems et al. 2008). The results demonstrated a correlation coefficient (R) between laboratories of 0.94 ($p<0.001$).

Concentrations of ATP (μM) are provided as the mean ± 1 standard deviation of 8 replicate wells. The slope of the 3-point cell dose response was obtained from the linear regression using least squares analysis (Prism version 5, GraphPad Software, LaJolla, CA). For correlations, the slope of the linear regression, goodness of fit (r^2) and correlation coefficient (R) are reported. Tests of significance for correlation were performed using the Pearson two-tailed test with an alpha of 0.05.

3. Results

The procedure for determining stem cell potency, quality and release criteria is a 3-step process. However, only the first step requires cell culture and provides all the information for the remaining steps of the procedure. The culture step involves a 3-point cell dose response for two stem cell populations (CFC-GEMM and HPP-SP) for both the RS and samples.

3.1 Step 1 – Measuring stem cell potency of mobilized peripheral blood

The first step in the procedure is illustrated in Figure 1. This shows the cell dose responses for the mature multipotential stem cell, CFC-GEMM (Figs. 1A and 1B), and the more primitive stem cell HPP-SP (Figs. 1C and 1D) from 4 different mPB samples cultured for 5 (Figs. 1A and 1C) and 7 days (Figs. 1B and 1D). The graphs demonstrate that an approximate 3-fold increase in ATP concentration occurs within 2 days when the incubation time is increased from 5 to 7 days. A 7 day incubation period allows for increased assay sensitivity as well as the ability to perform the assay to accommodate a work schedule. Since the increase is cell dose dependent, it demonstrates that the assay is directly measuring an increase in the number of cells as a result of cell proliferation. It should be noted however, that although measurements at both 5 and 7 days are on the exponential part of the growth curve for both HPP-SP and CFC-GEMM, measurement of proliferation on day 7 will exhibit slightly greater coefficients of variation (CVs) and will also include cells that have initiated differentiation. On day 5, little or no differentiation occurs (data not shown).

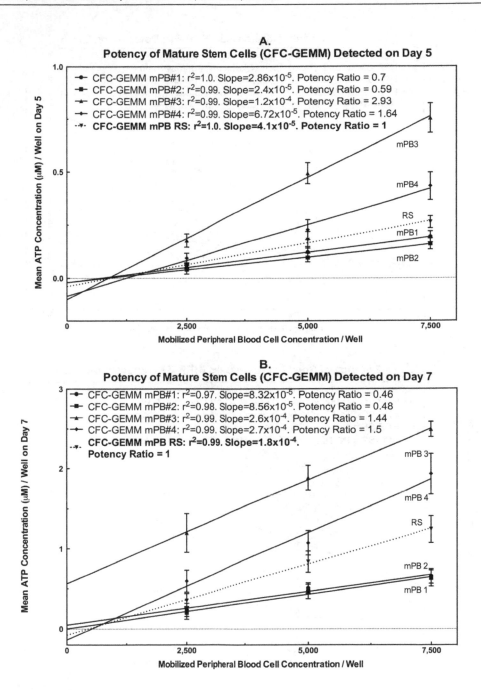

Fig. 1A and 1B. Measurement of Mobilized Peripheral Blood CFC-GEMM Stem Cell Potency on 5 and 7 Days of Culture.

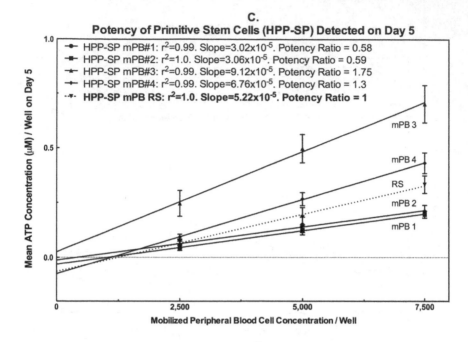

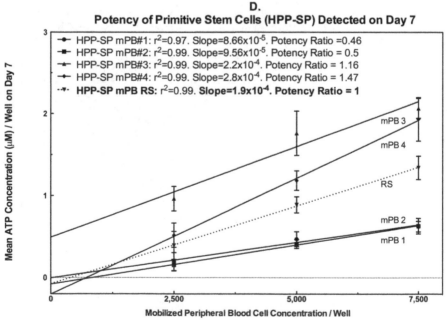

Fig. 1C and 1D. Measurement of Mobilized Peripheral Blood HPP-SP Stem Cell Potency on 5 and 7 Days of Culture.

In addition to the samples, a mPB RS was also included and allows the potency ratio to be calculated as follows:

Potency Ratio = Slope of the sample linear regression / Slope of the RS linear regression.

The potency ratio therefore provides information on the dose required to obtain the same response as the RS. Since the potency of the RS is always 1, samples with a potency ratio less than 1 will require larger cell doses to produce the same response, while potency ratios greater than 1 will require fewer cells to produce the same response as the RS.

3.2 Step 2 – The relationship between stem cell potency and quality

The results in Fig. 1 illustrate two fundamental concepts that are necessary for measuring stem cell potency and quality. The first concept is that the slope of the cell dose response should be greater for the more primitive stem cells (HPP-SP) than for the mature hematopoietic stem cells (CFC-GEMM), since the former have greater proliferation potential than the latter. The slope of the cell dose response therefore provides a direct measurement of stem cell proliferation potential. The greater the proliferation potential, the greater the potency. Thus, the slope of the cell dose response is also a direct measurement of potency. The second concept, also illustrated in Fig. 1, shows that as the slope increases at a specific cell dose, there is a concomitant increase in ATP concentration. This is a measure of stem cell quality.

The result of combining these two concepts is shown in Figures 2A and 2B for CFC-GEMM and HPP-SP stem cell populations, respectively. The figures show that when the ATP concentration at a specific cell dose (in this case 5,000 cells/well) is plotted against the slope of the cell dose response linear regression for both stem cell populations cultured for either 5 or 7 days, there is a direct correlation between stem cell potency and quality. As a result, both stem cell potency and quality have to be taken into account to determine if the stem cell product conforms to specific, but arbitrary, acceptance values and can therefore be released for use.

3.3 Step 3 – Using stem cell potency and quality to determine release criteria

Figure 3A and 3B shows the ability of CFC-GEMM and HPP-SP to proliferate at 5,000 cells/well after 5 and 7 days of culture, respectively. It had previously been found that, after 5 days in culture, an ATP concentration below 0.04µM indicated that cells could not sustain proliferation. At 7 days, this threshold was increased to 0.12µM. After 5 days of culture, the ATP concentration of samples 1 and 2 demonstrated minimal proliferation, but greater than the 0.04µM threshold. After 7 days of culture, proliferation of both samples had increased, together with samples 3 and 4. If release criteria were based solely on stem cell quality or proliferation ability, it would be assumed that all 4 samples might be acceptable for release. However, Fig. 2 demonstrates that both stem cell quality and potency have to be considered as part of the release criteria.

Figure 3C shows the cumulative potency ratios of both CFC-GEMM and HPP-SP after 5 days and 7 days (Fig. 3D) in culture. Since the potency of the CFC-GEMM and HPP-SP reference standards is always 1, samples 1 and 2 exhibited potency ratios significantly less than the reference standard. In contrast, samples 3 and 4 exhibited both high stem cell quality and potency after 5 and 7 days of culture. Based on these results, mPB samples 1 and 2 would be sub-optimal or rejected, while samples 3 and 4 would be acceptable for use.

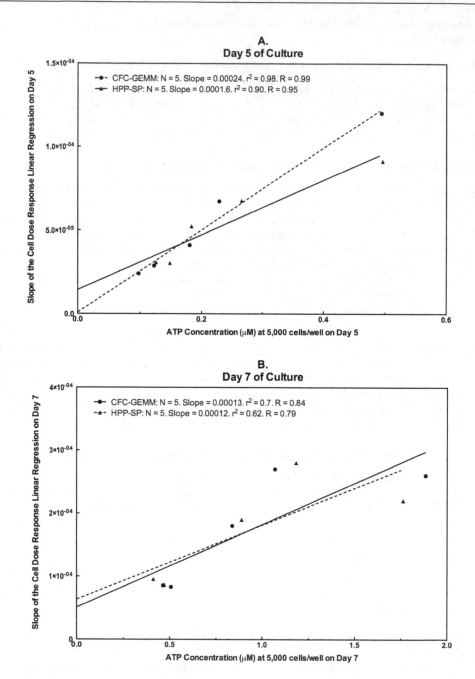

Fig. 2. Relationship Between Stem Cell Potency and Quality for Mobilized Peripheral Blood CFC-GEMM and HPP-SP Detected on Day 5 or 7 of Culture.

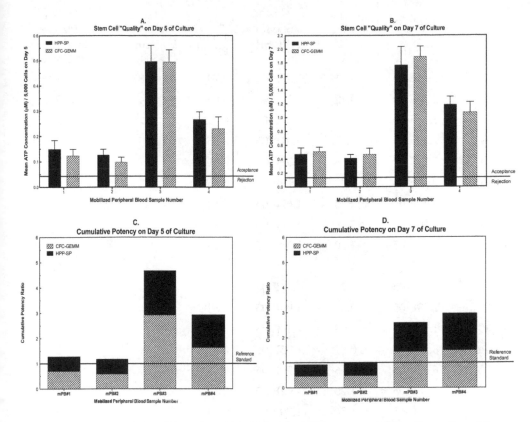

Fig. 3. Combining Mobilized Peripheral Blood Stem Cell Potency and Quality to Provide Release Criteria.

3.4 Umbilical cord blood stem cell potency, quality and release and the relationship to engraftment potential

A total of 28 UCB samples were analyzed for potency and quality using the same procedure described for mPB above, except that all assays were terminated after 5 days in culture, rather than performing both 5 and 7 day cultures. A 3-point cell dose response was performed for both the CFC-GEMM and HPP-SP stem cell populations and the slope of the linear regression was calculated for each cell dose response. The respective potency ratio for each CFC-GEMM and HPP-SP sample was then calculated using a UCB reference standard that was prepared from cord blood unit cells that did not meet the necessary criteria for storage. The slopes and potency ratios for each stem cell population are shown in Table 1. Also shown are the reported times to neutrophil and platelet engraftment. For one sample (sample 10), insufficient cells were obtained to perform a cell dose response for both stem cell populations. In two other samples (samples 18 and 25), insufficient cells were obtained after thawing to perform a HPP-SP stem cell dose response.

Sample Number	Slope for CFC-GEMM	Potency Ratio for CFC-GEMM	Slope for HPP-SP	Potency Ratio for HPP-SP	Days to Neutrophil Engraftment (>500/ul)	Days to Platelet Engraftment (>50k/ul)
1	2.94E-05	2.91	2.23E-05	0.70	28	237
2	3.14E-05	3.12	2.19E-05	0.69	14	2
3	1.41E-05	1.40	1.01E-05	0.31	6	45
4	2.09E-05	2.07	3.04E-05	0.95	30	49
5	2.19E-05	2.18	2.59E-05	0.81	17	39
6	9.28E-06	0.92	1.79E-05	0.56	12	9
7	2.25E-05	2.23	1.67E-05	0.52	17	45
8	2.50E-05	2.48	1.48E-05	0.46	22	39
9	1.52E-05	1.50	9.70E-06	0.30	56	13
10	IE	-	IE	-	43	103
11	1.77E-05	1.75	9.39E-06	0.29	34	7
12	2.83E-05	2.81	1.99E-05	0.62	20	26
13	1.09E-05	1.08	7.43E-06	0.23	NE	NE
14	8.12E-06	0.81	3.55E-06	0.11	19	183
15	6.69E-06	0.66	4.77E-06	0.15	31	122
16	1.26E-05	1.25	1.02E-05	0.32	13	39
17	1.81E-05	1.80	1.90E-05	0.60	5	40
18	3.07E-05	3.05	IE	-	NE	NE
19	2.01E-05	1.99	4.45E-05	1.39	27	38
20	2.52E-05	2.50	3.18E-05	1.00	22	62
21	1.54E-05	1.53	3.30E-05	1.03	29	55
22	2.31E-05	2.29	3.30E-05	1.03	18	23
23	1.20E-05	1.19	1.70E-05	0.53	28	70
24	1.63E-05	1.62	2.22E-05	0.70	15	46
25	1.46E-05	1.45	IE	-	26	39
26	2.12E-05	2.10	2.73E-05	0.85	28	61
27	1.37E-05	1.35	1.74E-05	0.54	37	126
28	1.50E-05	1.49	2.16E-05	0.68	114	113

IE = Insufficient cells to perform cell dose response. NE = No engraftment.

Table 1. Stem Cell Proliferation Potential / Potency Characteristics and Time to Engraftment of 28 Umbilical Cord Blood Samples.

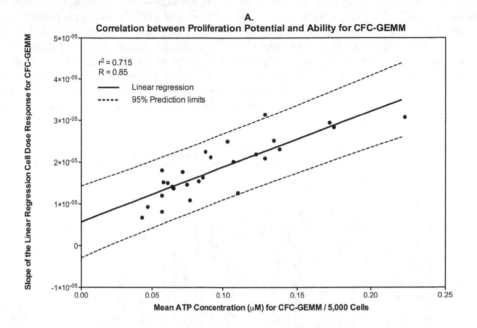

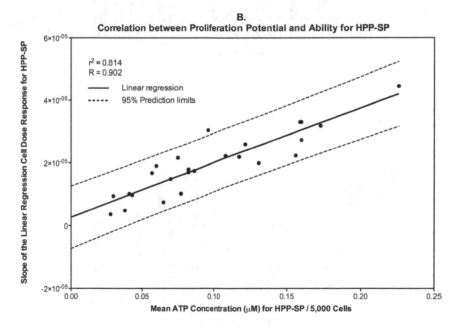

Fig. 4. Correlation Between Proliferation Potential (Potency) and Proliferation Ability (Quality) for CFC-GEMM and HPP-SP Stem Cells from Umbilical Cord Blood.

Figures 4A and 4B show the correlation of ATP concentrations at 5,000 cells/well with the slope of the UCB dose response for both CFC-GEMM and HPP-SP stem cell populations. The correlation coefficient (R) for HPP-SP was greater than that for CFC-GEMM, but the correlation for both stem cell populations was statistically significant (p < 0.001). The relationship between stem cell potency and quality is an indication that both parameters have to be taken into consideration when defining release criteria. Although stem cell quality could be ascertained for sample 10, insufficient cells were available to measure stem cell potency. Insufficient cells for samples 18 and 26 were also the reason why potency could not be determined for the HPP-SP stem cell population.

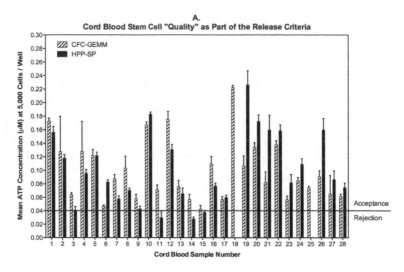

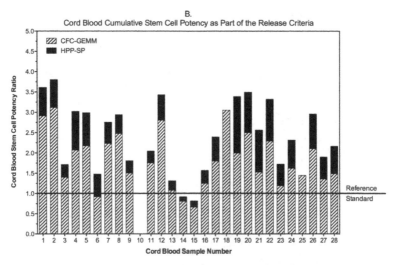

Fig. 5. Combining Umbilical Cord Blood Stem Cell Potency and Quality to Provide Release Criteria.

Figure 5A shows the stem cell quality (proliferation ability at a specific cell dose) and Fig. 5B, the cumulative stem cell potency ratio (proliferation potential measured as the slope of the linear regression of the cell dose response and compared to that of the reference standard) for each of the stem cell populations. Samples 18 and 25 only show the potency for the CFC-GEMM populations since insufficient cells were available to measure the potency of the more primitive HPP-SP population. For 21 of the samples, stem cell quality of both populations was greater than the arbitrary ATP concentration cutoff level of 0.04μM, below which cells cannot sustain proliferation. The same 21 samples also exhibited a cumulative potency above the RS potency of 1. Sample 6 exhibited a CFC-GEMM potency below the RS, while sample 13 demonstrated a CFC-GEMM potency slightly greater than the RS. However, the additional potency provided by the HPP-SP stem cell populations increased the cumulative potency above that of the RS.

It is now possible to consider the interpretation of the results. Samples 14 and 15 pose an interesting anomaly. The CFC-GEMM quality is below the ATP concentration cutoff point for both samples and slightly greater than the cutoff point for HPP-SP. However, both samples exhibit a cumulative potency below the RS. These results would indicate that both sample 14 and 15 would exhibit limited or no engraftment potential. From Table 1, the time to neutrophil engraftment for sample 14 was only 19 days while that for sample 15 was 31 days. Platelet engraftment was 183 and 122 days for sample 14 and 15, respectively. Therefore, these two samples did not agree with the reported clinical outcome. Table 1 also shows that samples 13 and 18 did not engraft. As described above, sample 13 exhibited a CFC-GEMM potency that was in a questionable range and may not have provided the necessary short-term engraftment and reconstitution. In contrast, sample 18, appeared to exhibit sufficient CFC-GEMM quality and potency, although insufficient cells did not allow information to be obtained for the primitive HPP-SP stem cell population. Despite the four sample outliers, the assay exhibits an accuracy of greater than 85%. Nevertheless, further studies that correlate *in vitro* data with more detailed clinical outcome for both engraftment and reconstitution would be prudent to ascertain a range for both stem cell quality and potency that would improve the accuracy of the assay.

3.5 Correlation between the ATP concentration and TNC, MNC, viability, CD34

There was no correlation between the ATP concentration for both cord blood stem cell populations with either dye exclusion viability or CD34+ counts. This was to be expected since neither viability nor CD34 membrane expression are cell functionality or proliferation markers. However, ATP concentration did correlate with both the TNC and MNC, but only when calculated on a per kilogram patient body weight basis. These results are shown in Fig. 6A for TNC and 6B for MNC. In both cases, the ATP concentration was calculated based on the patient body weight of the number of cells transplanted. The results in Fig. 6A demonstrate that when TNC is used, a strong correlation is obtained for the CFC-GEMM, but although still statistically significant, the primitive HPP-SP stem cell population exhibited a lower correlation coefficient. In contrast, Fig. 6B shows that the correlation between the ATP concentration and the MNC, both based on kilogram body weight, for CFC-GEMM and HPP-SP is highly significant with lower variation compared to the TNC values. The results clearly demonstrate that the greater the number of cells transplanted, the greater the number of stem cells transplanted that can exhibit proliferation ability. However, the results also demonstrates that using the mononuclear cell count rather than total nucleated cell count produces a better estimate for the stem cell response. However, cell counts alone cannot be used as a potency assay and cannot replace the information and value provided by a standardized cell functionality assay.

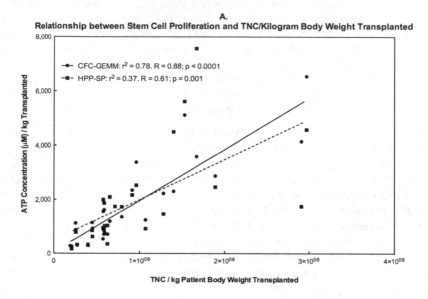

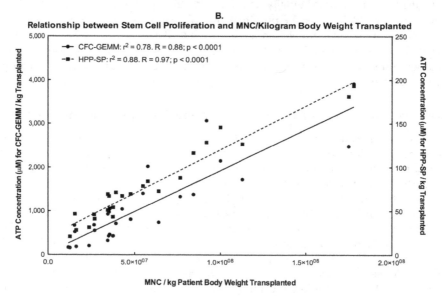

Fig. 6. Correlation between ATP Concentration as a Measure of Stem Cell Proliferation and the Number of Cord Blood Cells Transplanted Expressed as either Total Nucleated Cell Counts (TNC) or Mononuclear Cell Counts (MNC)/Kilogram Body Weight.

4. Discussion

For biopharmaceutical products, potency is measured by comparing the dose response to that of an established RS (Thorpe et al. 1999; Lansky, 1999; FDA, 2011). For these materials, a parallel dose response to that of the RS should be obtained (Thorpe et al, 1999; Gottscalk & Dunn, 2005; Jonkman & Sidik, 2009). Lack of parallelism indicates either contamination or a different material to that of the RS. When the dose response curves are parallel to the RS, the horizontal displacement to the left or right indicates a greater or lower potency, respectively. The dose of the compound can be compared and, if necessary, adjusted to that of the reference standard. In this way, the same dose can always be used with compound batches of different potency.

Cells, in particular, stem cells, pose significant differences and challenges to this paradigm. First, unlike biopharmaceutical products, where relatively large quantities of the material would be available to establish several batches of reference standards, it might be extremely difficult to establish cell reference standards (Strong et al. 2009; Rayment & Williams, 2010). There are several alternatives to establishing reference standards for cell therapeutics that have already been discussed above. However, a prerequisite for establishing reference standards and to compare results within and between laboratories is the use of a standardized and validated assay that is sufficiently robust so that it can be transferred and established in different laboratories. Lack of such an assay has been the reason why laboratories have not been able to directly compare processing, cryopreservation and thawing procedures for hematopoietic and other stem cell therapeutic products prior to use.

It might be argued that the present study should have been performed in parallel with the CFU assay. This has been the functional assay used previously in hematopoietic stem cell processing laboratories and is still used by the cord blood community today. More recently, the CFU assay has been suggested as a potency assay (Page et al. 2011a, 2011b), in addition to other parameters normally measured. These include total nucleated cell count (TNC), viability and CD34 membrane expression (FDA, 2009). There were three reasons for not performing parallel studies using the CFU assay. First, the ATP bioluminescence assay was originally derived from the methylcellulose CFU assay. Unlike the CFU assay, however, the ATP assay has undergone several major technical advances culminating in the assay used for the present study. It was also previously shown that even the methylcellulose-free format used in this study is not only equivalent to the original CFU assay, but is clearly a more reliable, reproducible and robust assay (Rich, 2007, Reems et al, 2008). Furthermore, lower sensitivity and precision (high variations) of the CFU assay, coupled with the lack of standardization (see below), would have resulted in inconclusive results. Second, unlike the CFU assay, the ATP assay can and has been validated in compliance with bioanalytical regulatory requirements (FDA, 2001). Furthermore, for an assay to be a potency assay, the regulatory agencies require demonstration of specific assay characteristics (FDA, 2011). Assay validation is just one of these characteristics, but to validate an assay, standards and controls are required. The CFU assay lacks standards and controls and cannot be validated according to regulatory requirements. Finally, it is often assumed that the CFU assay measures proliferation, whereas the CFU assay is actually a clonogenic differentiation assay. Proliferation is certainly involved in the formation of hematopoietic colonies. However, the colonies produced in methylcellulose are identified and counted by the ability of the cells producing the colonies to differentiate and mature. Therefore, the CFU assay detects differentiation ability and/or potential, but does not measure a parameter that directly correlates with the stem cell proliferation process. Based on these and other characteristics (discussed below), the CFU assay was not considered as a comparison assay for this study.

Many factors affect the quality and potency of a cellular product. First, proportions of different stem cell populations originally present in the umbilical cord blood, their quality and potency, are an inherent property of the tissue. Second, the procedures used to collect and store the cells prior to processing can affect quality and potency. Third, different stem cell processing, cryopreservation and thawing procedures not only affect quality and potency, but the proportion of stem cells remaining in the product. Finally, the decision process to use a particular product should be based on trusted results that can only be obtained from an assay(s) that is quantitative, standardized and validated to measure quality and potency of the active stem cell ingredients.

The stem cell potency assay described above is based on performing a minimum 3-point cell dose response and comparing the slope of the resulting linear regression to that of a RS of the same material. Comparison of cell dose response slopes to calculate the potency ratio was used for two reasons. First, measurement of potency of a biopharmaceutical compound usually relies on establishing parallelism between the sample and RS dose response curves. When the linear portions of the dose response curve are parallel, not only is this an indication that the sample and RS are of the same material, but also allows the potency ratio to be calculated from the horizontal displacement between the two dose response curves. If cells, and stem cells in particular, exhibit parallel cell dose response curves, this is an indication that both the sample and RS stem cells demonstrate a similar "stemness" or primitiveness. The resulting parallel displacement indicates a difference, not in potency, but in stem cell number between the sample and RS. Since hematopoiesis is a continuously proliferating system and the cells are continuously in flux, it follows that very few hematopoietic stem cell samples will exhibit exactly the same degree of primitiveness to the cells in the RS. Therefore potency measurement by parallelism will not provide a general procedure to calculate the potency ratio. Since an assay should show linearity within a specific cell concentration range, measuring the slope of the cell dose response not only demonstrates assay linearity characteristics, but also provides a direct measurement of stem cell primitiveness and proliferation potential, which in turn, is equivalent to stem cell potency. By comparing the slope of the sample cell dose response with that of the RS, the potency ratio can be calculated. Depending on the stem cell population detected, more primitive stem cells will show a steeper slope to that of mature stem cells. This procedure can then be used for any proliferating cell population. A 3-point cell dose response is the minimum number of data points that can be used to perform linear regression analysis. Although a larger number of points could also be used and would be more accurate, it was necessary to take into account that for hematopoietic tissues (and other cellular therapeutic products), cell availability is limited. Potency measurement should be performed just prior to use, since it is related to the dose that is to be administered. From a practical viewpoint, a cord blood potency determination would be performed on the limited number of cells thawed in a segment used for confirmatory testing prior to the cord blood unit being transplanted. Several publications have shown, using TNC, viability, CD34 and CFU, that segments of cryopreserved cord blood used for confirmatory testing are a representative sample of the cells in the cord blood unit (Goodwin et al. 2003; Solves et al. 2004, Rodriguez et al. 2005; Page et al. 2011b). However, in all of these cases, the potency of the active ingredients, i.e. the stem cells, were not taken into account.

A potency assay requires that all active ingredients be measured (FDA, 2011). This is relatively easy for a biopharmaceutical compound, but is impossible for a continuously proliferating system such as hematopoiesis. Although a hematopoietic stem cell tissue may contain many different cell types, the stem cells are the only cells responsible for engraftment and reconstitution. The stem cells are therefore the active ingredients for which the potency must be measured. Since the hematopoietic stem cell compartment consists of a continuum of stem cells and assays are not yet available to test each and every stem cell subpopulation, the regulatory requirement to measure all active ingredients, cannot be met at the present time. As an alternative, the quality and potency of a minimum of two different stem cell populations have been determined; the primitive HPP-SP and the more mature CFC-GEMM stem cell populations. As shown in Fig. 5, the potency of a single stem cell population would be insufficient and could lead to a false interpretation of the results. As also demonstrated in Fig. 5, even a minimum of two stem cell populations may result in a false interpretation, but the accuracy is significantly greater than if the potency of only one stem cell population was measured. It is certainly possible to reliably and reproducibly measure the quality and potency of more than two stem cell populations with present technology. However, this has to be weighed against the use of larger numbers of cells and the costs associated with testing. It should also be emphasized that potency and quality testing need to be performed on the cryopreserved sample intended for use. They provide predictive information for release. It is therefore reasonable to pose the question, is it preferable to use more cells for a predictive assay that might ensure stem cell functionality, engraftment potential and growth than to use fewer cells and not perform any assay?

In this respect, it is worth returning to the tests and assays presently used to characterize the cells in the processing laboratory. These are TNC, viability and viable CD34+ counts. These three parameters have been designated as measurements of potency for umbilical cord blood (FDA, 2009), despite the fact that they do not comply with the necessary regulations for a potency assay, especially since none of the parameters are functional assays and measure the active ingredients. Of the three parameters listed above, probably the most important is the TNC dose. However, the TNC count includes a large proportion of cells that play no role in engraftment. Inclusion of these cells actually results in a dilution of the active stem cell ingredients. In contrast to using TNC, removing most of the unnecessary cells to produce an MNC fraction that contained the pool of stem cells, it was possible to demonstrate that the MNC dose used for transplantation exhibited a greater correlation with the ATP dose for both the CFC-GEMM and HPP-SP stem cell populations (Fig. 6). This result illustrates that the ATP concentration can be used as a measure of stem cell dose, which in turn is related to the potency ratio.

The potency predicts the dose of the product for the intended use. The potency of a stem cell product should predict the dose of stem cells required to achieve engraftment. In other words, stem cell potency predicts engraftment potential. This should not be confused with, and is not the same as time to engraftment. If the slope of the stem cell linear regression dose response curves or the stem cell potency ratios provided in Table 1 is plotted against the time to engraftment, no correlation will be obtained. This is because potency is entirely dependent upon stem cell proliferation potential, while time to engraftment is dependent upon the differentiation and maturation of hematopoietic progenitor cells into neutrophils, platelets and erythrocytes. This is the reason why the presence and number of progenitor cell colonies counted in the CFU assay, especially GM-CFC and Mk-CFC, relates to the appearance and number of neutrophils and platelets in the circulation of the patient (Page et al. 2011a).

Although the number of UCB transplants has increased almost exponentially since the first published UCB transplant in 1989 (Gluckman et al. 1989), approximately 20% of patients receiving an unrelated UCB transplant exhibit graft failure (Page et al. 2011a, 2011b). This has, in part, been attributed to inadequate UCB potency (Page et al. 2011a, 2011b). Previous publications have focused on the need for standardized laboratory procedures (Rich, 1997; Wagner E et al. 2006; Brand A et al. 2008). A recent publication by Spellman et al. (2011) discusses problems facing the cord blood community and the guidelines and requirements for "standardized testing methodologies" to be established. The cell-based, ATP bioluminescence assay platform described in this communication to measure both stem cell potency and quality and, in addition, help define release criteria, constitutes the next generation of assays that addresses all of the necessary requirements including, but not limited to, standardized methodology, reproducibility with limited variability between testing sites, automated testing outputs, high throughput capability and rapid turnaround time.

5. Conclusions

It is often the case that an assay will be generic and adapted to fit the intended application. The present communication describes an assay that has been specifically designed and validated for the purpose of measuring stem cell quality and potency for hematopoietic cellular therapeutic products derived from mobilized peripheral blood, umbilical cord blood and even bone marrow (data not shown). A similar potency and quality assay has also been developed for mesenchymal stem cells. The assays incorporate an instrument-based, biochemical marker in the form of ATP, the concentration of which is directly proportional to the proliferation ability and potential of the stem cell populations being measured. The bioluminescence signal detection system is the most sensitive, non-radioactive readout available allowing the assay to incorporate external standards and controls. The implementation of a fully compliant potency and quality assay specific for hematopoietic stem cell products should not only help standardize cell processing procedures, but also reduce the risk of graft failure and improve safety and efficacy for the patient.

6. References

Botnick LE, Hannon EC, Hellman S. (1979). Nature of the hematopoietic stem cell compartment and its proliferative potential. Blood Cells. 5:195-210.

Brand A, Eichler H, Szczepiorkowski ZM, Hess JR, Kekomaki E, McKenna DH, PamphilionD, Reems J, Sacher RA, Takahashi TA, van der Watering LM (2008). Viability does not necessarily reflect the hematopoietic cell potency of a cord blood unit: results ofan interlaboratory exercise. Transfusion. 48:546-549.

Broxmeyer HE, Douglas GW, Hangoc C, Cooper S, Bard J, English D, Arny M, Thomas L, Boyse EA. (1989) Human umbilical cord blood as a potential source of transplantable hematopoietic stem/progenitor cells. Proc Natl Acad Sci USA 86:3828-3832.

Charbord P. (1994). Hemopoietic stem cells: analysis of some parameters critical for engraftment. Stem Cells. 12:545-62.

Civin CI, Almeida-Porada G, Lee MJ, Olweus J, Testappen LW, Zanjani ED. (1996). Sustained, retransplantable, multilineage engraftment of highly purified adult human bone marrow stem cells in vivo. Blood. 88:4102-9.

DeLong ER, Vernon WB, Bollinger RR. (1985). Sensitivity and specificity of a monitoring test. Biometrics. 41:947-58.

Duggan PR, Guo D, Luider J, Auer I, Klassen J, Chaudhry A, Morris D, Glueck S, Brown CB, Russell JA, Stewart DA. (2000). Predictive factors for long-term engraftment of autologous blood stem cells. Bone Marrow Transplant. 26:1299-304.

European Medicines Agency (EMA) (2008). Guideline on potency testing of cell based immunotherapy medicinal products for the treatment of cancer. http://www.tga.gov.au/pdf/euguide/bwp27147506en.pdf.

FDA Guidance for Industry. (2009). Minimally manipulated, unrelated allogeneic placental/umbilical cord blood intended for hematopoietic reconstitution for specified indication.
http://www.fda.gov/downloads/BiologicsBloodVaccines/GuidanceCompliance RegulatoryInformation/Guidances/Blood/UCM187144.pdf.

Gluckman E, Broxmeyer HA, Auerbach AD, Friedman HS, Douglas GW, Devergie A, Esperou H, Thierry D, Socie G, Lehn P, Scott Cooper BS, English D, Kurtzberg J, Bard J, Boyse EA. (1989). Hematopoietic reconstitution in a patient with Fanconi's anemia by means of umbilical-cord blood from an HLA-identical sibling. N Engl J Med. 321:1174-1178.

Goodwin HS, Grunzinger LM, Regan DM, McCormick KA, Johnson CE, Oliver DA, Muecki KA, Alonso JM, Wall DA. (2003). Long term cryostorage of UC blood units: ability of the integral segment to confirm both identity and hematopoietic potential. Cytotherapy. 5:80-86.

Gottschalk PG, Dunn JR. (2005). Measuring parallelism, linearity, and relative potency in bioassay and immunoassay data. J Biopharma Stat. 15:437-463.

Haas R, Ho AD, Bredthauer U, Cayeux S, Egerer G, Knauf W & Hunstein W. (1990). Successful autologous transplantation of blood stem cells mobilized with recombinant human granulocyte-macrophage colony-stimulating factor. Exp Hematol. 18:94-98.

Hall KM & Rich IN. (2009). Bioluminescence assays for assessing potency of cellular therapeutic products, In: Cellular Therapy: Principles, Methods and Regulations, Areman EM & Loper K, 581-591. AABB. ISBN 978-1-56395-296-8. Bethesda, MD.

Jonkman JN, Sidik, K. (2009). Equivalence testing for parallelism in the four-parameter logistic model. J Biopharma Stat. 19:818-37.

Koerbling M, Holle R, Haas R, Knauf W, Doerken B, Ho AS, Kuse R, Pralle H, Fliedner TM, Hunstein W. (1990). Autologous blood stem cell transplantation in patients with advanced Hodgkin's disease and prior radiation to the pelvic site. J Clin Oncol. 8:978-985.

Lansky D. (1999). Validation of bioassay for quality control. Dev Biol Stand. 97:157-68.

Leung W, Ramirez M, Civin CI. (1999). Quantity and quality of engrafting cells in cord blood and autologous mobilized peripheral blood. Biol Blood Marrow Transplant. 5:69-76.

National Marrow Donor Program (NMDP). http://www.marrow.org/PHYSICIAN/URD_Search_and_Tx/Number_of_Alloge neic_Tx_Perfor/index.html#grafts.

Olaharski AJ, Uppal H, Cooper M, Platz S, Zabka TS, Kolaja KL. (2009). In vitro to in vivo concordance of a high throughput assay for bone marrow toxicity across a diverse set of drug candidates. Toxicol Let 188:98-103.

Page KM, Zhang L, Mendizabai A, Weasse S, Carter S, Gentry T, Balber E, Kurtzberg J. (2011a). Total colony-forming units are a strong, independent predictor of neutrophil and platelet engraftment after unrelated umbilical cord blood transplantation: A single-center analysis of 435 cord blood transplants. Biol Blood Marrow Transplant. (Jan 28. Epub ahead of print).

Page KM, Zhang L, Mendizabai A, Weasse S, Carter S, Shoulars K, Gentry T, Balber E, Kurtzberg J. (2011b). The cord blood Apgar: a novel scoring system to optimize selection of banked cord blood grafts for transplantation. (2011b). Transfusion. (Aug. 2. Epub ahead of print).

Pasquini MC & Wang Z. (2010). Current use and outcome of hematopoietic stem cell transplantation. CIBMTR Summary Slides, 2010. http://www.cibmtr.org/ReferenceCenter/SlidesReports/SummarySlides/pages/index.aspx#CiteSummarySlides.

Picardi A, Arcese W. (2010). Quality assessment of cord blood units selected for unrelated transplantation: a transplant center perspective. Transfus Apher Sci. 42:289-97.

Querol S, Gomez SG, Pagliuca A, Torrabadella M, Madrigal JA. (2010). Quality rather than quantity: the cord blood bank dilemma. Bone Marrow Transplant. 45:970-8.

Rayment EA & Williams DJ. (2010). Concise rewiew: Mind the gap: challenges in characterizing and quantifying cell- and tissue-based therapies for clinical translation. Stem Cells. 28:996-1004.

Reems J-A, Hall KM, Gebru LH, Taber G, Rich IN. (2008). Development of a novel assay to evaluate the functional potential of umbilical cord blood progenitors. Transfusion. 48:620-628.

Rich IN & Hall KM. (2005). Validation and development of a predictive paradigm for hemotoxicity using a multifunctional bioluminescence colony-forming proliferation assay. Tox Sci. 87:427-41.

Rich IN, Kubanek B. (1982). The effect of reduced oxygen tension on colony formation of erythropoietic cells in vitro. Brit J Haematol. 52:579-88.

Rich IN. (1997). Standardization of the CFU-GM assay using hematopoietic growth factors. J. Hematother. 6:191-193.

Rich IN. (2003). In vitro hematotoxicity testing in drug development: A review of past, present, and future applications. Curr Opinion Drug Disc Devel. 6:100-109.

Rich IN. (2007). High-throughput in vitro hemotoxicity testing and in vitro cross-platform comparative toxicity. Expert Opin. Drug Metab Toxicol. 3:295-307.

Rodriguez L, Garcia J, Querol S. (2005). Predictive utility of the attached segment in the quality control of a cord blood graft. Biol Blood Marrow Transplant. 11:247-251.

Santos GW, Sensenbrenner LL, Burke PJ, Mullins GM, Vias WB, Tutschka PJ & Slavin RE. (1972). The use of cyclophosphamide for clinical transplantation. Transplant Proc. 4:559-564.

Santos GW. (1983). History of bone marrow transplantation. Clin Haematol. 12:611-639.

Sohn SK, Kim JG, Seo KW, Chae YS, Jung JT, Suh JS, Lee KB. (2002). GM-CSF-based mobilized effect in normal healthy donors for allogeneic peripheral blood stem cell transplantation. Bone Marrow Transplant. 30:81-86.

Solves P, Planelles D, Mirabet V, Blasco I, Carbonell-Uberos F, Soler MA, Roig RJ. (2004) Utility of bag segment and cryovial samples for quality and confirmatory HLA typing in umbilical cord blood banking. Clin Lab Haematol. 26:413-418.

Spellman S, Hurley CK, Brady C, Phillips-Johnson L, Chow R, Laughlin M, McMannis J, Reems J-A, Regan D, Rubinstein P, Kurtzberg J. (2011). Guidelines for the development and validation of new potency assays for the evaluation of umbilical cord blood. Cyotherapy (March, Epub ahead of print).

Strong M, Farrugia A & Rebulla P. (2009). Stem cell and cellular thereapy developments. Biologicals. 37:103-107.

Thomas ES, Buckner CD, Banaji M, Clift RA, Fefer A, Flournoy N, Goodell BW, Hickman RO, Lerner KG, Neiman PE, Sale GE, Sanders JE, Singer J, Stevens M, Storb R & Weiden PI. (1977).One hundred patients with acute leukemia treated by chemotherapy, total body irradiation, and allogeneic marrow transplantation. Blood. 49:511-533.

Thorpe R. Wadhwa M, Page C, Mire-Sluis A. (1999). Bioassays for the characterization and control of therapeutic cytokines; determination of potency. Dev Biol Stand. 97:61-71.

Till JE & McCulloch EA. (1971). A direct measurement of the radiation sensitivity of normal mouse bone marrow cells. Radiat Res. 175:145-149.

U.S. Food and Drug Administration (FDA) (2001). Guidance for Industry. Bioanalytical method validation.
    http://www.fda.gov/downloads/Drugs/GuidanceComplianceRegulatoryInfor mation/Guidances/ucm070107.pdf.

U.S. Food and Drug Administration (FDA) (2011). Guidance for Industry. Potency tests for cellular and gene therapy products.
    http://www.fda.gov/downloads/BiologicsBloodVaccines/GuidanceComplianceR egulatoryInformation/Guidances/CellularandGeneTherapy/UCM243392.pdf.

Wagner E. Duval M, Dalle JH, Morin H, Bizier S, Champagne J, Champagne MA. (2006) Assessment of cord blood unit characteristics on the day of transplant: comparison with data issued by cord blood banks. Transfusion. 46: 1190-1198.

Zubair AC, Kao G, Daley H, Schott D, Freedman A, Ritz J. (2006). CD34(+) CD38(-) and CD34(+) HLA-DR(-) cells in BM stem cell grafts correlate with short-term engraftment but have no influence on long-term hematopoietic reconstitution after autologous transplantation. Cytotherapy. 8:399-407.

9

Gene Therapy of Hematopoietic and Immune Systems: Current State and Perspectives

Maria Savvateeva[1], Fedor Rozov[1,2] and Alexander Belyavsky[1]
[1]Engelhardt Institute of Molecular Biology, Russian Academy of Sciences
[2]University of Oslo, Centre for Medical Studies Russia, Moscow
Russian Federation

1. Introduction

Hematopoietic stem cells (HSCs) present arguably the best entry point for gene therapy of hematopoietic and immune systems since genetically modified HSCs are long-lived and would eventually transfer the therapeutic constructs to all their descendants. However, gene therapy via HSCs, although conceptually simple, has proven to be a technically formidable problem that has yet to be solved successfully. Despite overtly positive results obtained in gene therapy experiments performed with mouse and larger animal models, these achievements did not translate into clinically acceptable outcomes for non-human primates and human patients, with exception of a few specific disease instances where a therapeutic gene brought about significant survival advantages to transduced cells (Cavazzana-Calvo et al., 2000, Schmidt et al, 2003). Major differences between outcomes of conceptually similar experiments in mice and primates underscore the notion that the fundamental principles governing functioning of hematopoietic system in small short-lived vs. larger long-lived animals differ significantly. Low degree of chimerism obtained in experiments with primates and humans is likely a result of intrinsically low efficiency of viral transduction of long-term repopulating (LTR) HSCs coupled with subsequent massive silencing of integrated constructs (Ellis, 2005; Horn et al, 2002). One may hypothesize that this situation reflects a better protection of hematopoietic system from external influences, in particular invasion of foreign genetic material, in longer-living animals.

However, our deepening knowledge of molecular mechanisms underlying functioning of HSCs within the organism provides hints as to what strategies may lead to the development of the efficient gene therapy via HSCs; some of these strategies are discussed below.

2. Improvements of vectors and ex vivo HSC transduction protocols

Numerous studies indicate that lentiviral vectors that are capable of transducing non-dividing cells may represent a more promising tool for introduction of genetic material into HSCs compared to retroviral vectors (Uchida et al, 1998, Case et al., 1999). This may be attributed to a largely quiescent nature of LTR HSCs, especially in larger animals (Cheshier et al., 1999, Shepherd et al., 2007). Since even lentiviral vectors transduce more efficiently dividing cells than quiescent ones (Trobridge et al., 2004), the current transduction protocols relied until recently on the use of culture conditions that induced entry of HSCs into cell cycle but incidentally failed to maintain their stem cell status (Bunting et al., 1999). This situation seems to have been ameliorated after introduction of transduction protocols that rely on the use of serum-free media that lack factors inducing SC differentiation (Mostoslavsky et al., 2005) and novel growth factors that better preserve cell stemness (Zhang C et al., 2008). It remains yet to see whether these improvements are sufficient to significantly increase the efficiency of HSC gene therapy in clinical settings.

3. Selection of genetically modified HSCs in vivo: Negative selection

As current efficiency of transduction of human LTR HSCs with viral vectors appears to be quite low and there are no clinically proven protocols for expansion of these cells ex vivo, the most promising solution at hand to this problem is an in vivo selection of modified cells after their transduction and re-transplantation back to a patient. Conceptually, one might distinguish negative and positive in vivo selection strategies. The first one can be defined as a strategy that is aimed at elimination of stem and progenitor cells that do not bear integrated functional constructs. Positive selection implies a strategy that does not target the construct-negative stem cells but rather provides selective survival and growth advantage to the cells that bear the inserted construct. The negative selection gains presently much of attention and seems to be better poised for a clinical advancement in the near future. Arguably, the most promising and advanced variant of negative selection is based on the use of O6-MGMT as a selection marker and various alkylating compounds as selection agents (Davis et al., 2000, Ragg et al., 2000). Using this approach and multiple rounds of selection in vivo, overall peripheral blood chimerism has been driven in mice and larger animal models to levels higher than 75%. However, the clinical applicability of this technique is as yet unclear, as recent experiments performed by two research teams with non-human primates using MGMT-mediated selection produced rather conflicting results. One team demonstrated successful implementation of this strategy in monkeys, although with selection efficiencies and chimerism rates highly variable between individual animals (Beard et al., 2010), whereas another team reported a rather negligible increase in chimerism rates upon selection in vivo (Larochelle et al., 2009).

Various implementations of negative selection strategy are listed in the Table 1.

4. Selection of genetically modified HSCs in vivo: Positive selection

Ongoing studies of the mechanisms controlling HSC self-maintenance and commitment continue to identify novel factors that bring about HSC expansion in vivo when over-expressed. A less than exhaustive set of these factors is listed in the Table 2. Arguably, the most extensively studied gene with such properties is the homeobox transcription factor HoxB4. Forced expression of HoxB4 in murine HSCs induces remarkable ex vivo and in vivo cell expansion without compromising their differentiation or inducing leukemic transformation (Sauvageau et al., 1995, Antonchuk et al., 2002). Similar effects were obtained using recombinant TAT-HOXB4 protein (Krosl et al., 2003). In some reports, HoxB4 and negative selection marker MGMT were used together to further increase percentage of modified HSCs (Chinnasamy et al., 2005). However, attempts to use HoxB4 for positive selection of HSCs in larger animals were much less successful, with a major expansion of short-term repopulating cells only (Zhang X et al., 2006). Besides, a significant number of leukemia occurrences apparently related to unregulated expression of HoxB4 were observed in these animals (Zhang X et al., 2008).

Slective marker	Selecting agent	Mode of action	References
O6-MGMT	BCNU, TMZ, other alkylating agents	MGMT protein functions to repair alkylated DNA caused by chemotherapeutic agents like BCNU or TMZ	Sawai et al, 2001; Zielske et al, 2003
Thymidylate synthase	5-fluorouracil (5-FU) 5-fluorodeoxy-uridine (5-FUdR)	Drug-resistant TS can protect bone marrow cells from 5-fluorouracil (5-FU) and related fluoropyrimidines that induce cessation of DNA and RNA synthesis, and subsequent cell death.	Bielas et al, 2009
Tyr22DHFR	Methotrexate	MTX acts on highly proliferative cells, blocking DNA synthesis through competitive inhibition of DHFR. Drug resistant dihydrofolate reductase such as Tyr22 (Tyr22DHFR) has the potential to selectively increase engraftment of gene-modified human hematopoietic cells	Gori et al, 2010
Multidrug resistance gene-1 (MDR)	Taxol, Paclitaxel	Overexpression of the multidrug resistance gene MDR1 in bone marrow cells results in protection from hematopoietic toxicity from chemotherapy drugs that are substrates for the MDR1 drug efflux pump	Cowan et al, 1999

Table 1. Strategies for negative selection of genetically modified HSC

Some other members of the HOX family, either alone or fused with specific cellular partners, are also able to induce expansion of hematopoietic progenitors in mice. Of particular importance is a fusion gene NUP98-HoxA10, which has a remarkable ability of multi-log expansion of murine repopulating cells ex vivo, exceeding that of HoxB4 (Ohta et al., 2007; Watts et al., 2011).

Recently, the powerful effect of overexpression of early acting transcription factor SALL4 on ex vivo expansion of human hematopoietic cells capable of long-term repopulation of NOD/SCID mice was demonstrated (Aguila et al., 2011). Significant ex vivo expansion could be also achieved using recombinant TAT-SALL4B protein.

There are at least a dozen of other genes that, when overexpressed, induce significant expansion of HSCs in mice in vivo. One of the most interesting groups of such factors are epigenetic regulators. Of particular interest is Bmi1, a member of Polycomb group, which is involved in regulation of maintenance of various adult stem cell types. Inactivation of Bmi1 leads to defect in HSC self-renewal (Park et al., 2003), whereas its enforced expression results a striking ex vivo expansion of multipotential progenitors and marked augmentation of HSC repopulating capacity in vivo (Iwama et al., 2004). In addition, enforced expression of Bmi1 in human CD34-positive cells leads to the ex vivo expansion of NOD/SCID repopulating cells (Rizo et al., 2008). Another Polycomb group gene that potentially could be used for positive selection is Ezh2; upon overexpression, it prevents HSC exhaustion (Kamminga et al., 2006). Forced expression of yet another epigenetic regulator, histone demethylase Fbxl10/Jhdm1b in HSCs abolishes exhaustion of the LTR HSCs following serial transplantation. This property of Ezh2 and Fbxl10/Jhdm1b makes them especially appropriate for schemes combining positive and negative selection since the latter one places very significant stress on hematopoietic system.

Another group of genes that might be used for positive selection are those that are frequently activated in predominant hematopoietic cell clones arising after retro- or lentiviral transduction, and are likely therefore to act as factors inducing in vivo expansion of these clones. The most prominent among such genes are MDS1/Evi-1 (Sellers et al., 2010; Métais & Dunbar, 2008), PRDM16 (Du et al., 2005; Ott et al., 2006) HMGA2 (Wang et al., 2010; Cavazzana-Calvo et al., 2010) and LMO2 (McCormack et al., 2003; McCormack et al., 2010). As a note of caution, forced expression of these genes may produce undesired effects; for example, expression of Evi-1 was reported to be associated with chromosomal instability (Stein et al., 2010).

In addition to protein factors, micro RNAs also have effect on HSC function and population size. In particular, miR-125a and miR-125b were shown to increase number of HSCs in vivo or enhance their repopulation capacity (Guo et al., 2010; Ooi et al., 2010).

Having focused on genes that expand stem cell population, one should not overlook another group of genes that exert an opposite effect, namely negative influence on HSC pool size. Thanks to RNA interference technology, suppression of gene expression in various cell types nowadays is nearly as simple as overexpression. If gene knockout or knockdown results in expansion of stem cell population, this property may potentially be used for positive selection. Among genes of interest in this respect are C/EBP alpha, Lnk and Nur77, to name a few. C/EBP alpha-deficient hematopoietic stem cells (HSCs) are hyperproliferative, have increased expression of Bmi-1 and enhanced competitive repopulating activity (Zhang et al. 2004; Heath et al., 2004). Inactivation of Lnk, inhibitory adaptor protein, leads to an expanded HSC pool with enhanced self-renewal (Bersenev et al., 2008). Mice with inactivation of both Nor-1 and Nur77 have abnormal expansion of HSCs and myeloid progenitors and develop lethal acute myeloid leukemia (AML).

Regardless of what gene is being used for positive selection, it is clear that its constitutive expression would eliminate one or more of the negative growth controls imposed on HSCs by organism, and thus increase risks of neoplastic transformation. Therefore, any clinically acceptable protocol for gene therapy using positive selection of transduced HSCs should be based on transient, tightly regulated gene expression. Given that positive selection, if correctly implemented, promises to provide significant advantages over negative selection schemes, further research into creation of robustly regulated expression systems for positive selection in HSCs seem to be fully warranted.

Gene	Observed effects	References
HOXB4	Overexpression of HoxB4 induces significant ex vivo and in vivo expansion of murine long-term repopulating HSCs.	Antonchuk et al., 2002; Sauvageau et al., 1995
NUP98-HOXA10	Enforced expression of NUP98-HOXA10 fusion protein results in significant expansion of murine repopulating cells ex vivo exceeding that of HoxB4.	Ohta et al., 2007; Watts et al., 2011
NF-Ya	Murine HSCs overexpressing NF-Ya demonstrate strongly increased in vivo repopulation.	Zhu et al., 2005
Bmi1	Enforced expression of Bmi1 leads to striking ex vivo expansion of multipotential progenitors and marked augmentation of HSC repopulating capacity in vivo.	Iwama et al., 2004; Rizo et al., 2008
Ezh2	Overexpression prevents exhaustion of long-term repopulating HSCs.	Kamminga et al., 2006
Fbxl10/Jhdm1b	Same as above.	Konuma et al., 2011
Jab1	Mice with Jab1 overexpression have expanded HSC pool and develop a myeloproliferative disease.	Mori et al., 2008
HMGA2	Frequently found in the vicinity of integrated constructs in gene therapy trials; HMGA2-expressing cells have growth advantage in competitive repopulation and serial transplantation.	Cavazzana-Calvo et al., 2010; Ikeda et al., 2011; Wang et al., 2010
Evi-1	Frequently found in the vicinity of integrated constructs in gene therapy trials.	Métais & Dunbar, 2008; Sellers et al., 2010
PRDM16	Frequently found in the vicinity of integrated constructs in gene therapy trials.	Du et al., 2005; Ott et al., 2006
Sall4	Enforced expression results in ex vivo expansion of long-term NOD/SCID repopulating cells.	Aguila et al., 2011
MicroRNAs miR-125a, miR-125b	Forced expression of miR-125a was capable of increasing the number of HSCs cells several-fold. Overexpression of miR-125b enhances HSC function, as judged by serial transplantation.	Guo et al., 2010; Ooi et al., 2010
Lnk	Mice with Lnk inactivation have an expanded HSC pool with enhanced self-renewal.	Bersenev et al., 2008
Nur77/NR4A1 & Nor-1/NR4A3	Mice with inactivation of both Nor-1 and Nur77 have abnormal expansion of HSCs and myeloid progenitors and develop lethal acute myeloid leukemia.	Mullican et al., 2007
C/EBPα	C/EBP alpha-deficient HSCs are hyperproliferative and have enhanced competitive repopulating activity.	Heath et al., 2004; Zhang P et al. 2004;
Latexin	Mouse strains expressing lower latexin levels have increased numbers of HSCs.	Liang et al., 2007

Table 2. Genes affecting in vivo expansion of HSCs

5. Expansion and selection of genetically modified HSCs ex vivo

Although much hope is currently invested into various schemes aimed at in vivo selection of gene-modified HSCs, a substantially simpler and arguably more elegant solution may be achieved if protocols for long-term culture and robust ex vivo expansion of HSCs could be developed. Very significant expansion of HSCs that occurs during embryonic development indicates that this might be eventually possible.

Over the last two decades, quite a few HSC culture protocols have been developed. The earlier established conditions involved cultivation in the presence of serum and cocktail of "classical" cytokines including SCF, IL3, IL6, FLT3L and TPO. Since bovine serum apparently contains factors that induce differentiation and/or apoptosis of HSCs, recent, more advanced protocols have been developed, which use defined, serum-free conditions that offer better reproducibility and minimize rapid loss of long-term repopulating HSCs during ex vivo culture and transduction with lenti- and retroviral vectors (Mostoslavsky et al., 2005).

In addition to classical cytokines, a number of new growth factors that have pronounced effect on HSC maintenance and expansion were identified in the last years. Among the most important are FGF1 (de Haan et al., 2003), IGFBP2 (Huynh et al., 2008), and several members of angiopoeitin-like family, in particular Angptl3 and 5 (Zhang et al., 2006).

Several major signaling pathways figuring prominently during embryonic development, in particular during specification of hematopoietic lineage, were shown to be important for adult HSC biology. Among those, Notch and Wnt pathways are currently considered as of the most immediate interest as far as HSC-niche interactions and ex vivo expansion are concerned. Stem and progenitor pool-enhancing properties of Notch signaling were demonstrated initially using constitutive Notch1 signaling in murine hematopoietic cells, which produced immortalized, cytokine-dependent stem cell-like cells (Varnum-Finney et al., 2000), and constitutive Notch4 signaling in human cord blood cells, which resulted in significant increase in cells repopulating immunodeficient mice (Vercauteren & Sutherland, 2004). Later on, culture of human CD34+ precursors with the immobilized Notch ligand Delta1 and cytokines was shown to result in a substantial increase in NOD/SCID-repopulating cells (Delaney et al., 2010); similar results were obtained for mouse cells with immobilized Jagged1 ligand (Toda et al., 2011).

As for Wnt signaling, initial studies indicated that overexpression of activated beta-catenin expanded the pool of HSCs in long-term cultures as judged by both phenotype and function. Wnt3a protein induced self-renewal of haematopoietic stem cells, whereas ectopic expression of inhibitors of the Wnt signalling pathway led to suppression of HSC growth in vitro and reduced reconstitution in vivo (Reya et al., 2003; Willert et al., 2003). Later publications demonstrated, though, that inactivation of the beta-catenin gene in bone marrow progenitors does not impair their ability to self-renew and reconstitute all hematopoietic lineages (Cobas et al., 2004), whereas activation of beta-catenin enforced cell cycle entry of hematopoietic stem cells, thus leading to exhaustion of the long-term stem cell pool (Sheller et al., 2006). Some recent studies demonstrate that it is the non-canonical Wnt signaling promoted by Wnt5a rather than the canonical one, that supports maintenance of competitive repopulating murine HSCs in culture (Buckley et al., 2011; Nemeth et al., 2007).

Yet another line of evidence indicates that activation of beta-catenin in the niche components rather than in HSCs may produce support of LTR cells ex vivo (Nemeth et al., 2009). Currently, there is little doubt that Wnt signaling plays important role in HSC biology, but the issue is apparently more complex than was implied by initial publications and remains highly controversial.

Other embryonic signaling pathways also might be exploited in HSC culture. Morphogens of the hedgehog family, namely Sonic and Indian hedgehogs, are able to support ex vivo expansion of human NOD/SCID repopulating cells (Bhardwaj et al., 2001; Kobune et al., 2004), despite the fact that in vivo Hedgehog signaling seems to not be necessary for adult murine hematopoietic stem cell function (Hofmann et al., 2009). BMP4, a member of BMP superfamily, is a critical component of the hematopoietic niche that regulates both HSC number and function (Goldman et al., 2009), and is able to expand NOD/SCID-repopulating cells in culture (Hutton et al., 2006).

In addition to the use of secreted proteins to for ex vivo HSC culture, one apparent trend of the last years is the application of low-molecular weight chemicals, in particular agonists or inhibitors of particular intracellular signaling pathways, for ex vivo culture. Thus, specific inhibitor of p38 kinase induces self-renewal and ex vivo expansion of HSCs as shown by the in vitro cobblestone area forming cell assay and serial transplantation (Wang et al., 2011). GSK-3β inhibitors, which stimulate Wnt signaling, were shown to promote engraftment of cultured HSCs (Ko et al., 2011; Trowbridge et al., 2006). Of significant clinical interest is the finding that ex vivo treatment with stabilized prostaglandin E2 enhances frequency of both hematopoietic progenitors and long-term repopulating HSCs present as analyzed by competitive transplantation (North et al., 2007). According to other data, only the short-term repopulating HSCs are expanded by this treatment, though (Frisch et al., 2009).

The initial studies demonstrating substantial degree of expansion of HSCs ex vivo relied the use of stromal cells as feeder layers (Moore et al., 1997). Based on the substantial progress in identification of HSC niches in bone marrow, there is currently a revival of interest in development of protocols for co-culture of HSC with stromal cell layers (Chou & Lodish, 2010; De Toni et al., 2011). These stromal cells produce a range of factors that significantly improve the maintenance and expansion of HSCs in culture, most likely by mimicking more or less successfully niche conditions. Very prominent components of the HSC niche are cell surface proteins, in particular cell adhesion molecules. The importance of cell-cell interactions was highlighted by the study by Wagner et al., 2007, indicating that maintenance of primitive hematopoietic progenitors by stromal lines is associated with expression of cell adhesion proteins rather than with secretory profiles of these lines. In particular, N-cadherin was shown to be an important component of the osteoblastic HSC niche (Zhang et al., 2003). However, importance of N-cadherin for HSC-niche interactions was later questioned (Kiel et al., 2007), thus rising substantial controversy. In an elegant in vitro study Lutolf et al. (2009) have shown that N-cadherin, as well as Wnt3a, are the only proteins among those tested that were capable of supporting self-renewal divisions of HSCs in vitro. N-cadherin expression was also shown to be important for maintenance of long-term repopulating cells in culture (Hosokawa et al., 2010). Ability of stromal cell line FMS/PA6-P to support primitive murine hematopoietic cells was found to depend critically on N-CAM expression (Wang et al., 2005). Yet another cell adhesion protein, namely mKirre, plays a prominent role in hematopoietic supportive capacity of OP9 stromal cells (Ueno et al., 2003).

Quite promising developments occur currently in the field of 3-D culture (Yuan et al., 2011; Tan et al., 2010; Miyoshi at el., 2011). Despite a relative paucity of data related to the 3-D culture of HSCs, available publications demonstrate significant advantages of this technique and indicate that in combination with correctly chosen or gene-modified stromal cell layers, 3-D culturing may eventually lead to creation of artificial niche that will be able to support substantial expansion of human HSCs ex vivo.

A question of paramount importance for the field is whether specific combinations of soluble factors will be able to attain a bone fide ex vivo expansion of HSCs, or this goal can only be achieved if specific cell surface proteins produced by the niche cells are also employed in the process, or perhaps the only way to the eventual success is the use of supporting stromal cell layers for ex vivo culture? As a number of molecules that contribute to the maintenance of HSCs in vitro and in vivo continues to rise, and there is a steady improvement in techniques for culturing HSCs, chances are that within a matter of a few years, key combination(s) of specific factors and modes of their application that can produce robust self-renewal and expansion of human HSC ex vivo will be identified. Table 3 provides a list, albeit incomplete, of factors and chemicals that, in addition to "classical" cytokines, are being used for maintenance and expansion of HSCs ex vivo.

6. Pre-conditioning and transplantation regimens

A common practice in the field of HSC gene therapy is a transduction of HSCs using viral vectors in the ex vivo setting. The advantages of this strategy include elimination of non-target transduction events, higher transduction efficiency and better control over the overall process. However, the opposite side of the coin in this case is the necessity for transduced cells to compete with the bone marrow-resident ones, which is likely to lower significantly the degree of chimerism after gene therapy. For efficient repopulation of hematopoietic system with gene-modified HSCs, extensive myeloablative treatments eliminating resident HSCs are usually performed. However, since these treatments are of generalized character and connected with substantial risks of morbidity and mortality, especially for elderly patients, they should preferably be avoided whenever possible. A combination of nonmyeloablative pre-conditioning of the recipient animals with in vivo selection strategy can be used to achieve substantial degrees of chimerism (Davis et al., 2000, Zielske et al., 2003). Additional ways to develop more appropriate pretreatment conditions involve the use of molecules that disrupt key signaling pathways within HSCs or niche components thus inducing HSC loss, as was shown for the case of inactivation of c-kit or mpl signaling by neutralizing antibodies (Czechowicz et al., 2007; Yoshihara et al., 2007), and for combined poly(I:C)/5-fluorouracil (5-FU) treatment (Sato et al., 2009). The other approach for nonmyeloablative HSC transplantation is based on disruption of HSC-niche interactions thus aiding in the stem cell mobilization (Chen et al., 2006). This alternative might grow into clinically relevant technique if the efficiency of current protocols for mobilization of HSCs is further improved. The more HSCs are mobilized into circulation and used for viral transduction, the higher is ratio of transduced vs. resident stem cells and better chances to achieve significant engraftment and chimerism of gene-modified cells without resorting to drastic myeloablative regimens. Although current combinations of mobilizing agents (Ramirez et al, 2009) demonstrate much higher mobilization rates than the initially used G-CSF, there is still a long way to go before this strategy may equal or surpass myeloablative pre-conditioning in its efficiency.

Factor	Observed effects	References
FGF1	FGF1 under serum-free conditions stimulates expansion of serially transplantable, long-term repopulating HSCs.	de Haan et al., 2003
Angptl2, 3 and 5	Proteins of angiopoeitin-like family provide 20- to 30-fold net expansion of long-term HSCs according to reconstitution analysis.	Zhang C et al., 2006
IGFBP2	IGFBP2 enhances ex vivo expansion of mouse HSCs.	Huynh et al., 2008
IL32	IL-32 significantly induces the proliferation of HSCs in culture.	Moldenhauer et al., 2011
Delta 1, Jagged1 (Notch ligands)	Culturing murine or human cells with surface-immobilized Notch ligands resulted in expansion of primitive hematopoietic population.	Delaney et al., 2010; Toda et al., 2011;
Wnt3a, Wnt10b (Wnt canonical pathway)	Wnt3a protein induces self-renewal of haematopoietic stem cells. Wnt10b enhances growth of hematopoietic precursors.	Willert et al., 2003; Congdon et al., 2010
Wnt5a (Wnt non-canonical pathway)	Wnt5a inhibits canonical Wnt signaling and supports maintenance of competitive repopulating murine HSCs in culture.	Nemeth et. al, 2007; Buckley et al., 2011
Shh, Ihh	Sonic hedgehog and Indian hedgehog support ex vivo expansion of human NOD/SCID repopulating cells.	Bhardwaj et al., 2001; Kobune et al., 2004
Bmp4	BMP4 expands NOD/SCID-repopulating cells in culture.	Hutton et al., 2006
TAT-HOXB4 fusion protein	TAT-HOXB4 protein produces significant ex vivo expansion of murine HSCs.	Krosl et al., 2003
TAT-NF-Ya fusion protein	TAT-NF-Ya protein treatment produces several-fold increase in the percentage of human cells repopulating immunodeficient mice.	Domashenko et al., 2010
TAT-SALL4B fusion protein	TAT-SALL4B fusion protein rapidly expands long-term NOD/SCID repopulating cells.	Aguila et al, 2011
Prostaglandin E2	Ex vivo incubation with PGE2 increases the frequency of long-term repopulating HSCs as measured by competitive transplantation.	North et al., 2007
SB203580	SB203580, specific p38 inhibitor, leads to increase in HSC self-renewal and ex vivo expansion.	Wang et al., 2011
StemRegenin 1	SR1, aryl hydrocarbon receptor antagonist, provides substantial increase in cells engrafting into immunodeficient mice.	Boitano et al., 2010
zVADfmk, zLLYfmk	Cord blood CD34+ cells cultured in presence of zVADfmk or zLLYfmk (inhibitors of caspases and calpains, respectively) have a higher ability for engraftment in NOD/SCID mice.	Imai et al., 2010; Sangeetha et al, 2010;
GSK-3 inhibitors	Pretreatment with GSK-3 inhibitors (BIO or CHIR-911) promotes engraftment and repopulation of ex vivo-expanded HSCs.	Ko et al., 2011; Trowbridge et al., 2006
Rapamycin	HSCs cultured in vitro in the presence of mTOR inhibitor rapamycin demonstrate enhanced engraftment.	Rohrabaugh et al., 2011
Copper helators	Copper chelator tetraethylenepentamine increases long-term ex vivo expansion and engraftment capabilities of blood progenitors.	Peled et al., 2004
N-cadherin	N-cadherin expression on stromal cells is important for maintenance of long-term repopulating cells in culture.	Hosokawa et al., 2010
N-CAM	N-CAM expression on stromal cells supports primitive murine hematopoietic cells.	Wang et al., 2005
mKirre	mKirre is responsible for hematopoietic supportive capacity of OP9 stromal cells.	Ueno et al., 2003

Table 3. Proteins and compounds affecting ex vivo maintenance and expansion of HSCs ("classical" cytokines not listed)

There are reports indicating that the engraftment of gene-modified stem cells might be significantly improved by their direct intra-bone transplantation (Mazurier et al., 2003). As irradiation commonly used for preconditioning also damages hematopoietic niche, in particular mesenchymal stem cells, HSC co-transplantation with MSCs was tested and showed promising results (Masuda et al., 2009).

Even a more radical departure from the accepted strategies for HSCs would be in situ transduction of HSCs using systemic or intra-bone delivery of viral vectors (McCauslin et al., 2003, Pan, 2009). Currently, this is a rather hypothetical approach due to serious safety concerns connected with potential off-target modifications of non-hematopoetic cells. However, this strategy alleviates the need for hazardous pre-conditioning treatments and will become a viable alternative with further development of modified viral envelops (Zhang X & Roth, 2010) that target vectors specifically to hematopoietic stem and progenitor cells while minimizing off-target events.

7. Safety: Vector genotoxicity, transposon vectors and other issues

The genotoxicity issue is currently the most immediate and direct safety concern related to the gene therapy using HSCs. Several otherwise successful gene therapy trials of severe combined immunodeficiency using retroviral vectors have resulted in occurrence of leukemia in a significant percentage of patients. Substantial efforts were thus devoted to elucidation of integration patterns and clonal population structure in the hematopoietic compartment after viral transduction, both in experimental models and in clinical trials. The obtained results, although not unanimous, demonstrate nevertheless a frequent occurrence of oligoclonal hematopoiesis after gene therapy, with viral integration sites tending to concentrate in the vicinity of a limited number of genes preferentially involved in growth and proliferation control such as above mentioned Evi-1, PRDM16 or HMGA2. Although upregulation of these genes rarely led to overt neoplastic transformation, it is nevertheless clear that the patients with oligoclonal hematopoiesis are at substantial risk of acquiring leukemias at some future time point.

Various strategies are being currently developed to minimize the risk of neoplastic transformations of HSCs after viral transduction. The most promising approaches include using lentiviral instead of retroviral vectors, and insulators to shield cellular oncogenes from activation by strong viral promoters (Puthenveetil et al., 2004). Insulators, however, tends to significantly reduce viral titers (Nielsen et al., 2009), relatively inefficient (Uchida et al., 2011) and do not provide guarantee against insertional activation of potential oncogenes such as HMGA2 (Cavazzana-Calvo et al., 2010). Another approach is to use promoters specific for differentiated cells that are expected to produce negligible activation of oncogenes in stem cells. However, such promoters tend to provide comparably lower expression levels, and although this might be improved by addition of strong enhancers (Gruh et al., 2008), it is far from certain that such combinations would not activate nearby cellular promoters.

Transposon vectors offer an exciting alternative to retro- and lentiviral vectors. The transposon-based gene delivery combines advantages of integrating viral vectors with those of plasmid vectors. Permanent genomic integration of transposon vectors provides long-term expression, whereas there are significantly fewer constraints on vector design and use of various function elements like insulators. Transposon systems are inherently less immunogenic than viral delivery systems, whereas their cargo capacity generally exceeds that of retro- and lentiviral vectors (Zayed et al., 2004). Initial experiments with transposons were plagued by low efficiency of integration, but continuous improvements in molecular design of transposases have significantly increased the efficiency of integration process (Mátés et al., 2009). Currently, transposons based on Sleeping Beauty (SB) system represent the most advanced version of this technology (reviewed by Ivics & Izsvák, 2011), although other system such as piggyBac are also being perfected (Yusa et al., 2011) and may offer some advantages, such as larger cargo capacity, over the SB system (Lacoste et al., 2009).

Although stable SB transposon-mediated gene transfer into hematopoietic cells was reported (Xue et al., 2009), efficient vector delivery to HSCs remains poorly resolved issue, which is currently being addressed by using electroporation or hybrid lentiviral-transposon vectors (Staunstrup et al., 2009). Although certain undesired effects such as SB transposase cytotoxicity were observed, it seems that they might be minimized by controllable mRNA delivery (Galla et al., 2011). Compared to lenti- and retroviral vectors that show preferential integration near active genes, SB transposon vectors demonstrate nearly random integration profiles (Moldt et al., 2011), although this property might not be shared by other transposon systems (Huang et al., 2010).

Another serious safety concern is a direct consequence of a current low efficiency of transduction of LTR HSCs, which necessitates the use of myeloablative pre-conditioning and negative selection strategies to eliminate competing endogenous HSCs and increase chimerism levels. Negative selection strategies using in particular alkylating drugs place a significant stress upon hematopoietic system. However, as demonstrated by Xie et al., 2010, repetitive hematopoietic stress by busulfan administration in a nonhuman primate may rapidly lead to reduction of polyclonality and eventually to cytopenia. In addition, potential long term mutagenic effects of alkylating agents are largely unknown, thus adding more uncertainty as to correct assessment of risks and benefits of this strategy. Apparently, in order to tackle efficiently the problem of low transduction efficiency, it is not sufficient to rely on the use of negative selection only, but is also important to achieve substantial improvements in ex vivo stem cell culturing, expansion and transduction efficiency. Promising approaches also involve use of positive ex vivo and in vivo selection and in situ transduction strategies.

8. Novel technologies

In the recent few years, a group of new exciting and very powerful technologies, namely cell reprogramming using specific combinations of transcription factors and/or micro RNAs appeared (Takahashi & Yamanaka, 2006; Miyoshi et al., 2011). Much hope is invested into development of strategies aiming at derivation of patient-specific induced pluripotent (iPS) cells similar to embryonic stem (ES) cells, with their subsequent differentiation into hematopoetic cells capable of long-term hematopoiesis. In addition to this indirect reprogramming strategy, methods for direct reprogramming that bypass derivation of iPS cells are also being elaborated. There is one report stating that ectopic expression of Oct4 transcription factor in human fibroblasts is sufficient to convert them into hematopoietic cells with in vivo engraftment capacity (Szabo et al., 2010). However, whether the published technique may result in production of bona fide hematopietic stem cells capable of long-term reconstitution, remains to be seen. It should be noted that such a goal has not yet been achieved for ES or iPS cells. If efficient reprogramming into HSCs were possible, the perspectives would look staggering. First of all, since starting primary cell populations such as mesenchymal stem/progenitor cells can be propagated for many generations and are amenable for selection of efficient vector integration events, it will be possible to obtain cell populations in which the majority of reprogrammed HCS-like cells bear functioning transgenes, thus increasing efficiency of gene therapy many-fold. Besides, if this technology were able to generate ex vivo significantly more reprogrammed cells with HSC properties than is possible to obtain from a patient, this would establish basis for a radically increase in a level of chimerism after transplantation, thus further improving the efficiency of gene therapy. Of course, the safety issues, in particular potential epigenetic and genome instability of reprogrammed cells that might result in neoplastic transformations, must be addressed especially carefully in this case.

9. Conclusion

Current protocols of gene therapy of hematopoietic and immune system, despite significant efforts by numerous teams worldwide, demonstrate as yet a relatively modest clinical efficiency. However, there are sufficient reasons to assume that many rather inconspicuous yet significant recent technical developments are preparing the field for a decisive breakthrough in the near future. In addition, new cutting- edge technologies such as direct cell reprogramming are entering the scene and may eventually present a radically different and a more efficient solution of the problem. Given all these considerations, the future of gene therapy of blood and immune system diseases looks definitely bright.

10. Acknowledgment

This work was supported by the Russian Foundation for Basic Research Grants 09-04-01312 to F.R. and 11-04-01814-a to A.B, and a grant of the RAS Program of Molecular Cellular Biology to A.B.

11. References

Aguila, J.R.; Liao, W. ; Yang, J., Avila, C.; Hagag, N.; Senzel, L. & Ma, Y. (2011). SALL4 is a robust stimulator for the expansion of hematopoietic stem cells. *Blood*, Vol.118, No.3, (July 2011), pp. 576-585, ISSN 0006-4971

Antonchuk, J.; Sauvageau, G. & Humphries, R.K. (2002). HOXB4-induced expansion of adult hematopoietic stem cells ex vivo. *Cell*, Vol.109, No.1, (April 2002), pp. 39–45, ISSN 0092-8674

Beard, B.C.; Trobridge, G.D.; Ironside, C.; McCune, J.S.; Adair, J.E. & Kiem, H.P. (2010). Efficient and stable MGMT-mediated selection of long-term repopulating stem cells in nonhuman primates. *The Journal of Clinical Investigation*, Vol.120, No.7, (July 2010), pp. 2345-2354, ISSN 0021-9738

Bersenev, A.; Wu, C.; Balcerek, J. & Tong, W. (2008). Lnk controls mouse hematopoietic stem cell self-renewal and quiescence through direct interactions with JAK2. *The Journal of Clinical Investigation*, Vol.118, No.8, (August 2008), pp. 2832-2844, ISSN 0021-9738

Bhardwaj, G.; Murdoch, B.; Wu, D.; Baker, D.P.; Williams, K.P.; Chadwick, K.; Ling, L.E.; Karanu, F.N. & Bhatia, M. (2001). Sonic hedgehog induces the proliferation of primitive human hematopoietic cells via BMP regulation. *Nature Immunology*, Vol.2, No.2, (February 2001), pp. 172-180, ISSN 1529-2908

Bielas, H.; Schmitt, M., Icreverzi, A.; Ericson,N. & Loeb, L. (2009). Molecularly evolved thymidylate synthase inhibits 5-fluorodeoxyuridine toxicity in human hematopoietic cells. *Human Gene Therapy*, Vol.20, No.12, (December 2009), pp. 703-707, ISSN 1043-0342

Bowman, J.E.; Reese, J.S.; Lingas, K.T. & Gerson, S.L. (2003). Myeloablation is not required to select and maintain expression of the drug-resistance gene, mutant MGMT, in primary and secondary recipients. *Molecular Therapy*, Vol. 8, No.1, (July 2003), pp. 42-50, ISSN 1525-0016

Buckley, S.M.; Ulloa-Montoya, F.; Abts, D.; Oostendorp, R.A.; Dzierzak, E.; Ekker, S.C. & Verfaillie, C.M. (2011). Maintenance of HSC by Wnt5a secreting AGM-derived stromal cell line. *Experimental Hematology*, (January 2011), Vol.39, No.1, pp. 114-123.e1-5, ISSN 0301-472X

Bunting, K.D.; Galipeau, J.; Topham, D.; Benaim, E. & Sorrentino, B.P. (1999). Effects of retroviral-mediated MDR1 expression on hematopoietic stem cell self-renewal and differentiation in culture. *Annals of the New York Academy of Sciences*, Vol.872, (April 1999), pp. 125-141, ISSN 0077-8923

Case, S.S.; Price, M.A.; Jordan, C.T.; Yu, X.J.; Wang, L.; Bauer, G.; Haas, D.L.; Xu, D.; Stripecke, R.; Naldini, L.; Kohn, D.B. & Crooks, G.M. (1999). Stable transduction of quiescent CD34+CD38- human hematopoietic cells by HIV-1-based lentiviral vectors. *Proceedings of the National Academy of Sciences of the United States of America*, Vol.96, No.6, (March 1999), pp. 2988–2993, ISSN 0027-8424

Cavazzana-Calvo, M.; Hacein-Bey, S.; de Saint Basile, G.; Gross, F.; Yvon, E.; Nusbaum, P.; Selz, F.; Hue, C.; Certain, S.; Casanova, J.L.; Bousso, P.; Deist, F.L. & Fischer, A. (2000). Gene therapy of human severe combined immunodeficiency (SCID)-X1 disease. *Science*, Vol.288, No.5466, (April 2000), pp. 669-672, ISSN 0036-8075

Cavazzana-Calvo, M.; Payen, E.; Negre, O.; Wang, G.; Hehir, K.; Fusil, F.; Down, J.; Denaro, M.; Brady, T.; Westerman, K.; Cavallesco, R.; Gillet-Legrand, B.; Caccavelli, L.; Sgarra, R.; Maouche-Chrétien, L.; Bernaudin, F.; Girot, R.; Dorazio, R.; Mulder, G.J.; Polack, A.; Bank, A.; Soulier, J.; Larghero, J.; Kabbara, N.; Dalle, B.; Gourmel, B.; Socie, G.; Chrétien, S.; Cartier, N.; Aubourg, P.; Fischer, A.; Cornetta, K.; Galacteros, F.; Beuzard, Y.; Gluckman, E.; Bushman, F.; Hacein-Bey-Abina, S. & Leboulch, P. (2010). Transfusion independence and HMGA2 activation after gene therapy of human β-thalassaemia. *Nature*, Vol. 467, No.7313, (September 2010), pp. 318-322, ISSN 0028-0836

Chen, J.; Larochelle, A.; Fricker, S.; Bridger, G.; Dunbar, C.E. & Abkowitz J.L. (2006). Mobilization as a preparative regimen for hematopoietic stem cell transplantation. *Blood*, Vol.107, No.9, (May 2006), pp. 3764-3771, ISSN 0006-4971

Cheshier, S.H.; Morrison, S.J.; Liao, X. & Weissman, I.L. (1999). In vivo proliferation and cell cycle kinetics of long-term self-renewing haematopoietic stem cells. *Proceedings of the National Academy of Sciences of the United States of America*, Vol.96, No.6, (March 1999), pp. 3120–3125, ISSN 0027-8424

Chinnasamy, D.; Milsom, M.D.; Shaffer, J.; Neuenfeldt, J.; Shaaban, A.F.; Margison, G.P.; Fairbairn, L.J. & Chinnasamy, N. (2006). Multicistronic lentiviral vectors containing the FMDV 2A cleavage factor demonstrate robust expression of encoded genes at limiting MOI. *Virology Journal*, Vol.3, (March 2006), pp. 14, ISSN 1743-422X

Chou, S. & Lodish, H.F. (2010). Fetal liver hepatic progenitors are supportive stromal cells for hematopoietic stem cells. *Proceedings of the National Academy of Sciences of the United States of America*, Vol.107, No.17, (April 2010), pp. 7799-7804, ISSN 0027-8424

Cobas, M.; Wilson, A.; Ernst, B.; Mancini, S.J.; MacDonald, H.R.; Kemler, R. & Radtke, F. (2004). Beta-catenin is dispensable for hematopoiesis and lymphopoiesis. *The Journal of Experimental Medicine*, Vol.199, No.2, (January 2004), pp. 221-229, ISSN 0022-1007

Cowan, K.H.; Moscow, J.A.; Huang, H.; Zujewski, J.A.; O'Shaughnessy, J.; Sorrentino, B.; Hines, K.; Carter, C.; Schneider, E.; Cusack, G.; Noone, M.; Dunbar, C.; Steinberg, S.; Wilson, W.; Goldspiel, B.; Read, E.J.; Leitman, S.F.; McDonagh, K.; Chow, C.; Abati, A.; Chiang, Y.; Chang, Y.N.; Gottesman, M.M.; Pastan, I. & Nienhuis, A. (1999). Paclitaxel chemotherapy after autologous stem-cell transplantation and engraftment of hematopoietic cells transduced with a retrovirus containing the multidrug resistance complementary DNA (MDR1) in metastatic breast cancer patients. *Clinical Cancer Research*, Vol.5, No.7, (July 1999), pp. 1619-1628, ISSN 1078-0432

Crcareva, A.; Saito, T.; Kunisato, A.; Kumano, K.; Suzuki, T.; Sakata-Yanagimoto, M.; Kawazu, M.; Stojanovic, A.; Kurokawa, M.; Ogawa, S.; Hirai, H. & Chiba, S. (2005). Hematopoietic stem cells expanded by fibroblast growth factor-1 are excellent targets for retrovirus-mediated gene delivery. *Experimental Hematology*, Vol.33, No.12, (December 2005), pp. 1459-1469, ISSN 0301-472X

Czechowicz, A.; Kraft, D.; Weissman, I.L. & Bhattacharya, D. (2007). Efficient transplantation via antibody-based clearance of hematopoietic stem cell niches. *Science*, Vol.318, No. 5854, (November 2007), pp. 1296-1299, ISSN 0036-8075

Davis, B.M.; Koç, O.N. & Gerson, S.L. (2000). Limiting number of G156A O6-methylguanine DNA methyltransferase-transduced marrow progenitors repopulate nonmyeloablated mice after drug selection. *Blood*, Vol. 95, No.10, (May 2000) pp. 3078–3084, ISSN 0006-4971

de Barros, A.P.; Takiya, C.M.; Garzoni, L.R.; Leal-Ferreira, M.L.; Dutra, H.S.; Chiarini, L.B.; Meirelles, M.N.; Borojevic, R. & Rossi, M.I. (2010). Osteoblasts and bone marrow mesenchymal stromal cells control hematopoietic stem cell migration and proliferation in 3D in vitro model. *PLoS One*, Vol.5, No.2, (February 2010), pp. e9093, ISSN 1932-6203

de Haan, G.; Weersing, E.; Dontje, B.; van Os, R.; Bystrykh, L.V.; Vellenga, E. & Miller, G. (2003). In vitro generation of long-term repopulating hematopoietic stem cells by fibroblast growth factor-1. *Developmental Cell*, Vol.4, No.2, (February 2003), pp. 241-251, ISSN 1534-5807

Delaney, C.; Heimfeld, S.; Brashem-Stein, C.; Voorhies, H.; Manger, R.L. & Bernstein, I.D. (2010). Notch-mediated expansion of human cord blood progenitor cells capable of rapid myeloid reconstitution. *Nature Medicine*, Vol.16, No.2, (February 2010), pp. 232-236, ISSN 1078-8956

De Toni, F.; Poglio, S.; Youcef, A.B.; Cousin, B.; Pflumio, F.; Bourin, P.; Casteilla, L. & Laharrague, P. (2011). Human Adipose-Derived Stromal Cells Efficiently Support Hematopoiesis In Vitro and In Vivo: A Key Step for Therapeutic Studies. *Stem Cells and Development*, (April 2011), advance online publication, ISSN 1547-3287

Domashenko, A.D.; Danet-Desnoyers, G.; Aron, A.; Carroll, M.P. & Emerson, S.G. (2010). TAT-mediated transduction of NF-Ya peptide induces the ex vivo proliferation and engraftment potential of human hematopoietic progenitor cells. *Blood*, Vol.116, No.15, (October 2010), pp. 2676-2683, ISSN 0006-4971

Du, Y.; Jenkins, N.A. & Copeland, N.G. (2005). Insertional mutagenesis identifies genes that promote the immortalization of primary bone marrow progenitor cells. *Blood*, Vol.106, No.12, (December 2005), pp. 3932-3939, ISSN 0006-4971

Ellis, J. (2005). Silencing and variegation of gammaretrovirus and lentivirus vectors. *Human Gene Therapy*, Vol.16, No.11, (November 2005), pp. 1241-1246, ISSN 1043-0342

Frisch, B.J.; Porter, R.L.; Gigliotti, B.J.; Olm-Shipman, A.J.; Weber, J.M.; O'Keefe, R.J.; Jordan, C.T. & Calvi, L.M. (2009). In vivo prostaglandin E2 treatment alters the bone marrow microenvironment and preferentially expands short-term hematopoietic stem cells. *Blood*, Vol.114, No.19, (November 2009), pp. 4054-4063, ISSN 0006-4971

Galla, M.; Schambach, A.; Falk, C.S.; Maetzig, T.; Kuehle, J.; Lange, K.; Zychlinski, D.; Heinz, N.; Brugman, M.H.; Göhring, G.; Izsvák, Z.; Ivics, Z. & Baum, C. (2011). Avoiding cytotoxicity of transposases by dose-controlled mRNA delivery. *Nucleic Acids Research*, Vol.39, No.16, (September 2011), pp. 7147-7160, ISSN 0305-1048

Goldman, D.C.; Bailey, A.S.; Pfaffle, D.L.; Al Masri, A.; Christian, J.L. & Fleming, W.H. (2009). BMP4 regulates the hematopoietic stem cell niche. *Blood*, Vol.114, No.20, (November 2009), pp. 4393-4401, ISSN 0006-4971

Gori, J.L.; McIvor, R. & Kaufman, D. (2010). Methotrexate supports in vivo selection of human embryonic stem cell derived-hematopoietic cells expressing dihydrofolate reductase. *Bioengineered Bugs*, Vol.1, No.6, (November 2010), pp. 434-436, ISSN 1949-1018

Guo, S.; Lu, J.; Schlanger, R.; Zhang, H.; Wang, J.Y.; Fox, M.C.; Purton, L.E.; Fleming, H.H.; Cobb, B.; Merkenschlager, M.; Golub, T.R. & Scadden, D.T. (2010). MicroRNA miR-125a controls hematopoietic stem cell number. *Proceedings of the National Academy of Sciences of the United States of America*, Vol.107, No.32, (August 2010), pp. 14229-14234, ISSN 0027-8424

Gruh, I.; Wunderlich, S.; Winkler, M.; Schwanke, K.; Heinke, J.; Blömer, U.; Ruhparwar, A.; Rohde, B.; Li, R.K.; Haverich, A. & Martin, U. (2008). Human CMV immediate-early enhancer: a useful tool to enhance cell-type-specific expression from lentiviral vectors. *The Journal of Gene Medicine*, Vol.10, No.1, (January 2008), pp. 21-32, ISSN 1099-498X

Heath, V.; Suh, H.C.; Holman, M.; Renn, K.; Gooya, J.M; Parkin, S.; Klarmann, K.D.; Ortiz, M.; Johnson, P. & Keller, J. (2004). C/EBPalpha deficiency results in hyperproliferation of hematopoietic progenitor cells and disrupts macrophage development in vitro and in vivo. *Blood*, Vol.104, No.6, (September 2004), pp. 1639-1647, ISSN 0006-4971

Hofmann, I.; Stover, E.H.; Cullen, D.E.; Mao, J.; Morgan, K.J.; Lee, B.H.; Kharas, M.G.; Miller, P.G.; Cornejo, M.G.; Okabe, R.; Armstrong, S.A.; Ghilardi, N.; Gould, S.; de Sauvage, F.J.; McMahon, A.P. & Gilliland, D.G. (2009). Hedgehog signaling is dispensable for adult murine hematopoietic stem cell function and hematopoiesis. *Cell Stem Cell*, Vol.4, No.6, (June 2009), pp. 559-567, ISSN 1934-5909

Horn, P.A.; Morris, J.C.; Bukovsky, A.A.; Andrews, R.G.; Naldini, L.; Kurre, P. & Kiem, H.P. (2002). Lentivirus-mediated gene transfer into hematopoietic repopulating cells in baboons. *Gene Therapy*, Vol.9, No.21, (November 2002), pp. 1464-1471, ISSN 0969-7128

Hosokawa, K.; Arai, F.; Yoshihara, H.; Iwasaki, H.; Nakamura, Y.; Gomei, Y. & Suda, T. (2010). Knockdown of N-cadherin suppresses the long-term engraftment of hematopoietic stem cells. *Blood*, Vol.116, No.4, (July 2010), pp. 554-563, ISSN 0006-4971

Huang, X.; Guo, H.; Tammana, S.; Jung, Y.C.; Mellgren, E.; Bassi, P.; Cao, Q.; Tu, Z.J.; Kim, Y.C.; Ekker, S.C.; Wu, X.; Wang, S.M. & Zhou, X. (2010). Gene transfer efficiency and genome-wide integration profiling of Sleeping Beauty, Tol2, and piggyBac transposons in human primary T cells. *Molecular Therapy*, Vol.18, No.10, (October 2010), pp. 1803-1813, ISSN 1525-0016

Hutton, J.F.; Rozenkov, V.; Khor, F.S.; D'Andrea, R.J. & Lewis, I.D. (2006). Bone morphogenetic protein 4 contributes to the maintenance of primitive cord blood hematopoietic progenitors in an ex vivo stroma-noncontact co-culture system. *Stem Cells and Development*, Vol.15, No.6, (December 2006), pp. 805-813, ISSN 1547-3287

Huynh, H.; Iizuka, S.; Kaba, M.; Kirak, O.; Zheng, J.; Lodish, H.F. & Zhang, C.C. (2008). Insulin-like growth factor-binding protein 2 secreted by a tumorigenic cell line supports ex vivo expansion of mouse hematopoietic stem cells. *Stem Cells*, Vol.26, No.6, (June 2008), pp. 1628-1635, ISSN 1066-5099

Ikeda, K.; Mason, P.J. & Bessler M. (2011). 3'UTR-truncated Hmga2 cDNA causes MPN-like hematopoiesis by conferring a clonal growth advantage at the level of HSC in mice. *Blood*, Vol.117, No.22, (June 2011), pp. 5860-5869, ISSN 0006-4971

Imai, Y.; Adachi, Y.; Shi, M.; Shima, C.; Yanai, S.; Okigaki, M.; Yamashima, T.; Kaneko, K. & Ikehara, S. (2010). Caspase inhibitor ZVAD-fmk facilitates engraftment of donor hematopoietic stem cells in intra-bone marrow-bone marrow transplantation. *Stem Cells and Development*, Vol.19, No.4, (April 2010), pp. 461-468, ISSN 1547-3287

Ivics, Z. & Izsvák, Z. (2011). Non-viral Gene Delivery with the Sleeping Beauty Transposon System. *Human Gene Therapy*, (August 2011), advance online publication, ISSN 1043-0342

Iwama, A.; Oguro, H.; Negishi, M.; Kato, Y.; Morita, Y.; Tsukui, H.; Ema, H.; Kamijo, T.; Katoh-Fukui, Y.; Koseki, H.; van Lohuizen, M. & Nakauchi, H. (2004). Enhanced self-renewal of hematopoietic stem cells mediated by the polycomb gene product Bmi-1. *Immunity*, Vol.21, No.6, (December 2004), pp. 843-851, ISSN 1074-7613

Khoury, M.; Drake, A.; Chen, Q.; Dong, D.; Leskov, I.; Fragoso, M.F.; Li, Y.; Iliopoulou, B.P.; Hwang, W.; Lodish, H.F. & Chen, J. (2011). Mesenchymal stem cells secreting angiopoietin-like-5 support efficient expansion of human hematopoietic stem cells without compromising their repopulating potential. *Stem Cells and Development*, Vol.20, No.8, (August 2011), pp. 1371-1381, ISSN 1547-3287

Kiel, M.J.; Radice, G.L. & Morrison, S.J. (2007). Lack of evidence that hematopoietic stem cells depend on N-cadherin-mediated adhesion to osteoblasts for their maintenance. *Cell Stem Cell*, Vol.1, No.2, (August 2007), pp. 204-217, ISSN 1934-5909

King, K.Y.; Baldridge, M.T.; Weksberg, D.C.; Chambers, S.M.; Lukov, G.L.; Wu, S.; Boles, N.C.; Jung, S.Y.; Qin, J.; Liu, D.; Songyang, Z.; Eissa, N.T.; Taylor, G.A. & Goodell, MA. (2011). Irgm1 protects hematopoietic stem cells by negative regulation of IFN signaling. *Blood*, Vol.118, No. 6, (August 2011), pp. 1525-33, ISSN 0006-4971

Ko, K.H.; Holmes, T.; Palladinetti, P.; Song, E.; Nordon, R.; O'Brien, T.A. & Dolnikov, A. (2011). GSK-3β inhibition promotes engraftment of ex vivo-expanded hematopoietic stem cells and modulates gene expression. *Stem Cells*, Vol.29, No.1, (January 2011), pp. 108-118, ISSN 1066-5099

Kobune, M.; Ito, Y.; Kawano, Y.; Sasaki, K.; Uchida, H.; Nakamura, K.; Dehari, H.; Chiba, H.; Takimoto, R.; Matsunaga, T.; Terui, T.; Kato, J.; Niitsu, Y. & Hamada, H. (2004). Indian hedgehog gene transfer augments hematopoietic support of human stromal cells including NOD/SCID-beta2m-/- repopulating cells. *Blood*, Vol.104, No.4, (August 2004), pp. 1002-1009, ISSN: 0006-4971

Konuma, T.; Nakamura, S.; Miyagi, S.; Negishi, M.; Chiba, T.; Oguro, H.; Yuan, J.; Mochizuki-Kashio, M.; Ichikawa, H.; Miyoshi, H.; Vidal, M. & Iwama, A. (2011). Forced expression of the histone demethylase Fbxl10 maintains self-renewing hematopoietic stem cells. *Experimental Hematology*, Vol.39, No.6, (June 2011), pp. 697-709.e5, ISSN 0301-472X

Krosl, J.; Austin, P.; Beslu, N.; Kroon, E.; Humphries, R.K. & Sauvageau, G. (2003). In vitro expansion of hematopoietic stem cells by recombinant TAT-HOXB4 protein. *Nature Medicine*, Vol.9, No.11, (November 2003), pp. 1428-1432, ISSN 1078-8956

Lacoste, A.; Berenshteyn, F. & Brivanlou, A.H. (2009). An efficient and reversible transposable system for gene delivery and lineage-specific differentiation in human embryonic stem cells. *Cell Stem Cell*, Vol.5, No.3, (September 2009), pp. 332-342, ISSN 1934-5909

Larochelle, A.; Choi, U.; Shou, Y.; Naumann, N.; Loktionova, N.A.; Clevenger, J.R.; Krouse, A.; Metzger, M.; Donahue, R.E.; Kang, E.; Stewart, C.; Persons, D.; Malech, H.L.; Dunbar, C.E. & Sorrentino, B.P. (2009). In vivo selection of hematopoietic progenitor cells and temozolomide dose intensification in rhesus macaques through lentiviral transduction with a drug resistance gene. *The Journal of Clinical Investigation*, Vol.119, No.7, (July 2009), pp. 1952-1963, ISSN 0021-9738

Lutolf, M.P.; Doyonnas, R.; Havenstrite, K.; Koleckar, K. & Blau, H.M. (2009). Perturbation of single hematopoietic stem cell fates in artificial niches. *Integrative biology*, Vol.1, No.1, (January 2009), pp. 59-69, ISSN 1757-9694

Masuda, S.; Ageyama, N.; Shibata, H.; Obara, Y.; Ikeda, T.; Takeuchi, K.; Ueda, Y.; Ozawa, K. & Hanazono, Y. (2009). Cotransplantation with MSCs improves engraftment of HSCs after autologous intra-bone marrow transplantation in nonhuman primates. *Experimental Hematology*, Vol.37, No.10, (October 2009), pp. 1250-1257.e1, ISSN 0301-472X

Mátés, L.; Chuah, M.K.; Belay, E.; Jerchow, B.; Manoj, N.; Acosta-Sanchez, A.; Grzela, D.P.; Schmitt, A.; Becker, K.; Matrai, J.; Ma, L.; Samara-Kuko, E.; Gysemans, C.; Pryputniewicz, D.; Miskey, C.; Fletcher, B.; VandenDriessche, T.; Ivics, Z. & Izsvák, Z. (2009). Molecular evolution of a novel hyperactive Sleeping Beauty transposase enables robust stable gene transfer in vertebrates. *Nature Genetics*, Vol.41, No.6, (June 2009), pp. 753-761, ISSN 1061-4036

Mazurier, F.; Doedens, M.; Gan, O.I. & Dick, J.E. (2003). Rapid myeloerythroid repopulation after intrafemoral transplantation of NOD-SCID mice reveals a new class of human stem cells. *Nature Medicine*, Vol.9, No.7, (July 2003), pp. 959-963, ISSN 1078-8956

McCauslin, C.S.; Wine, J.; Cheng, L.; Klarmann, K.D.; Candotti, F.; Clausen, P.A.; Spence, S.E. & Keller, J.R. (2003). In vivo retroviral gene transfer by direct intrafemoral injection results in correction of the SCID phenotype in Jak3 knock-out animals. *Blood*, Vol.102, No.3, (August 2003), pp. 843-848, ISSN 0006-4971

McCormack, M.P.; Forster, A.; Drynan, L.; Pannell, R. & Rabbitts, T.H. (2003). The LMO2 T-cell oncogene is activated via chromosomal translocations or retroviral insertion during gene therapy but has no mandatory role in normal T-cell development. *Molecular and Cellular Biology*, Vol.23, No.24, (December 2003), pp. 9003-9013, ISSN 0270-7306

McCormack, M.P.; Young, L.F.; Vasudevan, S.; de Graaf, C.A.; Codrington, R.; Rabbitts, T.H.; Jane, S.M. & Curtis, D.J. (2010). The Lmo2 oncogene initiates leukemia in mice by inducing thymocyte self-renewal. *Science*, Vol.327, No.5967, (February 2010), pp. 879-883, ISSN 0036-8075

Métais, J.Y. & Dunbar, C.E. (2008). The MDS1-EVI1 gene complex as a retrovirus integration site: impact on behavior of hematopoietic cells and implications for gene therapy. *Molecular Therapy*, Vol.16, No.3, (March 2008), pp. 439-449, ISSN 1525-0016

Milsom M.D.; Woolford L.B.; Margison G.P.; Humphries R.K. & Fairbairn L.J. (2004). Enhanced in vivo selection of bone marrow cells by retroviral-mediated coexpression of mutant O6-methylguanine-DNA-methyltransferase and HOXB4. *Molecular Therapy*, Vol.10, No.5, (November 2004), pp. 862-873, ISSN 1525-0016

Miyoshi, H.; Murao, M.; Ohshima, N. & Tun T. (2011). Three-dimensional culture of mouse bone marrow cells within a porous polymer scaffold: effects of oxygen concentration and stromal layer on expansion of haematopoietic progenitor cells. *Journal of Tissue Engineering and Regenerative Medicine*, Vol.5, No.2, (February 2011), pp. 112-118, ISSN 1932-6254

Miyoshi, N.; Ishii, H.; Nagano, H.; Haraguchi, N.; Dewi, D.L.; Kano, Y.; Nishikawa, S.; Tanemura, M.; Mimori, K.; Tanaka, F.; Saito, T.; Nishimura, J.; Takemasa, I.; Mizushima, T.; Ikeda, M.; Yamamoto, H.; Sekimoto, M.; Doki, Y. & Mori, M. (2011). Reprogramming of mouse and human cells to pluripotency using mature microRNAs. *Cell Stem Cell*, Vol.8, No.6, (June 2011), pp. 633-638, ISSN 1934-5909

Moldenhauer, A.; Futschik, M.; Lu, H.; Helmig, M.; Götze, P.; Bal, G.; Zenke, M.; Han, W. & Salama, A. (2011). Interleukin 32 promotes hematopoietic progenitor expansion and attenuates bone marrow cytotoxicity. *European Journal of Immunology*, Vol.41, No.6, (June 2011), pp. 1774-1786, ISSN: 0014-2980

Moldt, B.; Miskey., C.; Staunstrup, N.H.; Gogol-Döring, A.; Bak, R.O.; Sharma, N.; Mátés, L.; Izsvák, Z.; Chen, W.; Ivics, Z. & Mikkelsen, J.G. (2011). Comparative Genomic Integration Profiling of Sleeping Beauty Transposons Mobilized With High Efficacy From Integrase-defective Lentiviral Vectors in Primary Human Cells. *Molecular Therapy*, Vol.19, No.8, (August 2011), pp. 1499-1510, ISSN 1043-0342

Moore, K.A.; Ema, H. & Lemischka, I.R. (1997). In vitro maintenance of highly purified, transplantable hematopoietic stem cells. *Blood*, Vol.89, No.12, pp. 4337-4347, ISSN 0006-4971

Mori, M.; Yoneda-Kato, N.; Yoshida, A. & Kato, J.Y. (2008). Stable form of JAB1 enhances proliferation and maintenance of hematopoietic progenitors. *Journal of Biological Chemistry*, Vol.283, No.43, (October 2008), pp. 29011-29021, ISSN 0021-9258

Mostoslavsky, G.; Kotton, D.N.; Fabian, A.J.; Gray, J.T.; Lee, J.S. & Mulligan, R.C. (2005). Efficiency of transduction of highly purified murine hematopoietic stem cells by lentiviral and oncoretroviral vectors under conditions of minimal in vitro manipulation. *Molecular Therapy*, Vol.11, No.6, (June 2005), pp. 932-940, ISSN 1525-0016

Mullican, S.E.; Zhang, S.; Konopleva, M.; Ruvolo, V.; Andreeff, M.; Milbrandt, J. & Conneely, O.M. (2007). Abrogation of nuclear receptors Nr4a3 and Nr4a1 leads to development of acute myeloid leukemia. *Nature Medicine*, Vol.13, No.6, (June 2007), pp. 730-735, ISSN 1078-8956

Neff, T.; Beard, B.C.; Peterson, L.J.; Anandakumar, P.; Thompson, J. & Kiem, H.P. (2005). Polyclonal chemoprotection against temozolomide in a large-animal model of drug resistance gene therapy. *Blood*, Vol.105, No.3, (February 2005), pp. 997-1002, ISSN 0006-4971

Nemeth, M.J.; Topol, L.; Anderson, S.M.; Yang, Y. & Bodine, D.M. (2007). Wnt5a inhibits canonical Wnt signaling in hematopoietic stem cells and enhances repopulation. *Proceedings of the National Academy of Sciences of the United States of America*, Vol.104, No.39, (September 2007), pp. 15436-15441, ISSN 0027-8424

Nemeth, M.J.; Mak, K.K.; Yang, Y. & Bodine, D.M. (2009). beta-Catenin expression in the bone marrow microenvironment is required for long-term maintenance of primitive hematopoietic cells. *Stem Cells*, Vol.27, No.5, (May 2009), pp. 1109-1119, ISSN 1066-5099

Nielsen, T.T.; Jakobsson, J.; Rosenqvist, N. & Lundberg, C. (2009). Incorporating double copies of a chromatin insulator into lentiviral vectors results in less viral integrants. *BMC Biotechnology*, Vol.9, (February 2009), pp. 9-13, ISSN 1472-6750

North, T.E.; Goessling, W.; Walkley, C.R.; Lengerke, C.; Kopani, K.R.; Lord, A.M.; Weber, G.J.; Bowman, T.V.; Jang, I.H.; Grosser, T.; Fitzgerald, G.A.; Daley, G.Q.; Orkin, S.H. & Zon, L.I. (2007). Prostaglandin E2 regulates vertebrate haematopoietic stem cell homeostasis. *Nature*, Vol.447, No.7147, (June 2007), pp. 1007-1011, ISSN 0028-0836

Ohta, H.; Sekulovic, S.; Bakovic, S.; Eaves, C.J.; Pineault, N.; Gasparetto, M.; Smith, C.; Sauvageau, G. & Humphries, R.K. (2007). Near-maximal expansions of hematopoietic stem cells in culture using NUP98-HOX fusions. *Experimental Hematology*, Vol.35, No.5, (May 2007), pp. 817-830, ISSN 0301-472X

Ott, M.G.; Schmidt, M.; Schwarzwaelder, K.; Stein, S.; Siler, U.; Koehl, U.; Glimm, H.; Kühlcke, K.; Schilz, A.; Kunkel, H.; Naundorf, S.; Brinkmann, A.; Deichmann, A.; Fischer, M.; Ball, C.; Pilz, I.; Dunbar, C.; Du, Y.; Jenkins, N.A.; Copeland, N.G.; Lüthi, U.; Hassan, M.; Thrasher, A.J.; Hoelzer, D.; von Kalle, C.; Seger, R. & Grez, M. (2006). Correction of X-linked chronic granulomatous disease by gene therapy, augmented by insertional activation of MDS1-EVI1, PRDM16 or SETBP1. *Nature Medicine*, Vol.12, No.4, (April 2006), pp. 401-409, ISSN 1078-8956

Pan, D. (2009). In situ (in vivo) gene transfer into murine bone marrow stem cells. *Methods in Molecular Biology*, Vol.506, pp. 159-169, ISSN 1064-3745

Park, I.K.; Qian, D.; Kiel, M.; Becker, M.W.; Pihalja, M.; Weissman, I.L.; Morrison, S.J. & Clarke, M.F. (2003). Bmi-1 is required for maintenance of adult self-renewing haematopoietic stem cells. *Nature*, Vol.423, No.6937, (May 2003), pp. 302-305, ISSN 0028-0836

Peled, T.; Landau, E.; Mandel, J.; Glukhman, E.; Goudsmid, N.R.; Nagler, A. & Fibach, E. (2004). Linear polyamine copper chelator tetraethylenepentamine augments long-term ex vivo expansion of cord blood-derived CD34+ cells and increases their engraftment potential in NOD/SCID mice. *Experimental Hematology*, Vol.32, No.6, (June 2004), pp. 547-555, ISSN 0301-472X

Persons, D.A.; Allay, E.R.; Sawai, N.; Hargrove, P.W.; Brent, T.P.; Hanawa, H.; Nienhuis, A.W. & Sorrentino, B.P. (2003). Successful treatment of murine beta-thalassemia using in vivo selection of genetically modified, drug-resistant hematopoietic stem cells. *Blood*, Vol.102, No.2, (July 2003), pp. 506-513, ISSN 0006-4971

Podda, S.; Ward, M.; Himelstein, A.; Richardson, C.; de la Flor-Weiss, E.; Smith, L.; Gottesman, M.; Pastan, I. & Bank, A. (1992). Transfer and expression of the human multiple drug resistance gene into live mice. *Proceedings of the National Academy of Sciences of the United States of America*, Vol. 89, No.20, (October 1992), pp. 9676–9680, ISSN 0027-8424

Puthenveetil, G.; Scholes, J.; Carbonell, D.; Qureshi, N.; Xia, P.; Zeng, L.; Li, S.; Yu, Y.; Hiti, A.L.; Yee, J.K. & Malik, P. (2004). Successful correction of the human beta thalassemia major phenotype using a lentiviral vector. *Blood*, Vol.104, No.12, (December 2004), pp. 3445-3453, ISSN 0006-4971

Ragg, S.; Xu-Welliver, M.; Bailey, J.; D'Souza, M.; Cooper, R.; Chandra, S.; Seshadri, R.; Pegg, A.E. & Williams, D.A. (2000). Direct reversal of DNA damage by mutant methyltransferase protein protects mice against dose intensified chemotherapy and leads to in vivo selection of hematopoietic stem cells. *Cancer Research*, Vol.60, No.18, (September 2000), pp. 5187–5195, ISSN 0008-5472

Ramirez, P.; Rettig, M.P.; Uy, G.L.; Deych, E.; Holt, M.S.; Ritchey, J.K. & DiPersio, J.F. (2009). BIO5192, a small molecule inhibitor of VLA-4, mobilizes hematopoietic stem and progenitor cells. *Blood*, Vol.114, No.7, (August 2009), pp. 1340-1343, ISSN 0006-4971

Reya, T.; Duncan, A.W.; Ailles, L.; Domen, J.; Scherer, D.C.; Willert, K.; Hintz, L.; Nusse, R. & Weissman I.L. (2003). A role for Wnt signalling in self-renewal of haematopoietic stem cells. *Nature*, Vol.423, No.6938, (May 2003), pp. 409-414, ISSN 0028-0836

Richard, E.; Robert, E.; Cario-Andreé, M.; Ged, C.; Géronimi, F.; Gerson, S.L.; de Verneuil, H. & Moreau-Gaudry, F. (2004). Hematopoietic stem cell gene therapy of murine protoporphyria by methylguanine-DNA methyltransferase- mediated in vivo drug selection. *Gene Therapy*, Vol.11, No.22, (November 2004), pp. 1638-1647, ISSN 0969-7128

Rizo, A.; Dontje, B.; Vellenga, E.; de Haan, G. & Schuringa, J.J. (2008). Long-term maintenance of human hematopoietic stem/progenitor cells by expression of BMI1. *Blood*, Vol.111, No.5, (March 2008), pp. 2621-2630, ISSN 0006-4971

Rohrabaugh, S.L.; Campbell, T.B.; Hangoc, G. & Broxmeyer, H.E. (2011). Ex vivo rapamycin treatment of human cord blood CD34(+) cells enhances their engraftment of NSG mice. *Blood Cells, Molecules, & Diseases*, Vol.46, No.4, (April 2011), pp. 318-320, ISSN 1079-9796

Sangeetha, V.M.; Kale, V.P. & Limaye, LS. (2010). Expansion of cord blood CD34 cells in presence of zVADfmk and zLLYfmk improved their in vitro functionality and in vivo engraftment in NOD/SCID mouse. *PLoS One,* Vol.5, No.8, (August 2010), pp. e12221, ISSN 1932-6203

Sato, T.; Onai, N.; Yoshihara, H.; Arai, F.; Suda, T. & Ohteki, T. (2009). Interferon regulatory factor-2 protects quiescent hematopoietic stem cells from type I interferon-dependent exhaustion. *Nature Medicine,* Vol.15, No.6, (June 2009), pp. 696-700, ISSN 1078-8956

Sauvageau, G.; Thorsteinsdottir, U.; Eaves, C.J.; Lawrence, H.J.; Largman, C.; Lansdorp, P.M. & Humphries, R.K. (1995). Overexpression of HOXB4 in hematopoietic cells causes the selective expansion of more primitive populations in vitro and in vivo. *Genes & Development,* Vol.9, No.14, (July 1995), pp. 1753–1765, ISSN. 0890-9369

Sawai, N.; Zhou, S.; Vanin, E.; Houghton, P.; Brent, T. & Sorrentino, B. (2001). Protection and in Vivo Selection of Hematopoietic Stem Cells Using Temozolomide, O6-Benzylguanine, and an Alkyltransferase-Expressing Retroviral Vector. *Molecular Therapy,* Vol.3, No.1, (January 2001), pp. 78–87, ISSN 1525-0016

Scheller, M.; Huelsken, J.; Rosenbauer, F.; Taketo, M.M.; Birchmeier, W.; Tenen, D.G. & Leutz, A. (2006). Hematopoietic stem cell and multilineage defects generated by constitutive beta-catenin activation. *Nature Immunology,* Vol.7, No.10, (October 2006), pp. 1037-1047, ISSN 1529-2908

Schmidt, M.; Carbonaro, D.A.; Speckmann, C.; Wissler, M.; Bohnsack, J.; Elder, M.; Aronow, B.J.; Nolta, J.A.; Kohn, D.B. & von Kalle, C. (2003). Clonality analysis after retroviral-mediated gene transfer to CD34+ cells from the cord blood of ADA-deficient SCID neonates. *Nature Medicine,* Vol.9, No.4, (April 2003), pp. 463–468, ISSN 1078-8956

Sellers, S.; Gomes, T.J.; Larochelle, A.; Lopez, R.; Adler, R.; Krouse, A.; Donahue, R.E.; Childs, R.W. & Dunbar, C.E. (2010). Ex vivo expansion of retrovirally transduced primate CD34+ cells results in overrepresentation of clones with MDS1/EVI1 insertion sites in the myeloid lineage after transplantation. *Molecular Therapy,* Vol.18, No.9, (September 2010), pp. 1633-1639, ISSN 1525-0016

Shepherd, B.E.; Kiem, H.P.; Lansdorp, P.M.; Dunbar, C.E.; Aubert, G.; LaRochelle, A.; Seggewiss, R.; Guttorp, P. & Abkowitz, J.L. (2007). Hematopoietic stem-cell behavior in nonhuman primates. *Blood,* Vol.110, No.6, (September 2007) pp. 1806-1813, ISSN 0006-4971

Sorrentino, B.P.; Brandt, S.J.; Bodine, D.; Gottesman, M.; Pastan, I.; Cline, A. & Nienhuis A.W. (1992). Selection of drug-resistant bone marrow cells in vivo after retroviral transfer of human MDR1. *Science,* Vol.257, No.5066, (July 1992), pp. 99-103, ISSN 0036-8075

Staunstrup, N.H.; Moldt, B.; Mátés, L.; Villesen, P.; Jakobsen, M.; Ivics, Z.; Izsvák, Z. & Mikkelsen, J.G. (2009). Hybrid lentivirus-transposon vectors with a random integration profile in human cells. *Molecular Therapy,* Vol.17, No.7, (July 2009), pp. 1205-1214, ISSN 1525-0016

Stein, S.; Ott, M.G.; Schultze-Strasser, S.; Jauch, A.; Burwinkel, B.; Kinner, A.; Schmidt, M.; Krämer, A.; Schwäble, J.; Glimm, H.; Koehl, U.; Preiss, C.; Ball, C.; Martin, H.; Göhring, G.; Schwarzwaelder, K.; Hofmann, W.K.; Karakaya, K.; Tchatchou, S.; Yang, R.; Reinecke, P.; Kühlcke, K.; Schlegelberger, B.; Thrasher, A.J.; Hoelzer, D.; Seger, R.; von Kalle, C. & Grez, M. (2010). Genomic instability and myelodysplasia with monosomy 7 consequent to EVI1 activation after gene therapy for chronic granulomatous disease. *Nature Medicine*, Vol.16, No.2, (February 2010), pp. 198-204, ISSN 1078-8956

Szabo, E.; Rampalli, S.; Risueño, R.M.; Schnerch, A.; Mitchell, R.; Fiebig-Comyn, A.; Levadoux-Martin, M. & Bhatia, M. (2010). Direct conversion of human fibroblasts to multilineage blood progenitors. *Nature*, Vol.468, No.7323, (November 2010), pp. 521-526, ISSN 0028-0836

Takahashi, K. & Yamanaka, S. (2006). Induction of pluripotent stem cells from mouse embryonic and adult fibroblast cultures by defined factors. *Cell*, Vol.126, No.4, (August 2006), pp. 663-676, ISSN 0092-8674

Tan, J.; Liu, T.; Hou, L.; Meng, W.; Wang, Y.; Zhi, W. & Deng, L. (2010). Maintenance and expansion of hematopoietic stem/progenitor cells in biomimetic osteoblast niche. *Cytotechnology*, Vol.62, No.5, (October 2010), pp. 439-448, ISSN 0920-9069

Toda, H.; Yamamoto, M.; Kohara, H. & Tabata, Y. (2011). Orientation-regulated immobilization of Jagged1 on glass substrates for ex vivo proliferation of a bone marrow cell population containing hematopoietic stem cells. *Biomaterials*, Vol.32, No.29, (October 2011), pp. 6920-6928, ISSN 0142-9612

Trobridge, G. & Russell, D.W. (2004). Cell cycle requirements for transduction by foamy virus vectors compared to those of oncovirus and lentivirus vectors. *Journal of Virology*, Vol.78, No.5, (March 2004), pp. 2327–2335, ISSN 0022-538X

Trobridge, G.D.; Wu, R.A.; Beard, B.C.; Chiu, S.Y.; Muñoz, N.M.; von Laer, D.; Rossi, J.J. & Kiem, H.P. (2009). Protection of stem cell-derived lymphocytes in a primate AIDS gene therapy model after in vivo selection. *PLoS ONE*, Vol.4, No.11, (November 2009), pp. e7693, ISSN 1932-6203

Trowbridge, J.J.; Xenocostas, A.; Moon, R.T. & Bhatia, M. (2006). Glycogen synthase kinase-3 is an in vivo regulator of hematopoietic stem cell repopulation. *Nature Medicine*, Vol.12, No.1, (January 2006), pp. 89-98, ISSN 1078-8956

Uchida, N.; Sutton, R.E.; Friera, A.M.; He, D.; Reitsma, M.J.; Chang, W.C.; Veres, G.; Scollay, R. & Weissman, I.L. (1998). HIV, but not murine leukemia virus, vectors mediate high efficiency gene transfer into freshly isolated G0/G1 human hematopoietic stem cells. *Proceedings of the National Academy of Sciences of the United States of America*, Vol.95, No.20, (September 1998), pp. 11939–11944, ISSN 0027-8424

Uchida, N.; Washington, K.N.; Lap, C.J.; Hsieh, M.M. & Tisdale, J.F. (2011). Chicken HS4 insulators have minimal barrier function among progeny of human hematopoietic cells transduced with an HIV1-based lentiviral vector. *Molecular Therapy*, Vol.19, No.1, (January 2011), pp. 133-139, ISSN 1525-0016

Ueno, H.; Sakita-Ishikawa, M.; Morikawa, Y.; Nakano, T.; Kitamura, T. & Saito, M. (2003). A stromal cell-derived membrane protein that supports hematopoietic stem cells. *Nature Immunology*, Vol.4, No.5, (May 2003), pp. 457-463, ISSN 1529-2908

VandenDriessche, T.; Ivics, Z.; Izsvák, Z. & Chuah, M.K. (2009). Emerging potential of transposons for gene therapy and generation of induced pluripotent stem cells. *Blood*, Vol.114, No.8, (August 2009), pp. 1461-1468, ISSN 0006-4971

Varnum-Finney, B.; Xu, L.; Brashem-Stein, C.; Nourigat, C.; Flowers, D.; Bakkour, S.; Pear, W.S. & Bernstein, I.D. (2000). Pluripotent, cytokine-dependent, hematopoietic stem cells are immortalized by constitutive Notch1 signaling. *Nature Medicine*, Vol.6, No.11, (November 2000), pp. 1278-1281, ISSN 1078-8956

Vercauteren, S.M. & Sutherland, H.J. (2004). Constitutively active Notch4 promotes early human hematopoietic progenitor cell maintenance while inhibiting differentiation and causes lymphoid abnormalities in vivo. *Blood*, Vol.104, No.8, (October 2004), pp. 2315-2322, ISSN: 0006-4971

Wagner, W.; Roderburg, C.; Wein, F.; Diehlmann, A.; Frankhauser, M.; Schubert, R.; Eckstein, V. & Ho, A.D. (2007). Molecular and secretory profiles of human mesenchymal stromal cells and their abilities to maintain primitive hematopoietic progenitors. *Stem Cells*, Vol.25, No.10, (October 2007), pp. 2638-2647, ISSN 1066-5099

Wang, G.P.; Berry, C.C.; Malani, N.; Leboulch, P.; Fischer, A.; Hacein-Bey-Abina, S.; Cavazzana-Calvo, M. & Bushman, F.D. (2010). Dynamics of gene-modified progenitor cells analyzed by tracking retroviral integration sites in a human SCID-X1 gene therapy trial. *Blood*, Vol.115, No.22, (June 2010), pp. 4356-4366, ISSN 0006-4971

Wang, X.; Hisha, H.; Taketani, S.; Inaba, M.; Li, Q.; Cui, W.; Song, C.; Fan, T.; Cui, Y.; Guo, K.; Yang, G.; Fan, H.; Lian, Z.; Gershwin, M.E. & Ikehara, S. (2005). Neural cell adhesion molecule contributes to hemopoiesis-supporting capacity of stromal cell lines. *Stem Cells*, Vol.23, No.9, (October 2005), pp. 1389-1399, ISSN 1066-5099

Wang, Y.; Kellner, J.; Liu, L. & Zhou, D. (2011). Inhibition of p38 Mitogen-Activated Protein Kinase Promotes Ex Vivo Hematopoietic Stem Cell Expansion. *Stem Cells and Development*, Vol.20, No.7, (July 2011), pp. 1143-1152, ISSN 1547-3287

Watts, K.L.; Zhang, X.; Beard, B.C.; Chiu, S.Y.; Trobridge, G.D.; Humphries, R.K. & Kiem, H.P. (2011). Differential Effects of HOXB4 and NUP98-HOXA10hd on Hematopoietic Repopulating Cells in a Nonhuman Primate Model. *Human Gene Therapy*, (September 2011), advance online publication, ISSN 1525-0016

Willert, K.; Brown, J.D.; Danenberg, E.; Duncan, A.W.; Weissman, I.L.; Reya, T.; Yates, J.R. 3rd & Nusse, R. (2003). Wnt proteins are lipid-modified and can act as stem cell growth factors. *Nature*, Vol.423, No.6938, (May 2003), pp. 448-452, ISSN 0028-0836

Xie, J.; Larochelle, A.; Maric, I.; Faulhaber, M.; Donahue, R.E. & Dunbar, C.E. (2010). Repetitive busulfan administration after hematopoietic stem cell gene therapy associated with a dominant HDAC7 clone in a nonhuman primate. *Human Gene Therapy*, Vol.21, No.6, (June 2010), pp. 695-703, ISSN 1525-0016

Xue, X.; Huang, X.; Nodland, S.E.; Mátés, L.; Ma, L.; Izsvák, Z.; Ivics, Z.; LeBien, T.W.; McIvor, R.S.; Wagner, J.E. & Zhou, X. (2009). Stable gene transfer and expression in cord blood-derived CD34+ hematopoietic stem and progenitor cells by a hyperactive Sleeping Beauty transposon system. *Blood*, Vol.114, No.7, (August 2009), pp. 1319-1330, ISSN 0006-4971

Yoshihara, H.; Arai, F.; Hosokawa, K.; Hagiwara, T.; Takubo, K.; Nakamura, Y.; Gomei, Y.; Iwasaki, H.; Matsuoka, S.; Miyamoto, K.; Miyazaki, H.; Takahashi, T. & Suda, T. (2007). Thrombopoietin/MPL signaling regulates hematopoietic stem cell quiescence and interaction with the osteoblastic niche. *Cell Stem Cell*, Vol.1, No.6, (December 2007), pp. 685-697, ISSN 1934-5909

Yuan, Y.; Tse, K.T.; Sin, F.W.; Xue, B.; Fan, H.H.; Xie, Y. & Xie, Y. (2011). Ex vivo amplification of human hematopoietic stem and progenitor cells in an alginate three-dimensional culture system. *International Journal of Laboratory Hematology*, Vol.33, No.5, (October 2011), pp. 516-525, ISSN 1751-5521

Yusa, K.; Zhou, L.; Li, M.A.; Bradley, A. & Craig, N.L. (2011). A hyperactive piggyBac transposase for mammalian applications. *Proceedings of the National Academy of Sciences of the United States of America*, Vol.108, No.4, (January 2011), pp. 1531-1536, ISSN 0027-8424

Zayed, H.; Izsvák, Z.; Walisko, O. & Ivics, Z. (2004). Development of hyperactive sleeping beauty transposon vectors by mutational analysis. *Molecular Therapy*, Vol. 9, No.2, (February 2004), pp. 292-304, ISSN 1525-0016.

Zhang, C.C.; Kaba, M.; Ge, G.; Xie, K.; Tong, W.; Hug, C. & Lodish, H.F. (2006). Angiopoietin-like proteins stimulate ex vivo expansion of hematopoietic stem cells. *Nature Medicine*, Vol.12, No.2, (February 2006), pp. 240-245, ISSN 1078-8956

Zhang, J.; Niu, C.; Ye, L.; Huang, H.; He, X.; Tong, W.G.; Ross, J.; Haug, J.; Johnson, T.; Feng, J.Q.; Harris, S.; Wiedemann, L.M.; Mishina, Y. & Li, L. (2003). Identification of the haematopoietic stem cell niche and control of the niche size. *Nature*, Vol.425, No.6960, (October 2003), pp. 836-841, ISSN 0028-0836

Zhang, P.; Iwasaki-Arai, J.; Iwasaki, H.; Fenyus, M.L.; Dayaram, T.; Owens, B.M.; Shigematsu, H.; Levantini, E.; Huettner, C.S.; Lekstrom-Himes, J.A.; Akashi, K. & Tenen, D.G. (2004). Enhancement of hematopoietic stem cell repopulating capacity and self-renewal in the absence of the transcription factor C/EBP alpha. *Immunity*, Vol.21, No.6, (December 2004), pp. 853-863, ISSN 1074-7613

Zhang, X. & Roth, M.J. (2010). Antibody-directed lentiviral gene transduction in early immature hematopoietic progenitor cells. *The Journal of Gene Medicine*, Vol.12, No.12, (December 2010), pp. 945-955, ISSN 1099-498X

Zhang, X.B.; Beard, B.C.; Beebe, K.; Storer, B.; Humphries, R.K. & Kiem, H.P. (2006). Differential effects of HOXB4 on nonhuman primate short- and long-term repopulating cells. *PLoS Medicine*, Vol.3, No.5, (May 2006), pp. e173, ISSN 1549-1277

Zhang, X.B.; Beard, B.C.; Trobridge, G.D.; Wood, B.L.; Sale, G.E.; Sud, R.; Humphries, R.K. & Kiem H.P. (2008). High incidence of leukemia in large animals after stem cell gene therapy with a HOXB4-expressing retroviral vector. *The Journal of Clinical Investigation*, Vol.118, No.4, (April 2008), pp. 1502–1510, ISSN 0021-9738

Zhu, J.; Zhang, Y.; Joe, G.J.; Pompetti, R. & Emerson, S.G. (2005). NF-Ya activates multiple hematopoietic stem cell (HSC) regulatory genes and promotes HSC self-renewal. *Proceedings of the National Academy of Sciences of the United States of America*, Vol.102, No.33, (August 2005), pp. 11728-11733, ISSN 0027-8424

Zielske, S.P.; Reese, J.S.; Lingas, K.T.; Donze, J.R. & Gerson, S.L. (2003). In vivo selection of MGMT(P140K) lentivirus–transduced human NOD/SCID repopulating cells without pretransplant irradiation conditioning. *The Journal of Clinical Investigation*, Vol.12, No.10, (November 2003), pp. 1561-1570, ISSN 0021-9738

10

Bone Marrow Derived Pluripotent Stem Cells in Ischemic Heart Disease: Bridging the Gap Between Basic Research and Clinical Applications

Ahmed Abdel-Latif[1], Ewa Zuba-Surma[2] and Mariusz Z. Ratajczak[3]

[1]*Gill Heart Institute and Division of Cardiovascular Medicine,
University of Kentucky, and Lexington VA Medical Center, Lexington, KY*
[2]*Department of Medical Biotechnology, Faculty of Biochemistry,
Biophysics and Biotechnology, Jagiellonian University, Cracow,*
[3]*Stem Cell Biology Institute, James Graham Brown Cancer Center,
University of Louisville, Louisville, KY,*
[1,3]*USA*
[2]*Poland*

1. Introduction

The prevalence of ischemic heart disease and acute myocardial infarction (AMI) has increased to alarming rates in the United States and the western world (Roger *et al.*, 2011). Patients who survive the initial AMI suffer ischemic cardiomyopathy (ICM) which is often complicated by high mortality and poor overall prognosis (Braunwald *et al.*, 2000; McMurray *et al.*, 2005). Despite significant advances in medical therapy and revascularization strategies, the prognosis of patients with AMI and ischemic cardiomyopathy remains dismal (Levy D *et al.*, 2002; Roger VL *et al.*, 2004). The last decade has demonstrated significant progress and rapid translation of myocardial regenerative therapies particularly those utilizing stem cells isolated from adult tissues (Abdel-Latif *et al.*, 2007).

Studies examining the potential therapeutic use of bone marrow (BM)-derived cells in myocardial regeneration have overshadowed the growing evidence of innate cardiac reparatory mechanisms. Several studies have demonstrated the capability of cardiomyocytes to replenish through poorly understood innate mechanisms. Follow up of cardiac transplantation patients have demonstrated continuous replenishment of cardiomyocytes by recipient's derived cells through poorly understood mechanisms (Quaini *et al.*, 2002). There is growing evidence that BM-derived cells are responsible, at least in part, for organ chimerism including cardiomyocyte chimerism (de Weger *et al.*, 2008; Deb *et al.*, 2003). Animal studies have confirmed this to be a dynamic process responding to significant injury such as myocardial infarction and peaks in the peri-infarct zone (Hsieh *et al.*, 2007). Although this process appears to be robust enough to achieve the renewal of approximately 50% of all cardiomyocytes in the normal life span, very little is known about its underpinnings (Bergmann *et al.*, 2009).

Complex innate reparatory mechanisms are initiated by myocardial ischemia interacting with different elements of the immune system, the infarcted myocardium and bone marrow stem cells, culminating in BM-stem and progenitor cells' (SPCs) mobilization as we and others have demonstrated (Abdel-Latif *et al.*, 2010; Walter *et al.*, 2007; Wojakowski *et al.*, 2009). However, very little is known about the mechanisms and clinical significance of this mobilization. Animal studies show that mobilized BM-derived cells (BMCs) repopulate the infarct border, however the significance of this mobilization is unclear given the low rate of their differentiation into cardiomyocytes (Fukuhara *et al.*, 2005).

2. Isolation and functional characteristics of BM-derived pluripotent stem cells

The bone marrow acts as a reservoir for a heterogeneous pool of tissue-committed and non-committed stem cells. These populations contain progenitors that aid in the chimerism and cellular turnover of different organs as well as very rare populations of pluripotent and non-committed stem cells. The old dogma that adult tissues lack pluripotent stem cells (PSCs) has been continuously challenged during the last decade through multiple studies that isolated PSCs from adult humans' and animals' tissues. These populations were distinguished based on their morphology with small cell size, large nucleus demonstrating euchromatin and large nucleus to cytoplasm ratio. Furthermore, cell surface markers as well as nuclear transcription factors, such as SSEA1/4, Oct4 and Nanog, have been deployed.

Very small embryonic like stem cells (VSELs) represent a rare yet pluripotent population of adult stem cells. They have been initially described by Dr. Ratajczak's group in the murine BM based on their expression of Sca1 (murine stem cell marker) and lack of expression of CD45 (pan–leukocytic marker) and differentiated lineage (Lin) markers (Kucia *et al.*, 2006; Zuba-Surma *et al.*, 2008). Following their isolation from murine tissues, VSELs were subsequently isolated from human BM, umbilical cord blood (CB) and peripheral blood based on the lack of expression of Lin/CD45 and the expression of the stem cell markers CD133, CXCR4 and CD34. **Figure 1** illustrates the flow cytometry protocol for identifying and isolating VSELs from murine and human samples. VSELs were further characterized using a multi-dimensional approach comprising molecular, protein and cell imaging techniques to confirm their pluripotent features (Zuba-Surma *et al.* 2008). VSELs are morphologically similar to embryonic stem cells demonstrating small diameter compared to more committed progenitors/stem cells with large nucleus containing open-type chromatin surrounded with thin rim of cytoplasm and multiple mitochondria (Zuba-Surma *et al.* 2008).

VSELs exhibit multiple embryonic and pluripotent surface and nuclear embryonic markers such as Oct4, SSEA1/4, Nanog, and Rex1. In vivo and in vitro studies have demonstrated the capability of VSELs to differentiate into multiple cell lines across germ lines including cardiomyocytes (Kucia *et al.* 2006).

The bone marrow harbors other multi- and pluri-potent stem cell populations such as the mesenchymal stem cells (MSC) (Hattan *et al.*, 2005; Kawada *et al.*, 2004), multipotent adult progenitor cells (MAPC) (Jiang *et al.*, 2002), and marrow-isolated multilineage inducible cells (MIAMI) (D'Ippolito *et al.*, 2004). Similar populations with cardiac differentiation potential

Bone Marrow Derived Pluripotent Stem Cells in Ischemic Heart Disease: Bridging the Gap
Between Basic Research and Clinical Applications

207

have been also isolated from skeletal muscle and other tissues (Abdel-Latif *et al.*, 2008a). However, it is conceivable that different investigators have isolated, using different methods, the same or very similar populations and named them differently. It is also possible that these populations at least in part contain VSELs which might explain their pluripotent potential.

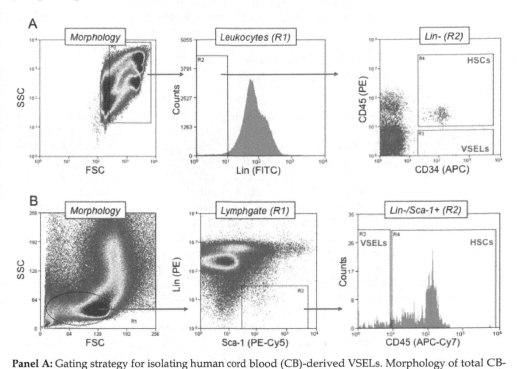

Panel A: Gating strategy for isolating human cord blood (CB)-derived VSELs. Morphology of total CB-derived nucleated cells is shown on dot-plot representing FSC and SSC parameters related to cell size and granularity/ complexity, respectively. All objects larger than 2μm are enclosed in region R1 and further visualized on histogram showing the expression of markers of mature hematopoietic cells (lineage markers; Lin). Cells not expressing differentiated hematopoietic markers (Lin- in region R2) are then analyzed for CD34 and CD45 expression. VSELs are identified as CD45-/Lin-/CD34+ cells (region R3), while hematopoietic stem cells (HSCs) as CD45+/Lin-/CD34+ cells (region R4).

Panel B: Sorting of murine bone marrow (BM)-derived VSELs. Morphology of total murine BM-derived nucleated cells is shown on dot-plot presenting FSC and SSC parameters and all objects in range of 2-10μm in diameter are included in region R1. Lymphocytic cells including stem cell fraction is further analyzed for Sca-1 and differentiated hematopoietic lineages markers (Lin) expression and only Sca-1+/Lin- cells are included in region R2. Cells from this region are further seperated based on CD45 expression. Murine VSELs are distinguished as CD45-/Lin-/Sca-1+ cells (region R3), while HSCs as CD45+/Lin-/Sca-1+ cells (region R4).

Fig. 1. Strategy for flow cytometric analysis of human and murine Very Small Embryonic-Like and hematopoietic stem cells. Briefly, BM is flushed from the femurs and tibias. Nucleated cells are isolated by lysis of red blood cells and cells are then gated on based on the cell size (>2 μm). Of note, lysis is preferred for isolating VSELs rather than Ficoll gradient that we have shown to lose some of the VSELs due to their small size.

3. BM-derived pluripotent stem cells are mobilized in the peripheral circulation following myocardial ischemia in animal models and humans

Myocardial ischemia, particularly large myocardial infarction, produce multiple stimuli include various chemokines, cytokines, kinins, bioactive lipids and members of the complement cascade, that lead to the mobilization and subsequent homing of BMSPCs. Indeed, several reports have confirmed that mobilization of stem cells originating from the BM occurs in response to myocardial ischemic injury (Grundmann et al., 2007; Kucia et al., 2004b; Leone et al., 2005; Massa et al., 2005; Shintani et al., 2001; Wojakowski et al., 2006) and heart failure (Valgimigli et al., 2004). Similar observations were noted in patients with acute neurological ischemia (Paczkowska et al., 2005) and patients with extensive skin burn (Drukala et al., 2011).

Stimuli responsible for the mobilization and homing of BMSCs in the setting of myocardial ischemia show similarities and differences with those involved in hematopoietic stem cells (HSCs) homing to the BM. The role of stromal cell derived factor (SDF-1) and its receptor (CXCR4) axis in the retention of hematopoietic stem/progenitor cells (HSPCs) in bone marrow is undisputed (Kucia et al., 2005; Lapidot et al., 2002), however, its role in the mobilization and homing of BM-SPCs to a highly proteolytic microenvironment, such as the ischemic/infarcted myocardium, is somewhat less certain. Studies have demonstrated that multiple members of the metalloproteinases (MMP) family, such as MMP2, MMP9 and MMP13, are upreagulated in the myocardium following infarction (Peterson et al., 2000). The elevated levels of the MMPs contribute to the degradation of chemokines such as SDF-1 and the byproduct of this degradation acts as an inhibitor the sole SDF-1 receptor, CXCR4 (McQuibban et al., 2001; McQuibban et al., 2002). In support of this hypothesis, Agrawal et al demonstrated that the conditional deletion of CXCR4 in cardiomyocytes did not influence the recovery of left ventricular (LV) function, reduce the scar size or alter the homing of MSCs to the myocardium following myocardial infarction (Agarwal et al., 2010). Thus, there is growing evidence that other mechanisms beside the SDF-1/CXCR4 axis are contributing to the mobilization and homing of BM-SPCs in AMI and other conditions (Jalili et al., 2010; Ratajczak et al., 2010). These data suggest an important interplay between the complement cascade, the immune system, cathelicidins, low levels of SDF-1, and sphingosine-1 phosphate (S1P) and other bioactive lipids in the mobilization and homing of HSPCs. Our preliminary data suggest that these complex interactions might be involved in the mobilization of BM-SPCs in acute myocardial ischemia as well (unpublished data). Clinically, pharmacological modulators of S1P receptors are already approved by the FDA and can be utilized to enhance BM-SPC mobilization in the setting of ischemic heart disease. Similarly, modulation of the complement cascade can be also utilized in this process similar to their role in the mobilization of HSPCs.

The first evidence for the mobilization of CD34+ mononuclear cells in AMI was demonstrated by Shintani et al (Shintani et al. 2001). The authors demonstrated successful in vitro differentiation of circulating BM-SPCs into endothelial cells that expressed CD31, VE-cadherin and the kinase insert domain receptor (KDR) (Shintani, et al. 2001). Leone et al demonstrated that the levels of circulating CD34+ cells in the setting of AMI were higher when compared to patients with mild chronic stable angina and healthy controls. The magnitude of CD34+ cell mobilization correlated with the recovery of regional and global LV function recovery as well as other functional LV parameters (Leone et al. 2005). Similarly,

Bone Marrow Derived Pluripotent Stem Cells in Ischemic Heart Disease: Bridging the Gap
Between Basic Research and Clinical Applications

209

Wojakowski *et al* demonstrated the mobilization of multiple BM-SPCs populations in patients with AMI and found significant correlation between the number of circulating CD34+ cells and plasma SDF-1 levels (Wojakowski *et al.*, 2004). In their following publication, the authors demonstrated the correlation between circulating BM-SPCs and ejection fraction at baseline and lower brain natriuretic peptide (BNP) levels (Wojakowski *et al.* 2006). Interestingly, the mobilization of BM-SPCs is reduced by the successful revascularization of the culprit vessel in acute STEMI (Müller-Ehmsen *et al.*, 2005). However, the majority of the above mentioned studies have focused on the mobilization of partially committed stem cells such as HSPCs and endothelial progenitor cells (EPCs).

We and others have demonstrated the mobilization of pluripotent stem cells (PSCs) including VSELs in the setting of myocardial ischemia (Abdel-Latif *et al.* 2010; Wojakowski *et al.* 2009). The number of circulating VSELs was highest in patients with ST-elevation myocardial infarction (STEMI), particularly in the early phases following the injury, when compared to patients with lesser degrees of ischemia such as non STEMI (NSTEMI) and those with chronic ischemic heart disease (Abdel-Latif *et al.* 2010). The mobilization of PSCs appears to be related to the extent of myocardial ischemia and the degree of myocardial damage. Moreover, the ability of patients to mobilize PSCs in the peripheral circulation in response to AMI decreases with age, reduced global LV ejection fraction (LVEF) and diabetes supporting the notion of an age/comorbidity related decline in the regenerative capacity (Abdel-Latif, *et al.* 2010; Wojakowski, *et al.* 2009). Indeed, animal models confirm the reduction of number as well as pluripotent features of BM-derived VSELs with age (Zuba-Surma *et al.* 2008). Similarly, studies have demonstrated the reduction of number as well as functional capacity of EPCs in diabetic patients (Fadini *et al.*, 2006).

The pluripotent features of mobilized VSELs, including the presence of octamer-binding transcription factor-4 (Oct4) and stage specific embryonic antigen-4 (SSEA4), were confirmed both on the RNA and protein levels. Utilizing the capabilities of the ImageStream system, we demonstrated that circulating VSELs during AMI have very similar embryonic features similar to their BM and CB counterparts including the small size (7-8 µm), large nucleus and high nuclear-to-cytoplasm ratio (**Figure 2**). Furthermore, circulating VSELs during AMI express markers of early cardiac and endothelial progenitors that suggest that the mobilization is rather specific and that circulating VSELs are destined to aid in the myocardial regeneration following injury (Abdel-Latif *et al.* 2010; Kucia *et al.* 2004b; Wojakowski *et al.* 2009).

The above evidence suggest an innate, yet poorly understood, reparatory mechanism that culminates in the mobilization of BMSCs including pluripotent and embryonic like stem cells in acute myocardial injury. This mobilization correlates with the recovery of LV function and other LV functional parameters. Therefore, mobilization of PSCs in myocardial ischemia is a relevant and clinically significant process. Future studies aiming at selective mobilization of PSCs rather than the non-selective actions of agents such as granulocyte colony stimulating factor (G-CSF) may prove beneficial in the field of myocardial regeneration.

Indeed, there is evidence that the mobilization of CXCR4+ cells in the setting of AMI is correlated with LVEF recovery as well as myocardial reperfusion when assessed with cardiac MRI in humans (Wojakowski, *et al.* 2006).

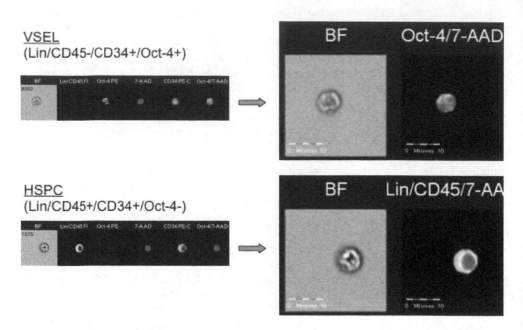

Fig. 2. Representative ImageStream images of VSEL and hematopoietic stem/ progenitor cell (HSPC) circulating in peripheral blood following acute ST-elevation myocardial infarction. Cells were stained against: 1) hematopoietic lineages markers (Lin) and CD45 to be detected in one channel (FITC, green), 2) marker of pluripotency Oct4 (PE, yellow) and 3) stem cell antigen CD34 (PE-Cy5, cyan). Nuclei are stained with 7-aminoactinomycin D (7-AAD, red). Scales represents 10 μm. VSELs are identified based on the lack of expression of both Lin and CD45 markers and positive staining for CD34 antigen and nuclear appearence of Oct-4 transcription factor (**Upper Panel**). HSCs are identified as cell expressing Lin and/ or CD45 markers as well as CD34 antigen; however, negative for Oct-4 (**Lower Panel**). BF: Bright field.

4. Therapeutic mobilization of BM-derived stem cells in myocardial regeneration

Hematologists have used the concept of BM-derived stem cell mobilization using pharmacological agents such as G-CSF for a long time. Based on the available clinical experience and safety profile of these therapies, pharmacological stem cell mobilization in the setting of AMI has gained increasing enthusiasm. Mobilized BM-SPCs are either harvested for further transplantation or allowed for spontaneous homing to the infarcted myocardium and has demonstrated various degrees of success (Engelmann *et al.*, 2006; Ince *et al.*, 2005; Zohlnhöfer *et al.*, 2006). Similar to BMCs transplantation studies, the heterogeneous methodologies of the included studies diluted the effect. The overall lack of efficacy with G-CSF BMCs mobilization in the setting of acute myocardial infarction is somewhat incongruent with the salutary effects of BMCs transplantation in humans and G-CSF therapy in animal models for myocardial regeneration.

Bone Marrow Derived Pluripotent Stem Cells in Ischemic Heart Disease: Bridging the Gap
Between Basic Research and Clinical Applications

211

The largest study utilizing G-CSF in the setting of acute myocardial infarction was the REVIVAL-2 trial that included 114 patients (Zohlnhöfer, *et al.* 2006). The study randomized AMI patients to 10 μg/kg of G-CSF vs. placebo and left ventricular functional parameters were assessed using cardiac MRI (CMR). The study demonstrated no significant difference in the tested parameters between patients treated with G-CSF or placebo. However, baseline characteristics in the study population showed normal or near normal LV function and therefore the expected benefit is minimal. Patient selection was a methodological flaw that plagued some of the studies that utilized G-CSF. Indeed, with careful examination of the available literature, patients with reduced LV function at baseline as well as those treated within the first 36 hours following AMI benefited the most (Abdel-Latif *et al.*, 2008b; Achilli *et al.*, 2010). On the other hand, safety concerns regarding a potentially increasing evidence of instent restenosis (Kang *et al.*, 2004) and recurrent ischemia (Hill *et al.*, 2005) have halted subsequent clinical trials. However, it is important to note that these safety concerns were not confirmed in large studies (Zohlnhöfer, *et al.* 2006) or in the cumulative meta-analyses (Abdel-Latif *et al.* 2008b).

Beyond the methodological flaws encountered in human trials, this lack of efficacy can be explained by multiple factors. While G-CSF and similar therapies mobilize a wide array of BMSPCs in the peripheral blood, homing factors may not be sufficient to guide them to the myocardial infarct zone. Indeed, the homing of c-Kit+ cells to the infarcted myocardium improved when G-CSF therapy was combined with local administration of SDF-1 (Askari *et al.*, 2003). The myocardial levels of chemoattractants peaks within 24-72 hours following injury (Kucia *et al.*, 2004a; Ma *et al.*, 2005; Wang *et al.*, 2006) and therefore delayed therapy in some human trials may have missed the homing window to the infarct zone. Similarly, the addition of Flt-3 to G-CSF therapy improved outcomes in animal models (Dawn *et al.*, 2008). Moreover, different cytokines are known to preferentially mobilize somewhat different subsets of BMCs (Hess *et al.*, 2002; Neipp *et al.*, 1998). Future studies investigating the characteristics of G-CSF-mobilized cells will be necessary to glean additional mechanistic insights in this regard.

Recently, a combined approach with stem cell mobilization and enhanced homing using therapies known to increase local SDF-1 or CXCR4 antagonists have been proposed and is currently being tested (Jujo *et al.*, 2010; Zaruba *et al.*, 2009). Going forward, the beneficial effects of BM-derived stem cell mobilization may be augmented by selective mobilization of undifferentiated BMSCs rather than differentiated inflammatory cells. It is also important to remember that some of the G-CSF arbitrated effects can be mediated by its direct effect on cardiomyocytes which are known to express G-CSF receptor (Shimoji *et al.*, 2010). G-CSF therapy may be inducing the proliferation of cardiomyocytes or the differentiation of resident cardiac stem cells. On a similar note, G-CSF therapy upregulates Akt (Ohtsuka *et al.*, 2004) and may result in reducing apoptosis of ischemic cardiomyocytes if utilized early following the acute event.

5. BM-derived stem cell transplantation for myocardial repair

The use of BM-derived cells in myocardial regeneration has moved rapidly from the basic research lab to the clinical arena. The results from these studies varied widely probably secondary to the heterogeneous methodologies used with an overall marginal benefit with

BM-derived cell transplantation compared to placebo. The majority of studies, however, utilized unselected populations of BMCs and these studies provide the longest follow-up of up to 5 years (Assmus *et al.*, 2010; Schachinger *et al.*, 2009). The underling mechanisms leading to the beneficial effect of transplanted BMCs are unclear. The observed benefits of BMCs transplantation is out of proportion of the observed rates of newly formed cardiomyocytes from BMCs' origin (Zuba-Surma *et al.*, 2011). Indeed, recent evidence suggest a primarily paracrine effect of BM-derived stem cells following their transplantation by recruiting and stimulating resident cardiac stem cells (CSCs) (Loffredo *et al.*, 2011). Furthermore, human purified CD34+ cells are a source of several growth factors including VEGF, cytokines and chemokines that may prevent apoptosis of dying cardiomyocytes and promote angiogenesis in damaged myocardium (Majka *et al.*, 2001). Cell membrane derived microvesicles or exosomes that are enriched in S1P may contribute to regeneration of myocardium and its re-vascularization (Baj-Krzyworzeka *et al.*, 2002). Hence, transplanted CD34+ cells may contribute to regeneration of damaged heart by paracrine signals and released microvesicles (Ratajczak *et al.*, 2008) and was recently confirmed by others (Sahoo *et al.*, 2011).

Long-term follow-up studies demonstrated 'catch-up phenomenon' of the placebo treated patients, thus leading to mixed results regarding the sustainability of the BMCs treatment benefit (Assmus, *et al.* 2010; Meyer *et al.*, 2009; Yousef *et al.*, 2009). The benefit of BMCs therapy is less robust among patients with chronic ischemic heart disease (IHD) (Assmus *et al.*, 2006; Strauer *et al.*, 2010). Similarly, smaller studies have demonstrated the antianginal effects of BMCs in patients with non-revascularizable severe coronary artery disease (Losordo *et al.*, 2007; Tse *et al.*, 2007).

Selected BM-derived stem cell subpopulations represent an attractive substrate for cellular therapies since they lack the inflammatory cells, which contribute to the ongoing inflammatory response at the site of myocardial infarction, contained in the unselected BMCs populations. Furthermore, highly purified stem cell populations are more likely to induce myocardial regeneration through paracrine effects or by directly differentiating into cardiomyocytes. The largest study utilizing selected BM-derived stem cell population is the REGENT study which compared selected to non-selected populations of BMCs in patients with acute ischemic heart disease and reduced LV function at baseline (Tendera *et al.*, 2009). While there were no significant differences between the groups, patients treated with selected CD34+/CXCR4+ cells showed trends of improvement in LV function when compared to controls. Other studies utilizing primitive populations of BM-SPCs such as CD133+ cells have reported improvement of LV function and perfusion (Bartunek *et al.*, 2005; Stamm *et al.*, 2004).

Nevertheless and despite the disparity in the methodologies of the conducted studies, the overall collective effect of BMCs' transplantation suggests small yet statistically significant benefit in myocardial regeneration (Abdel-Latif, *et al.* 2007; Martin-Rendon *et al.*, 2008). However, these trials have been hampered by their reliance on surrogate endpoints rather than patient important endpoints such as mortality, need for repeat revascularization, recurrent MI or re-hospitalization for congestive heart failure. While surrogate endpoints are important for mechanistic studies, patient-important endpoints are quintessential for a new therapy to achieve mainstream status.

Bone Marrow Derived Pluripotent Stem Cells in Ischemic Heart Disease: Bridging the Gap
Between Basic Research and Clinical Applications

213

6. Future directions

Growing evidence suggest that a multitude of BM-derived stem and pluripotent stem cells are mobilized in the peripheral blood following AMI. However, the clinical significance and the potential therapeutic use of this mobilization are still not fully understood. Circulating PSCs can be used as markers of ischemic injury in humans or as predictors of myocardial recovery following large ischemic damage. On the other hand, the therapeutic application of VSELs in myocardial regeneration has proven beneficial although the beneficial mechanisms remain elusive and are probably mainly paracrine in nature. Given the pluripotent potential of VSELs, their transplantation at smaller numbers (10,000 cells per mouse) have proven to be more beneficial than larger numbers of the more committed HSPCs (100,000 cells per mouse) indicating their greater therapeutic potential (Dawn *et al.* 2008). Current efforts directed at the ex-vivo expansion and priming of VSELs have proven to be a successful strategy in animal models and their clinical applications are pending (Dawn *et al.* 2008; Zuba-Surma, *et al.* 2011). Nuclear reprogramming has opened the door for creating patient-specific autologous pluripotent stem cells with multiple therapeutic opportunities (Takahashi *et al.*, 2006). Further studies are needed to examine the feasibility as well as the safety of inducible pluripotent stem cells (iPS) particularly their tumorigenicity and immunogenicity before they can be explored in human studies.

On the biotechnology frontier, multiple modifications of the transplanted cells (priming) and the host environment are being tested in humans to improve the efficiency of BM-SPCs' regenerative capacity. Transplanting three dimensional constructs that provide an enriched environment for the transplanted and resident stem cells are attractive modifications to the currently tested protocols [reviewed in (Mooney *et al.*, 2008)]. Similarly, the concept of multiple doses of stem cell to repair the complex process of myocardial remodeling following acute myocardial infarction is gaining traction and is very appealing. While the field of stem cell regenerative therapy for ischemic heart disease is still in its infancy, the accelerated advances in a wide array of biological and biotechnological areas have rapidly propelled the field from the bench to clinical applications.

7. Acknowledgments

Dr. Abdel-Latif is supported by the University of Kentucky Clinical and Translational Science Pilot Award and the University of Kentucky Clinical Scholar program.

Dr. Zuba-Surma is supported by the "Polish Foundation of Science" homing program grant number 2008/15.

Dr. Ratajczak is supported by NIH grant R01 CA106281, NIH R01 DK074720, and Stella and Henry Endowment.

We thank Dr. Karapetyan for her technical support for this review.

Conflict of interest: None.

8. References

Abdel-Latif A, Bolli R, Tleyjeh I, Montori V, Perin E, Hornung C, Zuba-Surma E, Al-Mallah M, and Dawn B (2007). Adult bone marrow-derived cells for cardiac repair: a systematic review and meta-analysis. *Arch Intern Med, 167:* 989-997.

Abdel-Latif A, Bolli R, Zuba-Surma EK, Tleyjeh IM, Hornung CA, and Dawn B (2008b). Granulocyte colony-stimulating factor therapy for cardiac repair after acute myocardial infarction: a systematic review and meta-analysis of randomized controlled trials. *Am Heart J, 156*: 216-226.

Abdel-Latif A, Zuba-Surma EK, Case J, Tiwari S, Hunt G, Ranjan S, Vincent RJ, Srour EF, Bolli R, and Dawn B (2008a). TGF-beta1 enhances cardiomyogenic differentiation of skeletal muscle-derived adult primitive cells. *Basic Res Cardiol, 103*: 514-524.

Abdel-Latif A, Zuba-Surma EK, Ziada KM, Kucia M, Cohen DA, Kaplan AM, Van Zant G, Selim S, Smyth SS, and Ratajczak MZ (2010). Evidence of mobilization of pluripotent stem cells into peripheral blood of patients with myocardial ischemia. *Exp Hematol, 38*: 1131-1142.

Achilli F, Malafronte C, Lenatti L, Gentile F, Dadone V, Gibelli G, Maggiolini S, Squadroni L, Di Leo C, Burba I, Pesce M, Mircoli L, Capogrossi MC, Di Lelio A, Camisasca P, Morabito A, Colombo G, and Pompilio G (2010). Granulocyte colony-stimulating factor attenuates left ventricular remodelling after acute anterior STEMI: results of the single-blind, randomized, placebo-controlled multicentre STem cEll Mobilization in Acute Myocardial Infarction (STEM-AMI) Trial. *Eur J Heart Fail, 12*: 1111-1121.

Agarwal U, Ghalayini W, Dong F, Weber K, Zou YR, Rabbany SY, Rafii S, and Penn MS (2010). Role of cardiac myocyte CXCR4 expression in development and left ventricular remodeling after acute myocardial infarction. *Circ Res, 107*: 667-676.

Askari AT, Unzek S, Popovic ZB, Goldman CK, Forudi F, Kiedrowski M, Rovner A, Ellis SG, Thomas JD, DiCorleto PE, Topol EJ, and Penn MS (2003). Effect of stromal-cell-derived factor 1 on stem-cell homing and tissue regeneration in ischaemic cardiomyopathy. *Lancet, 362*: 697-703.

Assmus B, Honold J, Schachinger V, Britten M, Fischer-Rasokat U, Lehmann R, Teupe C, Pistorius K, Martin H, Abolmaali N, Tonn T, Dimmeler S, and Zeiher A (2006). Transcoronary transplantation of progenitor cells after myocardial infarction. *N Engl J Med, 355*: 1222-1232.

Assmus B, Rolf A, Erbs S, Elsasser A, Haberbosch W, Hambrecht R, Tillmanns H, Yu J, Corti R, Mathey DG, Hamm CW, Suselbeck T, Tonn T, Dimmeler S, Dill T, Zeiher AM, and Schachinger V (2010). Clinical outcome 2 years after intracoronary administration of bone marrow-derived progenitor cells in acute myocardial infarction. *Circ Heart Fail, 3*: 89-96.

Baj-Krzyworzeka M, Majka M, Pratico D, Ratajczak J, Vilaire G, Kijowski J, Reca R, Janowska-Wieczorek A, and Ratajczak MZ (2002). Platelet-derived microparticles stimulate proliferation, survival, adhesion, and chemotaxis of hematopoietic cells. *Exp Hematol, 30*: 450-459.

Bartunek J, Vanderheyden M, Vandekerckhove B, Mansour S, De Bruyne B, De Bondt P, Van Haute I, Lootens N, Heyndrickx G, and Wijns W (2005). Intracoronary injection of CD133-positive enriched bone marrow progenitor cells promotes cardiac recovery after recent myocardial infarction: feasibility and safety. *Circulation, 112*: I178-183.

Bergmann O, Bhardwaj RD, Bernard S, Zdunek S, Barnabe-Heider F, Walsh S, Zupicich J, Alkass K, Buchholz BA, Druid H, Jovinge S, and Frisen J (2009). Evidence for cardiomyocyte renewal in humans. *Science, 324*: 98-102.

Braunwald E, and Bristow M (2000). Congestive heart failure: fifty years of progress. *Circulation, 102*: IV14-IV23.

Bone Marrow Derived Pluripotent Stem Cells in Ischemic Heart Disease: Bridging the Gap
Between Basic Research and Clinical Applications

215

D'Ippolito G, Diabira S, Howard G, Menei P, Roos B, and Schiller P (2004). Marrow-isolated adult multilineage inducible (MIAMI) cells, a unique population of postnatal young and old human cells with extensive expansion and differentiation potential. *J Cell Sci, 117*: 2971-2981.

Dawn B, Tiwari S, Kucia MJ, Zuba-Surma EK, Guo Y, Sanganalmath SK, Abdel-Latif A, Hunt G, Vincent RJ, Taher H, Reed NJ, Ratajczak MZ, and Bolli R (2008). Transplantation of bone marrow-derived very small embryonic-like stem cells attenuates left ventricular dysfunction and remodeling after myocardial infarction. *Stem Cells, 26*: 1646-1655.

de Weger RA, Verbrugge I, Bruggink AH, van Oosterhout MM, de Souza Y, van Wichen DF, Gmelig-Meyling FH, de Jonge N, and Verdonck LF (2008). Stem cell-derived cardiomyocytes after bone marrow and heart transplantation. *Bone Marrow Transplant, 41*: 563-569.

Deb A, Wang S, Skelding KA, Miller D, Simper D, and Caplice NM (2003). Bone marrow-derived cardiomyocytes are present in adult human heart: A study of gender-mismatched bone marrow transplantation patients. *Circulation, 107*: 1247-1249.

Drukala J, Paczkowska E, Kucia M, Mlynska E, Krajewski A, Machalinski B, Madeja Z, and Ratajczak MZ (2011). Stem Cells, Including a Population of Very Small Embryonic-Like Stem Cells, are Mobilized Into Peripheral Blood in Patients After Skin Burn Injury. *Stem Cell Rev.*

Engelmann M, Theiss H, Hennig-Theiss C, Huber A, Wintersperger B, Werle-Ruedinger A, Schoenberg S, Steinbeck G, and Franz W (2006). Autologous bone marrow stem cell mobilization induced by granulocyte colony-stimulating factor after subacute ST-segment elevation myocardial infarction undergoing late revascularization: final results from the G-CSF-STEMI (Granulocyte Colony-Stimulating Factor ST-Segment Elevation Myocardial Infarction) trial. *J Am Coll Cardiol, 48*: 1712-1721.

Fadini GP, Sartore S, Schiavon M, Albiero M, Baesso I, Cabrelle A, Agostini C, and Avogaro A (2006). Diabetes impairs progenitor cell mobilisation after hindlimb ischaemia-reperfusion injury in rats. *Diabetologia, 49*: 3075-3084.

Fukuhara S, Tomita S, Nakatani T, Yutani C, and Kitamura S (2005). Endogenous bone-marrow-derived stem cells contribute only a small proportion of regenerated myocardium in the acute infarction model. *J Heart Lung Transplant, 24*: 67-72.

Grundmann F, Scheid C, Braun D, Zobel C, Reuter H, Schwinger R, and Müller-Ehmsen J (2007). Differential increase of CD34, KDR/CD34, CD133/CD34 and CD117/CD34 positive cells in peripheral blood of patients with acute myocardial infarction. *Clin Res Cardiol, 96*: 621-627.

Hattan N, Kawaguchi H, Ando K, Kuwabara E, Fujita J, Murata M, Suematsu M, Mori H, and Fukuda K (2005). Purified cardiomyocytes from bone marrow mesenchymal stem cells produce stable intracardiac grafts in mice. *Cardiovasc Res, 65*: 293-295.

Hess DA, Levac KD, Karanu FN, Rosu-Myles M, White MJ, Gallacher L, Murdoch B, Keeney M, Ottowski P, Foley R, Chin-Yee I, and Bhatia M (2002). Functional analysis of human hematopoietic repopulating cells mobilized with granulocyte colony-stimulating factor alone versus granulocyte colony-stimulating factor in combination with stem cell factor. *Blood, 100*: 869-878.

Hill JM, Syed MA, Arai AE, Powell TM, Paul JD, Zalos G, Read EJ, Khuu HM, Leitman SF, Horne M, Csako G, Dunbar CE, Waclawiw MA, and Cannon RO, 3rd (2005). Outcomes and risks of granulocyte colony-stimulating factor in patients with coronary artery disease. *J Am Coll Cardiol, 46*: 1643-1648.

Hsieh PC, Segers VF, Davis ME, MacGillivray C, Gannon J, Molkentin JD, Robbins J, and Lee RT (2007). Evidence from a genetic fate-mapping study that stem cells refresh adult mammalian cardiomyocytes after injury. *Nat Med, 13*: 970-974.

Ince H, Petzsch M, Kleine H, Eckard H, Rehders T, Burska D, Kische S, Freund M, and Nienaber C (2005). Prevention of left ventricular remodeling with granulocyte colony-stimulating factor after acute myocardial infarction: final 1-year results of the Front-Integrated Revascularization and Stem Cell Liberation in Evolving Acute Myocardial Infarction by Granulocyte Colony-Stimulating Factor (FIRSTLINE-AMI) Trial. *Circulation, 112*: I73-80.

Jalili A, Shirvaikar N, Marquez-Curtis L, Qiu Y, Korol C, Lee H, Turner AR, Ratajczak MZ, and Janowska-Wieczorek A (2010). Fifth complement cascade protein (C5) cleavage fragments disrupt the SDF-1/CXCR4 axis: further evidence that innate immunity orchestrates the mobilization of hematopoietic stem/progenitor cells. *Exp Hematol, 38*: 321-332.

Jiang Y, Jahagirdar B, Reinhardt R, Schwartz R, Keene C, Ortiz-Gonzalez X, Reyes M, Lenvik T, Lund T, Blackstad M, Du J, Aldrich S, Lisberg A, Low W, Largaespada D, and Verfaillie C (2002). Pluripotency of mesenchymal stem cells derived from adult marrow. *Nature, 418*: 41-49.

Jujo K, Hamada H, Iwakura A, Thorne T, Sekiguchi H, Clarke T, Ito A, Misener S, Tanaka T, Klyachko E, Kobayashi K, Tongers J, Roncalli J, Tsurumi Y, Hagiwara N, and Losordo DW (2010). CXCR4 blockade augments bone marrow progenitor cell recruitment to the neovasculature and reduces mortality after myocardial infarction. *Proc Natl Acad Sci U S A, 107*: 11008-11013.

Kang HJ, Kim HS, Zhang SY, Park KW, Cho HJ, Koo BK, Kim YJ, Soo Lee D, Sohn DW, Han KS, Oh BH, Lee MM, and Park YB (2004). Effects of intracoronary infusion of peripheral blood stem-cells mobilised with granulocyte-colony stimulating factor on left ventricular systolic function and restenosis after coronary stenting in myocardial infarction: the MAGIC cell randomised clinical trial. *Lancet, 363*: 751-756.

Kawada H, Fujita J, Kinjo K, Matsuzaki Y, Tsuma M, Miyatake H, Muguruma Y, Tsuboi K, Itabashi Y, Ikeda Y, Ogawa S, Okano H, Hotta T, Ando K, and Fukuda K (2004). Nonhematopoietic mesenchymal stem cells can be mobilized and differentiate into cardiomyocytes after myocardial infarction. *Blood, 104*: 3581-3587.

Kucia M, Dawn B, Hunt G, Guo Y, Wysoczynski M, Majka M, Ratajczak J, Rezzoug F, Ildstad ST, Bolli R, and Ratajczak MZ (2004a). Cells expressing early cardiac markers reside in the bone marrow and are mobilized into the peripheral blood after myocardial infarction. *Circ Res, 95*: 1191-1199.

Kucia M, Dawn B, Hunt G, Guo Y, Wysoczynski M, Majka M, Ratajczak J, Rezzoug F, Ildstad ST, Bolli R, and Ratajczak MZ (2004b). Cells expressing early cardiac markers reside in the bone marrow and are mobilized into the peripheral blood following myocardial infarction. *Circ Res, 95*: 1191-1199.

Kucia M, Reca R, Campbell FR, Zuba-Surma E, Majka M, Ratajczak J, and Ratajczak MZ (2006). A population of very small embryonic-like (VSEL) CXCR4(+)SSEA-1(+)Oct-4+ stem cells identified in adult bone marrow. *Leukemia, 20*: 857-869.

Kucia M, Reca R, Miekus K, Wanzeck J, Wojakowski W, Janowska-Wieczorek A, Ratajczak J, and Ratajczak MZ (2005). Trafficking of normal stem cells and metastasis of cancer stem cells involve similar mechanisms: pivotal role of the SDF-1-CXCR4 axis. *Stem Cells, 23*: 879-894.

Bone Marrow Derived Pluripotent Stem Cells in Ischemic Heart Disease: Bridging the Gap
Between Basic Research and Clinical Applications

217

Lapidot T, and Kollet O (2002). The essential roles of the chemokine SDF-1 and its receptor CXCR4 in human stem cell homing and repopulation of transplanted immune-deficient NOD/SCID and NOD/SCID/B2m(null) mice. *Leukemia : official journal of the Leukemia Society of America, Leukemia Research Fund, U.K, 16*: 1992-2003.

Leone A, Rutella S, Bonanno G, Abbate A, Rebuzzi A, Giovannini S, Lombardi M, Galiuto L, Liuzzo G, Andreotti F, Lanza G, Contemi A, Leone G, and Crea F (2005). Mobilization of bone marrow-derived stem cells after myocardial infarction and left ventricular function. *Eur Heart J, 26*: 1196-1204.

Levy D, Kenchaiah S, Larson MG, Benjamin EJ, Kupka MJ, Ho KK, Murabito JM, and RS. V (2002). Long-term trends in the incidence of and survival with heart failure. *N Engl J Med, 347*: 1442-1444.

Loffredo FS, Steinhauser ML, Gannon J, and Lee RT (2011). Bone marrow-derived cell therapy stimulates endogenous cardiomyocyte progenitors and promotes cardiac repair. *Cell Stem Cell, 8*: 389-398.

Losordo DW, Schatz RA, White CJ, Udelson JE, Veereshwarayya V, Durgin M, Poh KK, Weinstein R, Kearney M, Chaudhry M, Burg A, Eaton L, Heyd L, Thorne T, Shturman L, Hoffmeister P, Story K, Zak V, Dowling D, Traverse JH, Olson RE, Flanagan J, Sodano D, Murayama T, Kawamoto A, Kusano KF, Wollins J, Welt F, Shah P, Soukas P, Asahara T, and Henry TD (2007). Intramyocardial transplantation of autologous CD34+ stem cells for intractable angina: a phase I/IIa double-blind, randomized controlled trial. *Circulation, 115*: 3165-3172.

Ma J, Ge J, Zhang S, Sun A, Shen J, Chen L, Wang K, and Zou Y (2005). Time course of myocardial stromal cell-derived factor 1 expression and beneficial effects of intravenously administered bone marrow stem cells in rats with experimental myocardial infarction. *Basic Res Cardiol, 100*: 217-223.

Majka M, Janowska-Wieczorek A, Ratajczak J, Ehrenman K, Pietrzkowski Z, Kowalska MA, Gewirtz AM, Emerson SG, and Ratajczak MZ (2001). Numerous growth factors, cytokines, and chemokines are secreted by human CD34(+) cells, myeloblasts, erythroblasts, and megakaryoblasts and regulate normal hematopoiesis in an autocrine/paracrine manner. *Blood, 97*: 3075-3085.

Martin-Rendon E, Brunskill SJ, Hyde CJ, Stanworth SJ, Mathur A, and Watt SM (2008). Autologous bone marrow stem cells to treat acute myocardial infarction: a systematic review. *European heart journal, 29*: 1807-1818.

Massa M, Rosti V, Ferrario M, Campanelli R, Ramajoli I, Rosso R, De Ferrari G, Ferlini M, Goffredo L, Bertoletti A, Klersy C, Pecci A, Moratti R, and Tavazzi L (2005). Increased circulating hematopoietic and endothelial progenitor cells in the early phase of acute myocardial infarction. *Blood, 105*: 199-206.

McMurray J, and Pfeffer M (2005). Heart failure. *Lancet, 365*: 1877-1889.

McQuibban GA, Butler GS, Gong JH, Bendall L, Power C, Clark-Lewis I, and Overall CM (2001). Matrix metalloproteinase activity inactivates the CXC chemokine stromal cell-derived factor-1. *The Journal of biological chemistry, 276*: 43503-43508.

McQuibban GA, Gong JH, Wong JP, Wallace JL, Clark-Lewis I, and Overall CM (2002). Matrix metalloproteinase processing of monocyte chemoattractant proteins generates CC chemokine receptor antagonists with anti-inflammatory properties in vivo. *Blood, 100*: 1160-1167.

Meyer GP, Wollert KC, Lotz J, Pirr J, Rager U, Lippolt P, Hahn A, Fichtner S, Schaefer A, Arseniev L, Ganser A, and Drexler H (2009). Intracoronary bone marrow cell transfer after myocardial infarction: 5-year follow-up from the randomized-controlled BOOST trial. *European heart journal, 30*: 2978-2984.

Mooney DJ, and Vandenburgh H (2008). Cell delivery mechanisms for tissue repair. *Cell Stem Cell, 2*: 205-213.

Müller-Ehmsen J, Scheid C, Grundmann F, Hirsch I, Turan G, Tossios P, Mehlhorn U, and Schwinger R (2005). The mobilization of CD34 positive mononuclear cells after myocardial infarction is abolished by revascularization of the culprit vessel. *Int J Cardiol, 103*: 7-11.

Neipp M, Zorina T, Domenick MA, Exner BG, and Ildstad ST (1998). Effect of FLT3 ligand and granulocyte colony-stimulating factor on expansion and mobilization of facilitating cells and hematopoietic stem cells in mice: kinetics and repopulating potential. *Blood, 92*: 3177-3188.

Ohtsuka M, Takano H, Zou Y, Toko H, Akazawa H, Qin Y, Suzuki M, Hasegawa H, Nakaya H, and Komuro I (2004). Cytokine therapy prevents left ventricular remodeling and dysfunction after myocardial infarction through neovascularization. *The FASEB journal : official publication of the Federation of American Societies for Experimental Biology, 18*: 851-853.

Paczkowska E, Larysz B, Rzeuski R, Karbicka A, Jałowiński R, Kornacewicz-Jach Z, Ratajczak M, and Machaliński B (2005). Human hematopoietic stem/progenitor-enriched CD34(+) cells are mobilized into peripheral blood during stress related to ischemic stroke or acute myocardial infarction. *Eur J Haematol, 75*: 461-467.

Peterson JT, Li H, Dillon L, and Bryant JW (2000). Evolution of matrix metalloprotease and tissue inhibitor expression during heart failure progression in the infarcted rat. *Cardiovascular research, 46*: 307-315.

Quaini F, Urbanek K, Beltrami AP, Finato N, Beltrami CA, Nadal-Ginard B, Kajstura J, Leri A, and Anversa P (2002). Chimerism of the transplanted heart. *N Engl J Med, 346*: 5-15.

Ratajczak MZ, Lee H, Wysoczynski M, Wan W, Marlicz W, Laughlin MJ, Kucia M, Janowska-Wieczorek A, and Ratajczak J (2010). Novel insight into stem cell mobilization-plasma sphingosine-1-phosphate is a major chemoattractant that directs the egress of hematopoietic stem progenitor cells from the bone marrow and its level in peripheral blood increases during mobilization due to activation of complement cascade/membrane attack complex. *Leukemia, 24*: 976-985.

Ratajczak MZ, Zuba-Surma EK, Shin DM, Ratajczak J, and Kucia M (2008). Very small embryonic-like (VSEL) stem cells in adult organs and their potential role in rejuvenation of tissues and longevity. *Exp Gerontol, 43*: 1009-1017.

Roger VL, Weston SA, Redfield MM, Hellermann-Homan JP, Killian J, Yawn BP, and SJ. J (2004). Trends in heart failure incidence and survival in a community-based population. *JAMA, 292*: 344-350.

Roger VL, Go AS, Lloyd-Jones DM, Adams RJ, Berry JD, Brown TM, Carnethon MR, Dai S, de Simone G, Ford ES, Fox CS, Fullerton HJ, Gillespie C, Greenlund KJ, Hailpern SM, Heit JA, Ho PM, Howard VJ, Kissela BM, Kittner SJ, Lackland DT, Lichtman JH, Lisabeth LD, Makuc DM, Marcus GM, Marelli A, Matchar DB, McDermott MM, Meigs JB, Moy CS, Mozaffarian D, Mussolino ME, Nichol G, Paynter NP, Rosamond WD, Sorlie PD, Stafford RS, Turan TN, Turner MB, Wong ND, and Wylie-Rosett J (2011). Heart disease and stroke statistics--2011 update: a report from the American Heart Association. *Circulation, 123*: e18-e209.

Bone Marrow Derived Pluripotent Stem Cells in Ischemic Heart Disease: Bridging the Gap
Between Basic Research and Clinical Applications

219

Sahoo S, Klychko E, Thorne T, Misener S, Schultz KM, Millay M, Ito A, Liu T, Kamide C, Agarwal H, Perlman H, Qin G, Kishore R, and Losordo DW (2011). Exosomes From Human CD34+ Stem Cells Mediate Their Proangiogenic Paracrine Activity. *Circ Res*.

Schachinger V, Assmus B, Erbs S, Elsasser A, Haberbosch W, Hambrecht R, Yu J, Corti R, Mathey DG, Hamm CW, Tonn T, Dimmeler S, and Zeiher AM (2009). Intracoronary infusion of bone marrow-derived mononuclear cells abrogates adverse left ventricular remodelling post-acute myocardial infarction: insights from the reinfusion of enriched progenitor cells and infarct remodelling in acute myocardial infarction (REPAIR-AMI) trial. *Eur J Heart Fail, 11*: 973-979.

Shimoji K, Yuasa S, Onizuka T, Hattori F, Tanaka T, Hara M, Ohno Y, Chen H, Egasgira T, Seki T, Yae K, Koshimizu U, Ogawa S, and Fukuda K (2010). G-CSF promotes the proliferation of developing cardiomyocytes in vivo and in derivation from ESCs and iPSCs. *Cell Stem Cell, 6*: 227-237.

Shintani S, Murohara T, Ikeda H, Ueno T, Honma T, Katoh A, Sasaki K, Shimada T, Oike Y, and Imaizumi T (2001). Mobilization of endothelial progenitor cells in patients with acute myocardial infarction. *Circulation, 103*: 2776-2779.

Stamm C, Kleine HD, Westphal B, Petzsch M, Kittner C, Nienaber CA, Freund M, and Steinhoff G (2004). CABG and bone marrow stem cell transplantation after myocardial infarction. *Thorac Cardiovasc Surg, 52*: 152-158.

Strauer BE, Yousef M, and Schannwell CM (2010). The acute and long-term effects of intracoronary Stem cell Transplantation in 191 patients with chronic heARt failure: the STAR-heart study. *Eur J Heart Fail, 12*: 721-729.

Takahashi K, and Yamanaka S (2006). Induction of pluripotent stem cells from mouse embryonic and adult fibroblast cultures by defined factors. *Cell, 126*: 663-676.

Tendera M, Wojakowski W, Ruzyllo W, Chojnowska L, Kepka C, Tracz W, Musialek P, Piwowarska W, Nessler J, Buszman P, Grajek S, Breborowicz P, Majka M, and Ratajczak MZ (2009). Intracoronary infusion of bone marrow-derived selected CD34+CXCR4+ cells and non-selected mononuclear cells in patients with acute STEMI and reduced left ventricular ejection fraction: results of randomized, multicentre Myocardial Regeneration by Intracoronary Infusion of Selected Population of Stem Cells in Acute Myocardial Infarction (REGENT) Trial. *European heart journal, 30*: 1313-1321.

Tse HF, Thambar S, Kwong YL, Rowlings P, Bellamy G, McCrohon J, Thomas P, Bastian B, Chan JK, Lo G, Ho CL, Chan WS, Kwong RY, Parker A, Hauser TH, Chan J, Fong DY, and Lau CP (2007). Prospective randomized trial of direct endomyocardial implantation of bone marrow cells for treatment of severe coronary artery diseases (PROTECT-CAD trial). *European heart journal, 28*: 2998-3005.

Valgimigli M, Rigolin G, Fucili A, Porta M, Soukhomovskaia O, Malagutti P, Bugli A, Bragotti L, Francolini G, Mauro E, Castoldi G, and Ferrari R (2004). CD34+ and endothelial progenitor cells in patients with various degrees of congestive heart failure. *Circulation, 110*: 1209-1212.

Walter DH, Rochwalsky U, Reinhold J, Seeger F, Aicher A, Urbich C, Spyridopoulos I, Chun J, Brinkmann V, Keul P, Levkau B, Zeiher AM, Dimmeler S, and Haendeler J (2007). Sphingosine-1-phosphate stimulates the functional capacity of progenitor cells by activation of the CXCR4-dependent signaling pathway via the S1P3 receptor. *Arterioscler Thromb Vasc Biol, 27*: 275-282.

Wang Y, Haider H, Ahmad N, Zhang D, and Ashraf M (2006). Evidence for ischemia induced host-derived bone marrow cell mobilization into cardiac allografts. *Journal of molecular and cellular cardiology, 41*: 478-487.

Wojakowski W, Tendera M, Kucia M, Zuba-Surma E, Paczkowska E, Ciosek J, Halasa M, Krol M, Kazmierski M, Buszman P, Ochala A, Ratajczak J, Machalinski B, and Ratajczak MZ (2009). Mobilization of bone marrow-derived Oct-4+ SSEA-4+ very small embryonic-like stem cells in patients with acute myocardial infarction. *J Am Coll Cardiol, 53*: 1-9.

Wojakowski W, Tendera M, Michałowska A, Majka M, Kucia M, Maślankiewicz K, Wyderka R, Ochała A, and Ratajczak M (2004). Mobilization of CD34/CXCR4+, CD34/CD117+, c-met+ stem cells, and mononuclear cells expressing early cardiac, muscle, and endothelial markers into peripheral blood in patients with acute myocardial infarction. *Circulation, 110*: 3213-3220.

Wojakowski W, Tendera M, Zebzda A, Michalowska A, Majka M, Kucia M, Maslankiewicz K, Wyderka R, Król M, Ochala A, Kozakiewicz K, and Ratajczak M (2006). Mobilization of CD34(+), CD117(+), CXCR4(+), c-met(+) stem cells is correlated with left ventricular ejection fraction and plasma NT-proBNP levels in patients with acute myocardial infarction. *Eur Heart J, 27*: 283-289.

Yousef M, Schannwell CM, Kostering M, Zeus T, Brehm M, and Strauer BE (2009). The BALANCE Study: clinical benefit and long-term outcome after intracoronary autologous bone marrow cell transplantation in patients with acute myocardial infarction. *Journal of the American College of Cardiology, 53*: 2262-2269.

Zaruba MM, Theiss HD, Vallaster M, Mehl U, Brunner S, David R, Fischer R, Krieg L, Hirsch E, Huber B, Nathan P, Israel L, Imhof A, Herbach N, Assmann G, Wanke R, Mueller-Hoecker J, Steinbeck G, and Franz WM (2009). Synergy between CD26/DPP-IV inhibition and G-CSF improves cardiac function after acute myocardial infarction. *Cell Stem Cell, 4*: 313-323.

Zohlnhöfer D, Ott I, Mehilli J, Schömig K, Michalk F, Ibrahim T, Meisetschläger G, von Wedel J, Bollwein H, Seyfarth M, Dirschinger J, Schmitt C, Schwaiger M, Kastrati A, Schömig A, and Investigators. R- (2006). Stem cell mobilization by granulocyte colony-stimulating factor in patients with acute myocardial infarction: a randomized controlled trial. *JAMA, 295*: 1003-1010.

Zuba-Surma EK, Guo Y, Taher H, Sanganalmath SK, Hunt G, Vincent RJ, Kucia M, Abdel-Latif A, Tang XL, Ratajczak MZ, Dawn B, and Bolli R (2011). Transplantation of expanded bone marrow-derived very small embryonic-like stem cells (VSEL-SCs) improves left ventricular function and remodelling after myocardial infarction. *Journal of cellular and molecular medicine, 15*: 1319-1328.

Zuba-Surma EK, Kucia M, Abdel-Latif A, Dawn B, Hall B, Singh R, Lillard JW, Jr., and Ratajczak MZ (2008). Morphological characterization of very small embryonic-like stem cells (VSELs) by ImageStream system analysis. *J Cell Mol Med, 12*: 292-303.

Permissions

The contributors of this book come from diverse backgrounds, making this book a truly international effort. This book will bring forth new frontiers with its revolutionizing research information and detailed analysis of the nascent developments around the world.

We would like to thank Rosana Pelayo, for lending her expertise to make the book truly unique. She has played a crucial role in the development of this book. Without her invaluable contribution this book wouldn't have been possible. She has made vital efforts to compile up to date information on the varied aspects of this subject to make this book a valuable addition to the collection of many professionals and students.

This book was conceptualized with the vision of imparting up-to-date information and advanced data in this field. To ensure the same, a matchless editorial board was set up. Every individual on the board went through rigorous rounds of assessment to prove their worth. After which they invested a large part of their time researching and compiling the most relevant data for our readers. Conferences and sessions were held from time to time between the editorial board and the contributing authors to present the data in the most comprehensible form. The editorial team has worked tirelessly to provide valuable and valid information to help people across the globe.

Every chapter published in this book has been scrutinized by our experts. Their significance has been extensively debated. The topics covered herein carry significant findings which will fuel the growth of the discipline. They may even be implemented as practical applications or may be referred to as a beginning point for another development. Chapters in this book were first published by InTech; hereby published with permission under the Creative Commons Attribution License or equivalent.

The editorial board has been involved in producing this book since its inception. They have spent rigorous hours researching and exploring the diverse topics which have resulted in the successful publishing of this book. They have passed on their knowledge of decades through this book. To expedite this challenging task, the publisher supported the team at every step. A small team of assistant editors was also appointed to further simplify the editing procedure and attain best results for the readers.

Our editorial team has been hand-picked from every corner of the world. Their multi-ethnicity adds dynamic inputs to the discussions which result in innovative outcomes. These outcomes are then further discussed with the researchers and contributors who give their valuable feedback and opinion regarding the same. The feedback is then collaborated with the researches and they are edited in a comprehensive manner to aid the understanding of the subject.

Apart from the editorial board, the designing team has also invested a significant amount of their time in understanding the subject and creating the most relevant covers. They scrutinized every image to scout for the most suitable representation of the subject and create an appropriate cover for the book.

The publishing team has been involved in this book since its early stages. They were actively engaged in every process, be it collecting the data, connecting with the contributors or procuring relevant information. The team has been an ardent support to the editorial, designing and production team. Their endless efforts to recruit the best for this project, has resulted in the accomplishment of this book. They are a veteran in the field of academics and their pool of knowledge is as vast as their experience in printing. Their expertise and guidance has proved useful at every step. Their uncompromising quality standards have made this book an exceptional effort. Their encouragement from time to time has been an inspiration for everyone.

The publisher and the editorial board hope that this book will prove to be a valuable piece of knowledge for researchers, students, practitioners and scholars across the globe.

List of Contributors

A. Herrera-Merchan, I. Hidalgo, L. Arranz and S. Gonzalez
Stem Cell Aging Group, Foundation Spanish National Cardiovascular Research Centre, Carlos III. (CNIC), Madrid, Spain

Rosana Pelayo and Eduardo Vadillo
Oncology Research Unit, Oncology Hospital, Mexican Institute for Social Security, Mexico City, Mexico

Elisa Dorantes-Acosta
Oncology Research Unit, Oncology Hospital, Mexican Institute for Social Security, Mexico City, Mexico
Leukemia Clinic, Mexican Children's Hospital 'Federico Gómez', Mexico City, Mexico

Ezequiel Fuentes-Pananá
Research Unit on Parasitic and Infectious Diseases, Pediatric Hospital, Mexican Institute for Social Security, Mexico City, Mexico

Sérgio Paulo Bydlowski and Felipe de Lara Janz
University of Sao Paulo School of Medicine, Laboratory of Genetics and Molecular Hematology, São Paulo, SP, Brazil

Carolina García-de-Alba, Moisés Selman and Annie Pardo
Instituto Nacional de Enfermedades Respiratorias, Universidad Nacional Autónoma de México, México

Jenhani Faouzi
Cellular Immunology and Cytometry and Cellular Therapy Laboratory, National Blood Transfusion Center, Tunisia
Immunology Unit research, Faculty of Pharmacy, Monastir, Tunisia

Ben Nasr Moufida
Immunology Unit research, Faculty of Pharmacy, Monastir, Tunisia

Carla McCrave
Children's Mercy Hospital in Kansas City, MO, USA

Pilar Blanco-Lobo, Omar J. BenMarzouk-Hidalgo and Pilar Pérez-Romero
Unit of Infectious Disease, Microbiology and Preventive Medicine, Instituto de Biomedicina de Sevilla (IBiS)/CSIC/Universidad de Sevilla, University Hospital Virgen del Rocio, Sevilla, Spain

Karen M. Hall, Holli Harper and Ivan N. Rich
HemoGenix, Inc, USA

Maria Savvateeva and Alexander Belyavsky
Engelhardt Institute of Molecular Biology, Russian Academy of Sciences, Russian Federation

Fedor Rozov
Engelhardt Institute of Molecular Biology, Russian Academy of Sciences, Russian Federation
University of Oslo, Centre for Medical Studies Russia, Moscow, Russian Federation

Ahmed Abdel-Latif
Gill Heart Institute and Division of Cardiovascular Medicine, University of Kentucky, and
Lexington VA Medical Center, Lexington, KY, USA

Ewa Zuba-Surma
Department of Medical Biotechnology, Faculty of Biochemistry, Biophysics and Biotechnology,
Jagiellonian University, Cracow, Poland

Mariusz Z. Ratajczak
Stem Cell Biology Institute, James Graham Brown Cancer Center, University of Louisville,
Louisville, KY, USA